MCQs in Clinical Medicine

Dedicated to my wife Jayashree and son Anoop

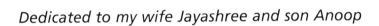

For W. B. Saunders

Commissioning Editor: Ellen Green
Project Editor: Janice Urquhart
Project Controller: Nancy Arnott
Design direction: Judith Wright

MCQs in Clinical Medicine

Ragavendra R. Baliga
MB BS MD DNB MRCP
Division of Cardiology,
University of Texas Southwestern Medical School,
Dallas, Texas, USA

SECOND EDITION

W. B. SAUNDERS

Edinburgh • London • Philadelphia • Toronto • St Louis • Sydney • Tokyo 1999

W. B. SAUNDERS
An imprint of Harcourt Publishers Limited

First edition 1994
Second edition 1999

ISBN 0–7020–2296–9

British Library Cataloguing in Publication Data
A catalogue record for this book is available from the British Library.

Library of Congress Cataloging in Publication Data
A catalog record for this book is available from the Library of Congress.

Medical knowledge is constantly changing. As new information
becomes available, changes in treatment, procedures, equipment and
the use of drugs become necessary. The author and the publishers
have, as far as it is possible, taken care to ensure that the information
given in this text is accurate and up to date. However, readers are
strongly advised to confirm that the information, especially with regard
to drug usage, complies with current legislation and standards of
practice.

The
publisher's
policy is to use
paper manufactured
from sustainable forests

Printed in China

Preface

Multiple choice questions are popular with examining bodies because they allow accurate ranking of examinees in a convenient manner. They are used for both undergraduate (MB BS, LRCP, PLAB, USMLE) and postgraduate (MRCP Part I and MRCGP) examinations in general internal medicine. Merely reading a medical text may not necessarily prepare students for such examinations. This book which contains over 1600 questions (each with five statements), derived from the 4th edition of Kumar and Clark's *Clinical Medicine*, should meet the needs of aspiring candidates. Although no explanations accompany the answers at the end of the book, most questions contain a cross reference to *Clinical Medicine* to allow ready reference to the original text.

To make best use of the book I would recommend that the student reads the corresponding chapter in the original text before answering these questions. However, candidates using other texts should also find this book a useful revision guide. None of these questions have hidden meanings and are not meant to confuse the reader. Each statement or stem has 5 items, and the answer to each item is independent of every other item. While testing yourself you must decide on one of the three options, viz. 'True', 'False' or 'Don't Know'. To time yourself you must attempt to complete 60 stems in two and a half hours or two and a half minutes for each stem. To prepare for postgraduate examinations I recommend that the original textbook be read several times until the reader gets over 99% of the questions right.

I thank Dr. Parveen Kumar and Dr. Michael Clark for allowing me to use their book to derive these MCQs.

I thank Prof. James Scott, FRCP, FRS for writing the Foreword. I would like to thank Prof. Rodney Falk, MD, FRCP at Boston University Medical Center for his support when I needed it most.

At University of Southwestern Medical Center I would like to thank Prof. Sanders Williams, MD, Chief of Cardiology and Dr. Clyde Yancy, MD, Director of Heart Transplantation, for awarding me the first heart failure/cardiac transplant fellowship of the department. I thank Prof. John Rutherford, MD, Dean for Clinical Affairs, for his advice. I would like to thank Dr. Eric Eichhorn for training me in cardiac catheterization. I thank Dr. Thomas Andrews, MD for working towards my board eligibility. I would like to thank Dr. Mark Drazner, MD for his counsel and advice during my fellowship and finally Dr. Michael Solomon, MD for very patiently initiating me to the UT Southwestern method of managing congestive heart failure.

I would like to thank Margaret MacDonald, Ellen Green and Janice Urquhart, Senior Editor at Harcourt Brace, particularly Janice for her patience when I failed to meet her deadlines. Finally I would like to thank Jenny Bew for painstakingly copyediting this book.

I dedicate this book to my wife Jayashree and my son Anoop for their support throughout the book's preparation

Ragavendra R. Baliga   Dallas, Texas

Foreword to the first edition

Multiple choice questions in general internal medicine are now an integral part of both undergraduate (MB BS and PLAB) and postgraduate examinations (MRCP Part 1 and MRCGP).

Examining bodies use such questions to test more than factual recall; they are used to assess the understanding and application of essential facts. Simply reading a medical text will not prepare a candidate adequately for these examinations and to be well prepared the individual will have to solve several MCQs. These questions can also be used to determine areas of weakness and of expertise in general internal medicine. Although no bank of questions can be all-embracing, this book which contains over 1600 multiple choice questions in *MCQs in Clinical Medicine* should be a valuable revision guide for aspiring students.

Prospective candidates, however, must be forewarned that merely solving multiple choice questions is not a satisfactory method of enhancing their medical knowledge. Sincere and dedicated students should use both this book and the clinical text on which it is based, Kumar and Clark's *Clinical Medicine*, as complementary approaches to enhance their understanding of clinical medicine.

Professor James Scott FRCP FRS
Imperial College of Science, Technology and Medicine,
Hammersmith Hospital,
London

Contents

Infectious Diseases, Tropical Medicine and Sexually Transmitted Diseases

1.1 Common infectious diseases worldwide include (Table 1.1):
- (a) Chagas' disease
- (b) Diarrhoeal disease
- (c) Malaria
- (d) Schistosomiasis
- (e) Whooping cough

1.2 The following associations between microorganisms and body sites that serve as permanent reservoirs are correct (pages 1–2):
- (a) Gall bladder – hepatitis B
- (b) Skin – *Staphylococcus epidermidis*
- (c) Nasopharynx – meningococci
- (d) Intestinal tract – *giardia* Sp.
- (e) Intestinal tract – *Entamoeba histolytica*

1.3 The following associations between animal reservoirs and microorganisms are correct (page 2):
- (a) Battery-farmed chickens – salmonellae
- (b) Battery-farmed chickens – *Campylobacter jejuni*
- (c) Domestic cats – *Toxoplasma gondii*
- (d) Wild animals – *Giardia* sp.
- (e) Cattle – *Cryptosporidium parvum*

1.4 The following associations between environmental reservoirs and microorganisms are correct (page 2):
- (a) Water – hepatitis B
- (b) Water – hepatitis A
- (c) Water – *Giardia* sp.
- (d) Soil – clostridia
- (e) Soil – *Bacillus anthracis*

1.5 The following associations are correct (page 2):
- (a) Airborne spread – influenza
- (b) Person-to-person spread – impetigo
- (c) Infection by entry of larvae through skin – hookworm
- (d) Faeco-oral spread – shigellosis
- (e) Spread by inoculation – HIV

1.6 The following associations between diseases and their insect vectors are correct (page 2):
(a) Babesiosis – ticks
(b) Malaria – sandfly
(c) Leishmaniasis – sandfly
(d) Chagas' disease – mosquito
(e) Yellow fever – bugs

1.7 The following statements are correct (pages 2–3):
(a) Amoebiasis only naturally affects humans.
(b) Individuals with Duffy blood group negative have decreased susceptibility to *Plasmodium vivax* malaria.
(c) Anaerobic organisms rarely colonize the colon.
(d) Aerobic organisms are generally found in the mouth.
(e) Reovirus selectively enters the body through the specialized epithelial cells known as M cells, which cover the Peyer's patches.

1.8 The following pathogens are located intracellularly (page 3):
(a) *Toxoplasma*
(b) *Leishmania*
(c) *Entamoeba histolytica*
(d) *Plasmodium*
(e) Staphylococci

1.9 The following associations between bacterial exotoxins and their mechanisms of action are correct (page 3):
(a) Inhibition of protein synthesis – Diphtheria exotoxin
(b) Neurotoxicity – *Clostridium perfringens*
(c) Neurotoxicity – *Cl. tetani*
(d) Enterotoxicity – *Escherichia coli*
(e) Neurotoxicity – *Cl. botulinum*

1.10 Endotoxin (page 3):
(a) is a lipopolysaccharide
(b) is found in the cell wall of Gram-negative bacteria
(c) causes intravascular coagulation
(d) effects are mediated predominantly by the release of tumour necrosis factor
(e) causes hypotension

1.11 The following statements are correct (page 4):
(a) Endogenous pyrogen is secreted by the thermoregulatory centre.
(b) The thermoregulatory centre is located in the posterior hypothalamus.
(c) Interleukin-1 is released from blood monocytes and phagocytes.
(d) Interleukin-1 acts on the thermoregulatory centre by inhibiting prostaglandin synthesis.

(e) The antipyretic action of salicylates is brought about, in part, through their inhibitory effects on prostaglandin synthetase.

1.12 During acute infection the following changes occur in protein metabolism (page 4):
(a) There is a diversion of synthesis away from somatic and circulating proteins towards acute-phase proteins.
(b) Protein synthesis is directed towards immunoglobulin production.
(c) There is a marked decrease in nitrogen losses.
(d) There is a decrease in the production of phagocytic leucocytes.
(e) There is an increase in the production of fibrinogen.

1.13 The following associations are correct (page 6):
(a) Sheep farmers – hydatid disease
(b) Sewer workers – leptospirosis
(c) Leather workers – anthrax
(d) Budgerigars – *Toxocara canis* infection
(e) Dogs – psittacosis

1.14 Common causes of fever in a traveller returning to the UK include (Table 1.2):
(a) Malaria
(b) Dysentery
(c) Typhoid
(d) Hepatitis A
(e) Urinary tract infection

1.15 The following associations between disease and differential count are correct (page 6):
(a) Polymorphonuclear leucocytosis – bacterial infections
(b) Neutropenia – brucellosis
(c) Lymphocytosis-whooping cough
(d) Eosinophilia – parasitic infections
(e) Atypical lymphocytes – infectious mononucleosis

1.16 The following statements about investigations in infection are correct (page 6):
(a) Liver biochemistry is often slightly abnormal in infections.
(b) Blood cultures are no longer routinely required before giving antibiotics because they are usually negative.
(c) A single raised titre of IgG specific to a pathogen is diagnostic of recent infection.
(d) Abscesses can be imaged by radionuclide scanning using radiolabelled ciprofloxacin.
(e) Rotavirus can be identified using immunological antigen capture techniques.

1.17 The following associations between disease and mode of tissue diagnosis are correct (page 6):
  (a) Bone marrow biopsy – leishmaniasis
  (b) Liver biopsy – tuberculosis
  (c) Bone marrow biopsy – infectious mononucleosis.
  (d) Splenic aspiration – leishmaniasis
  (e) Transbronchial biopsy – *Pneumocystis carinii*

1.18 Pyrexia is a feature of the following conditions (Information Box 1.1, page 7):
  (a) Leukaemia
  (b) Lymphoma
  (c) Renal carcinoma
  (d) Drugs
  (e) SLE

1.19 The following statements are correct (pages 7–8):
  (a) Bacteraemia is the transient presence of organisms in the blood.
  (b) Septicaemia refers to organisms actually multiplying in the blood.
  (c) Primary septicaemia is used to describe the situation when the focus of infection is not apparent.
  (d) Pyaemia is a situation in a septicaemia when organisms and neutrophil polymorphs embolize to many sites, causing abscesses.
  (e) Pyrexia means organisms are present in the body.

1.20 The following associations between common sites of infection and infective agents responsible for secondary septicaemia in a previously healthy adult are correct (Table 1.3):
  (a) Skin – Gram-positive cocci
  (b) Urinary tract – Gram-negative rods
  (c) Respiratory tract – *Streptococcus pneumoniae*
  (d) Gall bladder – *Escherichia coli*
  (e) Pelvic organs – *Neisseria gonorrhoeae*

1.21 In septicaemic shock (page 8):
  (a) high-dose steroids should be administered
  (b) suspected to be due to *Staphylococcus aureus* a combination of flucloxacillin and an aminoglycoside should be used pending cultures
  (c) due to bowel sepsis a broad-spectrum cephalosporin should be used pending culture
  (d) due to *Pseudomonas* a penicillin drug effective against it and an aminoglycoside such as tobramycin should be used
  (e) suspected anaerobic infections metronidazole should be added

1.22 The following associations in septicaemic patients are correct (Table 1.4):
  (a) Urinary catheter – *Escherichia coli*
  (b) Intravenous catheter – *Staphylococcus aureus*

(c) Postoperative wound infection – anaerobes
(d) Urinary catheter – *Serratia*
(e) Burns – *Candida albicans*

1.23 Recognized features of septicaemia include (Table 1.5):
(a) Hypertension
(b) Pulmonary oedema
(c) Acute respiratory distress syndrome
(d) Disseminated intravascular coagulation
(e) Shock

1.24 Correct statements about the choice of antibiotic include (page 9):
(a) The spectrum of antibacterial activity of the chosen drug should ideally be as broad as possible.
(b) In the majority of infections there is firm evidence that bactericidal drugs are more effective than bacteriostatic drugs.
(c) Ticarcillin is safe in chronic renal failure.
(d) In bacterial endocarditis bacteriostatic drugs are preferred to bactericidal drugs.
(e) In patients with neutropenia bacteriostatic drugs are preferred to bactericidal drugs.

1.25 Drugs which should be avoided altogether in renal impairment include (page 9):
(a) Nalidixic acid
(b) Tetracycline
(c) Vancomycin
(d) Erythromycin
(e) Ampicillin

1.26 The following associations regarding antibiotic chemoprophylaxis are correct (Table 1.6):
(a) Rheumatic fever – benzyl penicillin
(b) Meningococcal meningitis – rifampicin
(c) *Haemophilus* meningitis – rifampicin
(d) Tuberculosis – isoniazid
(e) Malaria – chloroquine

1.27 Combination antibiotic therapy is used in the empirical treatment of (page 10):
(a) Tuberculosis
(b) Meningitis
(c) Sarcoidosis
(d) Septicaemia
(e) Endocarditis

1.28 The following statements about combination antibiotic therapy are correct (page 8):
(a) Combinations of bactericidal and bacteriostatic drugs may impair their therapeutic efficacy.
(b) Combinations of bactericidal drugs are additive.
(c) Combinations of bactericidal drugs may be synergistic.
(d) Combinations of bacteriostatic drugs are generally only additive.
(e) In septicaemic shock combination therapy should be avoided.

1.29 The following associations between antibiotics and their sites of action on the bacterium are correct (page 9–17):
(a) Rifampicin – RNA synthesis
(b) Quinolones – DNA synthesis
(c) Sulphonamides – folic acid antagonists
(d) Polymyxins – disrupt cell membranes
(e) Amphotericin – inhibition of sterol synthesis

1.30 The following statements about antibiotic resistance are correct (page 10):
(a) Single point mutations in *E. coli* lead to acquired resistance.
(b) Transformation is the introduction of large fragments of DNA into a bacterium via a bacteriophage (a virus) DNA vector.
(c) Transduction is the introduction of 'naked' DNA into the bacterium by transfer.
(d) Conjugation involves the passage of extrachromosomal DNA (a plasmid) containing the resistance factor
(R factor) from one cell to another during direct contact.
(e) Penicillins are ineffective against Gram-negative bacteria because they fail to penetrate the outer bacterial membrane.

1.31 The following statements about penicillin are correct (page 11):
(a) It has a β lactam ring fused to a thiazolidine ring.
(b) Changes in the side chain of benzylpenicillin render the phenoxymethyl derivative to be absorbed orally.
(c) The presence of an amino group in the phenyl radical of benzyl penicillin increases the antimicrobial spectrum.
(d) Modification of the side chain can render the drug insensitive to bacterial penicillinase.
(e) Pencillin blocks cell wall mucopeptide formation.

1.32 The following statements about penicillin are correct (pages 11–12):
(a) Benzylpenicillin can be given orally.
(b) Flucloxacillin is used in infections caused by penicillinase-producing staphylococci.
(c) Penicillins inactivate aminoglycosides when mixed in the same solution.
(d) Clavulanic acid is a powerful inhibitor of bacterial β-lactamases.
(e) Carbenicillin is not reliable for treating *Pseudomonas* infections.

1.33 The following associations are correct (pages 10–17):
    (a) Benzylpenicillin – actinomycosis
    (b) Erythromycin – legionella
    (c) Tetracyclines – chlamydia
    (d) Benzylpenicillin – urinary tract infections
    (e) Metronidazole – *Trichomonas vaginalis*

1.34 The following statements about penicillin are correct (pages 10–12):
    (a) Methicillin-resistant *Staphylococcus aureus* (MRSA) produce a high-affinity penicillin-binding protein which retains its peptidase activity even in the presence of high concentrations of methicillin.
    (b) Phenoxymethylpenicillin is used chiefly in the treatment of acute rheumatic fever.
    (c) Ampicillin is better absorbed than amoxycillin when given by mouth.
    (d) Azlocillin is very reliable in the treatment of staphylococcal disease.
    (e) The combination of piperacillin with tazobactam (Tazocin) is ineffective in appendicitis.

1.35 The following statements are correct (page 12):
    (a) Second- and third-generation cephalosporins have a broad spectrum of activity.
    (b) First-generation cephalosporins are active against Gram-negative cocci.
    (c) Increased nephrotoxicity is seen when cephalosporins are used with aminoglycosides.
    (d) Cephalosporins inhibit bacterial wall synthesis.
    (e) Cephalosporins are resistant to staphylococcal penicillinases.

1.36 The following statements are correct (pages 10–16):
    (a) Aztreonam activity is limited to anaerobic Gram-positive bacilli.
    (b) Imipenam has the broadest spectrum of activity of all known antibiotics.
    (c) Tetracyclines are bactericidal.
    (d) Fusidic acid is mainly used for penicillinase-producing *Staph. aureus*.
    (e) Erythromycin should be avoided in patients with penicillin allergy.

1.37 The following associations are correct (pages 10–17):
    (a) Penicillin – tubulo interstitial nephritis
    (b) Aminoglycosides – neuromuscular blockade with curariform drugs
    (c) Co-trimaxazole – death in the elderly
    (d) Aminoglycosides – enhance ototoxicity when given with some diuretics
    (e) Chloramphenicol – enhances the activity of anticoagulants

1.38 The following associations are correct (pages 10–17):
    (a) Tetracyclines – enhance existing renal failure
    (b) Tetracyclines – 'grey baby syndrome'
    (c) Erythromycin estolate – cholestatic jaundice

(d) Chloramphenicol – brownish discoloration of growing teeth
(e) Chloramphenicol – bone marrow suppression

1.39 The following indications for antibiotic therapy are correct (pages 10–17):
(a) Chloramphenicol – *Salmonella typhi*
(b) Sulphamethoxazole with trimethoprim – *Pneumocystis carinii* infection
(c) Ciprofloxacin – *Chlamydia trachomitis* urethritis
(d) Vancomycin – *Clostridium difficile*-related pseudomembranous enterocolitis
(e) Benzylpenicillin – prophylaxis for rheumatic fever

1.40 The following indications are correct (page 17):
(a) Ketoconazole – invasive aspergillosis.
(b) Griseofulvin – chronic fungal infections of the nail
(c) Nystatin – oral candidiasis
(d) Nystatin – systemic fungal infections.
(e) Clotrimazole – ringworm

1.41 The following indications are correct (Table 1.11):
(a) Idoxuridine – herpes simplex virus keratitis
(b) Vidarabine – varicella zoster infections
(c) Acyclovir – HIV
(d) Zidovudine – HIV
(e) Ganciclovir – cytomegalovirus

1.42 The following examples of passive immunization infection are correct (Table 1.12):
(a) Measles – human normal immune globulin
(b) Rubella – human normal immune globulin
(c) Varicella zoster – horse serum
(d) Tetanus – human tetanus immune globulin
(e) Diphtheria – horse serum

1.43 Examples of live vaccine include (Table 1.13):
(a) Salk vaccine
(b) Rabies
(c) Measles
(d) BCG
(e) Mumps

1.44 The following statements about staphylococci are correct (pages 20–22):
(a) Staphylococci are Gram-negative cocci.
(b) Staphylococci produce enterotoxin.
(c) Twenty-five percent of the population are permanent carriers.
(d) About one-fifth of all human infections are autogenous.
(e) Diabetics show increased resistance to staphylococcal infections.

1.45 Conditions produced by direct invasion of *Staph. aureus* include (Table 1.15):
- (a) Carbuncles
- (b) Lung abscess
- (c) Food poisoning
- (d) Endocarditis
- (e) Scalded skin syndrome

1.46 Correct statements about acute osteomyelitis in young children include (pages 10–21):
- (a) It is almost always due to staphylococcal infection.
- (b) It occurs predominantly in females.
- (c) It usually affects the vertebra.
- (d) A history of trauma is often present.
- (e) The diaphysis is initially involved.

1.47 Correct statements about toxic shock syndrome include (page 21):
- (a) It is seen most frequently before menarche.
- (b) It is the same as scalded skin syndrome.
- (c) Men and children are exempt.
- (d) Blood cultures are negative.
- (e) It is frequent in women who use high-absorbancy polyacrylate-containing tampons.

1.48 Correct statements about MARSA staphylococci include (page 21):
- (a) Immediate isolation of infected individuals is necessary.
- (b) They are resistant to aminoglycosides.
- (c) Outbreaks of infection are commoner in tertiary referral centres.
- (d) It is commoner in those with surgical wounds.
- (e) Treatment is with teicoplanin.

1.49 Streptococci are virulent because of (pages 22–23):
- (a) the fact that they are Gram-positive organisms
- (b) cell wall M protein
- (c) production of hyaluronidase
- (d) production of DNAses
- (e) production of streptokinase

1.50 The following associations are correct (pages 22–23):
- (a) Group A β-haemolytic streptococci – rarely cause human infections.
- (b) Group B streptococci – neonatal sepsis
- (c) Group C streptococci – pharyngitis
- (d) Group D streptococci – endocarditis
- (e) Group D streptococci – septicaemia

1.51 Non-suppurative diseases caused by streptococci include (Table 1.16):
- (a) Rheumatic fever
- (b) Glomerulonephritis

(c) Scarlet fever
(d) Tonsillitis
(e) Cellulitis

1.52 Recognized features of scarlet fever include (page 22):
(a) Peritonsillar abscess
(b) Otitis media
(c) Circumoral pallor
(d) Strawberry tongue
(e) Extensive desquamation of the skin

1.53 Diagnostic tests to establish streptococcal infection include (page 22):
(a) Isolation of the organism on throat swabs
(b) Latex agglutination of throat swabs
(c) Elevated anti-streptolysin O
(d) Elevated anti-DNAse B levels
(e) Complement fixation test

1.54 Correct statements about the management of streptococcal infections include (page 22):
(a) Treatment is directed at preventing the non-suppurative complications of streptococcal infection.
(b) Penicillin is the drug of choice.
(c) Erythromycin is ineffective.
(d) Tonsillectomy is essential in preventing further attacks.
(e) Chemoprophylaxis with penicillin should be given in epidemics.

1.55 Recognized features of erysipelas include (page 23):
(a) It is a rapidly progressive infection of the skin
(b) Abrupt onset
(c) Erythematous lesion, usually on the face
(d) Regional lymphadenopathy
(e) Treatment with penicillin is rapidly effective

1.56 Neisseria (page 23):
(a) are Gram-positive organisms
(b) are diplococci
(c) cause chronic renal failure
(d) cause gonorrhoea
(e) cause meningitis

1.57 Recognized manifestations of *N. meningitidis* include (page 23):
(a) Polyarthritis
(b) Pericarditis
(c) Nephritis
(d) Waterhouse – Friderichsen syndrome
(e) Myocardial infarction

1.58 Recognized features of meningococcaemia include (page 24):
(a) Purpuric rash
(b) Shock
(c) Disseminated intravascular coagulation
(d) Haemorrhage into the adrenal glands
(e) Coma

1.59 Correct statements about the treatment and prevention of meningococcal infection include (page 24):
(a) Benzylpenicillin is the treatment of choice
(b) Chloramphenicol is effective
(c) Steroids should be used in meningitis
(d) Penicillin eradicates the carrier state
(e) Family contacts are protected by rifampicin

1.60 Correct statements about *Corynebacteria diphtheriae* include (pages 24–25):
(a) It is a Gram-negative organism.
(b) It is a club-shaped bacillus.
(c) Three morphological varieties – mitis, intermedius and gravis – are recognized.
(d) Only those exposed to bacteriophage β, which carries the tox$^+$ gene, are capable of toxin production.
(e) Humans are the only natural hosts

1.61 Clinical features of diphtheria include (pages 24–25):
(a) Respiratory obstruction of the larynx
(b) Myasthenia gravis
(c) Myocarditis
(d) Palatal palsy
(e) Encephalitis

1.62 Correct statements about the treatment and prevention of diphtheria include (pages 24–25):
(a) Therapy can wait until the bacteriological results of culture studies and toxin production are available.
(b) Antitoxin therapy is the only specific treatment.
(c) It can be effectively prevented by active immunization in childhood.
(d) Those with a positive culture from a throat swab should be treated with penicillin or erythromycin.
(e) Those with a positive culture from a throat swab should receive active immunization or a booster dose of toxoid.

1.63 Listeriosis (page 25):
(a) predominantly occurs perinatally
(b) causes abortions
(c) organism can multiply in a refrigerator if temperatures are not kept below 4°C

(d) is treated with ampicillin and gentamicin
(e) is associated with a high mortality

1.64 Clostridium (page 25):
    (a) is a Gram-negative organism
    (b) is an aerobe
    (c) is a bacillus
    (d) forms spores
    (e) is a normal commensal in the human gastrointestinal tract

1.65 Clinical features of tetanus include (page 26):
    (a) Trismus or lockjaw
    (b) Opisthotonus
    (c) Altered mental state
    (d) Cardiac arrhythmias
    (e) Labile blood pressure

1.66 Death in tetanus results from (page 26):
    (a) Aspiration
    (b) Hypoxia
    (c) Respiratory failure
    (d) Cardiac arrest
    (e) Exhaustion

1.67 Poor prognostic factors in tetanus include (page 26):
    (a) Long incubation period
    (b) Short onset time
    (c) Extremes of age
    (d) Cephalic tetanus
    (e) Narcotic addicts who inject drugs subcutaneously

1.68 Correct statements about tetanus neonatorum include (page 26):
    (a) It occurs as a result of infection of the umbilical stump.
    (b) It is associated with almost 100% mortality.
    (c) Poor sucking is a feature.
    (d) Failure to thrive is a feature.
    (e) Grimacing is a feature.

1.69 Diseases which can mimic tetanus include (page 26):
    (a) Phenothiazine overdosage
    (b) Strychnine poisoning
    (c) Meningitis
    (d) Tetany
    (e) Diazepam overdosage

1.70 Correct statements about the prevention of tetanus include (page 26):
    (a) Tetanus is eminently preventable.

(b) Alum absorbed toxoid is superior to plain toxoid in active immunization.
(c) After the initial course, booster doses of toxoid are required at 5-year intervals.
(d) Infant immunization schedules in the UK include tetanus.
(e) Protection by human antitetanus toxin is lifelong.

1.71 *Clostridium botulinum* (page 27):
(a) is found in the soil
(b) spores can survive heating to 100°C
(c) proliferates in preserved canned foods
(d) produces several toxins which are known to consistently produce disease in humans
(e) destroys the myocardium

1.72 Correct statements about the clinical features of *Cl. botulinum* include (page 27):
(a) Fever is usual.
(b) Conciousness is altered.
(c) Nausea, vomiting and diarrhoea are early symptoms.
(d) Respiratory insufficiency may occur.
(e) Neurological symptoms dominate the clinical picture.

1.73 Neurological manifestations of *Cl. botulinum* infection include (page 27):
(a) Laryngeal paralysis
(b) Pharyngeal paralysis
(c) Generalized paralysis
(d) Strabismus
(e) Urinary retention

1.74 Correct statements about the treatment and prognosis of *Cl. botulinum* infection include (page 27):
(a) Artificial ventilation should be avoided.
(b) Antitoxins should be administered.
(c) Antibiotics form the cornerstone of treatment.
(d) Guanidine improves botulism-induced paralysis.
(e) The overall mortality is less than 10%.

1.75 Features of gas gangrene include (page 27):
(a) It occurs in lacerated wounds.
(b) It is caused by *Cl. perfringens.*
(c) Crepitus of the affected muscles.
(d) Systemic signs are rare.
(e) Marked tachycardia.

1.76 Correct statements about pseudomembranous colitis include (page 27):
(a) Clindamycin has been most frequently implicated.

(b) Bloody diarrhoea is common.
(c) It has been known to occur as long as a month after discontinuing antibiotics.
(d) Normal sigmoidoscopy excludes it.
(e) It has been caused by the toxin of *Cl. difficile.*

1.77 Antibiotics implicated in pseudomembranous colitis include (page 27):
(a) Clindamycin
(b) Ampicillin
(c) Cephalosporins
(d) Lincomycin
(e) Tetracycline

1.78 Correct statements regarding anthrax include (page 28):
(a) Farmers are not susceptible to *Bacillus anthracis.*
(b) Cutaneous anthrax is characterized by a central black eschar.
(c) Penicillin is the drug of choice.
(d) Any infected animal that dies should be burned.
(e) Mass vaccination of animals may prevent widespread contamination.

1.79 The following associations are correct (page 28):
(a) *Bacillus cereus* – food poisoning
(b) *Cl. difficile* – pseudomembranous colitis
(c) Cat-scratch disease – neuroretinitis
(d) Brucella – splenomegaly
(e) Bordetella – whooping cough

1.80 Correct statements about brucellosis include (pages 28–29):
(a) Blood cultures are positive in most of the patients during the acute phase.
(b) Serological tests are of greater value than blood cultures in chronic disease.
(c) A negative 2-mercaptoethanol test excludes chronic brucellosis.
(d) Human vaccine is useful in prevention.
(e) Pasteurization of milk prevents the disease.

1.81 Features of whooping cough include (page 29):
(a) In the catarrhal stage the patient is rarely infectious
(b) The paroxysms of coughing usually terminate in vomiting
(c) Lymphocytosis
(d) Conjunctival petechiae
(e) Ulceration of the frenulum of the tongue

1.82 Complications of whooping cough include (page 29):
(a) Bronchitis
(b) Rectal prolapse
(c) Inguinal hernia

    (d) Cerebral anoxia
    (e) Lobar pneumonia

1.83 Correct statements about the management and prevention of whooping cough include (page 30):
    (a) Erythromycin will reduce the severity of the infection if administered late in the paroxysmal stage.
    (b) In the catarrhal stage antibiotics have little role in altering the course of the illness.
    (c) Affected individuals should be isolated to prevent contact with others.
    (d) Antitoxin is effective.
    (e) Any susceptible infant should receive prophylactic erythromycin.

1.84 Clinical features of *Haemophilus influenzae* include (Table 1.18):
    (a) Meningitis
    (b) Endocarditis
    (c) Septic arthritis
    (d) Epiglottitis
    (e) Otitis media

1.85 High-risk factors for *Haemophilus influenzae* infection include (page 30):
    (a) Children
    (b) Alcoholics
    (c) Sickle cell disease
    (d) Splenectomy
    (e) Hypogammaglobulinaemia

1.86 Correct statements about the treatment and prevention of *Haemophilus* infection include (page 30):
    (a) Delay in treatment may result in high mortality.
    (b) Chloramphenicol is the drug of choice.
    (c) Ampicillin is contraindicated.
    (d) Conjugate vaccines are ineffective in preventing infection.
    (e) Rifampicin is helpful in preventing infection in close contacts.

1.87 Correct statements about cholera include (page 31):
    (a) The El Tor biotype has replaced the classic biotype as the major cause of cholera.
    (b) A chronic gall bladder state results in most of the affected adults.
    (c) The clinical effects are due to the fact that it is an invasive organism.
    (d) Achlorhydria facilitates the passage of the organism into the small intestine.
    (e) Stimulation of adenylate cyclase causes massive secretion of isotonic fluid in the intestinal system.

1.88 Recognized features of cholera include (page 31):
(a) Transmission is by the faeco-oral route.
(b) The majority of patients with cholera have a mild illness that cannot be distinguished from diarrhoea due to other infective causes.
(c) Circulatory collapse.
(d) 'Rice-water' stools.
(e) It carries a high mortality.

1.89 Correct statements about the treatment and prevention of cholera include (page 31):
(a) Effective rehydration has reduced mortality.
(b) Oral rehydration should be avoided.
(c) Tetracycline has no effect on the duration of illness.
(d) Ciprofloxacin should be avoided.
(e) Immunization with currently available vaccines results in excellent immunity.

1.90 Recognized causes of traveller's diarrhoea include (Table 1.22):
(a) Shigella
(b) Salmonella
(c) Rotavirus
(d) *Giardia intestinalis*
(e) *Entamoeba histolytica*

1.91 Correct statements about the treatment and prevention of *E. coli* infection include (page 33):
(a) Oral fluid and electrolytes are the mainstay of therapy.
(b) Many *E. coli* gut infections are self-limiting and require no antibiotic therapy.
(c) Ciprofloxacin is effective in colitis.
(d) Gentamicin is effective in septicaemia.
(e) Trimethoprim is effective prophylaxis against traveller's diarrhoea.

1.92 Clinical syndromes caused by *salmonella* sp. include (page 34):
(a) Enterocolitis
(b) Osteomyelitis
(c) Food poisoning
(d) Enteric fever
(e) Yellow fever

1.93 Correct statements about typhoid fever include (page 34):
(a) It is caused by *Salmonella typhimurium.*
(b) It is characterized by remittent fever with a step-ladder pattern of increase.
(c) The onset is insidious.
(d) The majority of complications occur in the third week.
(e) The fourth week of illness is characterized by a gradual return to health.

1.94 Clinical features of typhoid fever include (page 34):
  (a) Relative bradycardia
  (b) Maculopapular rash
  (c) Splenomegaly
  (d) Haemolytic anaemia
  (e) Acute cholecystitis

1.95 Correct statements about the diagnosis of typhoid fever include (page 35):
  (a) Leucopenia is present.
  (b) Blood cultures are more often positive in the first week than the third week.
  (c) Urine cultures are helpful in the second week.
  (d) Stool cultures are helpful during the second to fourth weeks.
  (e) A fourfold increase in titre of the Widal test is suggestive of salmonella infection.

1.96 Correct statements about the carrier state in typhoid fever include (page 35):
  (a) It is said to be chronic when individuals excrete *Salmonella* for at least 1 year.
  (b) It is suggested by the presence of increased Vi agglutinin in the serum.
  (c) Ampicillin and probenicid are used in the eradication of the carrier state.
  (d) It is suggested by increased titres of the Widal test.
  (e) Cholecystectomy is the only mode of treatment in those not responding to antibiotics.

1.97 Correct statements about the treatment of typhoid fever include (page 35):
  (a) Chloramphenicol is the drug of choice.
  (b) Co-trimoxazole should be avoided.
  (c) Intestinal perforation may occur despite therapy.
  (d) Intestinal perforation can often be managed conservatively.
  (e) Ampicillin is useful.

1.98 Correct statements about the prevention and control of typhoid fever include (page 35):
  (a) The parenteral monovalent typhoid vaccine gives complete protection.
  (b) The parenteral monovalent typhoid vaccine protects for over 3 years.
  (c) The vaccine based on the Vi polysaccharide antigen rarely provides protection for more than a year.
  (d) Live oral vaccine provides protection for 2 years.
  (e) The typhoid vaccine protects against paratyphoid fever.

1.99 Causes of food poisoning include (Table 1.21):
  (a) *Clostridium perfringens*
  (b) *Campylobacter jejuni*
  (c) Dinoflagellate plankton toxin in shellfish

(d) Scrombotoxin in spoiled fish
(e) Red kidney bean toxin from partially cooked beans

1.100 Shigellosis (page 35):
(a) is a self-limiting illness
(b) when due to *Sh. dysenteriae* can be confused with cholera
(c) is transmitted by the faeco-oral route
(d) is more prevalent in areas with poor hygiene
(e) has an unusually long incubation period

1.101 Features of shigellosis include (page 35):
(a) Bloody diarrhoea
(b) Tenesmus
(c) Haemolytic uraemic syndrome
(d) Colonic perforation
(e) Arthritis

1.102 Correct statements about *Campylobacter jejuni* include (page 35):
(a) It causes ulceration of the mucosa.
(b) It occurs after eating infected chicken.
(c) In a majority of the cases the infection has a fulminant course.
(d) Treatment with erythromycin has been shown to alter the natural history of the infection.
(e) It is a rare cause of acute gastroenteritis in the UK.

1.103 Complications of *Campylobacter jejuni* include (page 35):
(a) Pancreatitis
(b) Cholecystitis
(c) Reactive arthritis
(d) Guillain – Barré syndrome
(e) Haemolytic uraemic syndrome

1.104 Clinical features of *Yersinia enterocolitica* and *Y. pseudotuberculosis* include (page 36):
(a) Mesenteric adenitis
(b) Ulcerative colitis
(c) Terminal ileitis
(d) Reiter's syndrome
(e) Erythema nodosum

1.105 Correct statements about plague include (page 36):
(a) It is caused by *Yersinia pestis*.
(b) The major reservoirs are woodland rodents, which transmit infection to domestic rats.
(c) The vector is the rat flea, *Xenopsylla cheopis*.

    (d) Humans are bitten by the rat flea when there is a sudden decline in the rat population.
    (e) Clinical manifestations are attributed to the exotoxin.

1.106 Clinical features of plague include (page 36):
    (a) Cardiac failure
    (b) Angina
    (c) Suppurative lymphadenopathy
    (d) Shock
    (e) Disseminated intravascular coagulation

1.107 Correct statements about the prevention and control of plague include (page 37):
    (a) It is largely dependent on control of the flea population.
    (b) Rodents should not be killed until the fleas are under control.
    (c) Tetracycline is used as a chemoprophylactic agent.
    (d) A partially effective formalin-killed vaccine is available for use by travellers to endemic areas.
    (e) Patients with pneumonic plague cannot spread the infection because the rat flea is required as a vector.

1.108 The following associations are correct (pages 37–38):
    (a) Bartonellosis – haemolytic anaemia
    (b) Glanders – mainly affects horses
    (c) Meliodosis – caused by soil saprophyte
    (d) Pasteurellosis – focal soft-tissue infection
    (e) Tularaemia – infection from eating uncooked meat

1.109 *Bacteroides fragilis* (page 38):
    (a) is an obligate aerobe
    (b) is a normal commensal in the human large gut
    (c) produces endotoxin
    (d) causes Fournier's gangrene
    (e) infection following colorectal surgery is prevented by metronidazole

1.110 Correct statements about actinomycetes include (page 39):
    (a) It is a fungus.
    (b) The cervicofacial variety usually occurs following dental infection.
    (c) *Actinomyces* is a normal mouth and intestine commensal.
    (d) Pelvic actinomycosis appears to be increasing with the wider use of intrauterine contraceptive devices.
    (e) Surgery as well as penicillin therapy is usually required

1.111 Clinical features of nocardiosis include (page 39):
    (a) Haemoptysis
    (b) Empyema
    (c) Madura foot

(d) Mycetoma

(e) Systemic symptoms are common

1.112 Recognized fungal causes of mycetoma include (page 39):

(a) *Actinomadura*

(b) *Streptomyces* sp.

(c) *Madurella mycetomi*

(d) *Petriellidium boydii*

(e) *Nocardia* sp.

1.113 Mycobacteria (page 40):

(a) are acid-fast bacilli

(b) are aerobic

(c) produce extracellular lecithinase

(d) contain cord factor in the cell wall which are responsible for producing granulomas

(e) produce exotoxin

1.114 Correct statements about the pathology of TB include (page 40):

(a) The primary infection usually spares the lungs.

(b) In primary infection lymph node involvement is rare.

(c) In most people the primary infection heals, leaving some surviving TB bacilli.

(d) TB in the adult is usually the result of reactivation of old disease.

(e) The primary infection can involve the ileocaecal region.

1.115 The following associations are correct (Table 1.25):

(a) *Mycobacterium leprae* – cattle tuberculosis

(b) *M. avium intracellulare* – tuberculosis in HIV infection

(c) *M. tuberculosis* – scrofula

(d) *M. scrofulaceum* – Johne's disease

(e) *M. kansasii* – human tuberculosis

1.116 Patients susceptible to TB include (page 40):

(a) The elderly

(b) Those with diabetes mellitus

(c) Those on corticosteroid therapy

(d) After gastrectomy

(e) Alcohol abusers

1.117 Recognized clinical features of tuberculosis include (page 40):

(a) Lupus pernio

(b) Addison's disease

(c) Constrictive pericarditis

(d) Hypertrophic cardiomyopathy

(e) Phlyctenular keratoconjunctivitis

1.118 Properties of *Mycobacterium leprae* include (page 41):
   (a) It grows in tissue culture.
   (b) It does not grow in the foot-pad of mice.
   (c) It loses acid fastness following pyridine extraction.
   (d) It oxidizes 3,4-dihydroxyphenlyalanine to pigmented products.
   (e) It is unable to invade peripheral nerves.

1.119 Recognized features of leprosy include (page 42):
   (a) Tuberculoid leprosy is a localized disease that occurs in individuals with a high degree of cell-mediated immunity.
   (b) In lepromatous leprosy cell-mediated immunity is intact.
   (c) Hypopigmented skin patches with loss of sensation.
   (d) Tuberculoid lesions are known to heal spontaneously.
   (e) The earlobes are spared in lepromatous leprosy.

1.120 Correct statements about lepra reactions include (page 43):
   (a) Dharmendra lepromin is used to elicit it.
   (b) The late reaction is known as the Mitusuda reaction.
   (c) The type II reaction is a humoral antibody response to an antigen – antibody complex.
   (d) Thalidomide is used in treatment.
   (e) Treatment is urgent.

1.121 Correct statements about the diagnosis and treatment of leprosy include (page 43):
   (a) The bacteriological index is an objective way of evaluating the response to treatment.
   (b) A patient with a morphological index of 0% is highly infectious.
   (c) Bacteriostatic drugs should be avoided.
   (d) The erythromycin derivative clarithromycin is currently under evaluation in human infection.
   (e) In multibacillary leprosy triple therapy should be given for a minimum of 2 years.

1.122 The following associations regarding spirochaetal infection are correct (Table 1.26):
   (a) Syphilis – *Treponema pertenue*
   (b) Cancrum oris – *Borrelia vincenti*
   (c) Lyme disease – *Spirillum minus*
   (d) Rat-bite fever – *Streptobacillus moniliformis*
   (e) Relapsing fever – *Borrelia* sp.

1.123 Recognized features of leptospirosis include (page 45):
   (a) It is common in those who take part in water sports.
   (b) The liver is usually not affected.
   (c) The majority recover in the immune phase.

(d) Penicillins should be avoided.

(e) The heart may be involved.

1.124 Features of Lyme disease include (page 47):

(a) It is transmitted by ticks.

(b) Meningoencephalitis.

(c) Erythema chronicum migrans.

(d) The diagnosis is usually confirmed by isolation of the spirochaetes from blood.

(e) Intravenous benzylpenicillin should be given early in the course of the disease.

1.125 The following associations between rickettsial infections and their vectors are correct (Table 1.27):

(a) Epidemic typhus – ticks

(b) Rocky Mountain spotted fever – human lice

(c) Scrub typhus – larval mite

(d) Q-fever – ticks

(e) Endemic typhus fever – flea

1.126 The following statements regarding rickettsial infections are correct (pages 48–49):

(a) The recrudescence of epidemic typhus is known as Brill–Zinser disease.

(b) The main lesion produced is a vasculitis.

(c) Rocky Mountain spotted fever is common in Europe.

(d) Tetracycline is used in the treatment of acute Q-fever.

(e) Endocarditis is a feature of Q-fever.

1.127 The following associations are correct (pages 51–52):

(a) Human herpes virus type 8 – Kaposi's sarcoma

(b) Herpes simplex virus – encephalitis

(c) Primary varicella zoster infection – shingles

(d) Epstein–Barr virus – cervical lymphadenopathy

(e) Uterine cytomegalovirus – microcephaly

1.128 Correct statements about the clinical features of chickenpox include (pages 52–53):

(a) Characteristic absence of a prodromal illness.

(b) The skin lesions occur on the face, scalp and trunk and to a much lesser extent on the extremities.

(c) It is characteristic to see skin lesions at all stages of development on the same area of skin.

(d) The primary infection almost never occurs twice in the same individual.

(e) The illness can be debilitating in adults.

1.129 Recognized complications of chickenpox include (pages 52–53):
  (a) Acute truncal cerebellar ataxia
  (b) Pneumonia
  (c) Disseminated infection with multiorgan involvement
  (d) Cardiac failure
  (e) Infectious mononucleosis

1.130 Correct statements about treatment of chickenpox and shingles include (page 53):
  (a) Chickenpox requires no treatment in healthy children.
  (b) An infection results in lifelong immunity.
  (c) The disease can be fatal in the immunocompromised.
  (d) Anyone over the age of 16 years with chickenpox should be considered for acyclovir therapy if they present within 72 hours.
  (e) Acyclovir treatment in shingles has been shown to reduce the burden of zoster-associated pain when treatment is given in the acute phase.

1.131 Recognized clinical manifestations of cytomegalovirus include (pages 53–54):
  (a) Hepatitis
  (b) Atypical lymphocytes
  (c) It does not affect healthy adults
  (d) Retinitis
  (e) It can be transmitted by kissing

1.132 Recognized laboratory features of Epstein–Barr virus infection include (page 54):
  (a) Atypical mononuclear cells
  (b) A positive Paul–Bunnell reaction in the second week
  (c) IgM antibodies
  (d) A positive Monospot test
  (e) Varicella zoster antibodies

1.133 Indications for corticosteroid therapy in Epstein–Barr virus infections include (page 54):
  (a) Guillain–Barré syndrome
  (b) Encephalitis
  (c) Splenic rupture
  (d) Thrombocytopenia
  (e) Haemolysis

1.134 The following associations are correct (pages 54–55):
  (a) The human BK virus, polyomavirus – urine of renal transplant recipients
  (b) Human parvovirus B19 produces – aplastic crisis in sickle cell disease
  (c) Epstein–Barr virus – Burkitt's lymphoma
  (d) Epstein–Barr virus – nasopharyngeal carcinoma
  (e) Epstein–Barr virus – cat-scratch disease

1.135 Factors that predispose to the development of paralysis in poliomyelitis include (pages 56–57):
   (a) Female sex
   (b) Exercise early in the illness
   (c) Recent tonsillectomy
   (d) HLA-3
   (e) Intramuscular injection

1.136 Clinical features of poliomyelitis include (pages 56–57):
   (a) Sensory involvement
   (b) Symmetrical paralysis
   (c) Cranial nerve involvement
   (d) Quadriplegia in adults
   (e) Myocarditis

1.137 The following associations are correct (page 58):
   (a) Bornholm disease – picornavirus
   (b) Gastroenteritis – rotavirus
   (c) Gastroenteritis – Norwalk virus
   (d) Forchheimer spots – rubella
   (e) Haemorrhagic manifestations – yellow fever

1.138 The following are RNA viruses (Table 1.31):
   (a) Poxvirus
   (b) Rubella virus
   (c) Measles virus
   (d) Herpes virus
   (e) Human immunodeficiency virus

1.139 Correct statements about rotavirus include (page 58):
   (a) Adults are more often affected than children.
   (b) Geriatric patients are typically spared.
   (c) The diagnosis can be established by ELISA.
   (d) Rhesus–human reassortment vaccines have been shown to give levels of protection in children in developing countries.
   (e) Antibiotics should be prescribed as soon as the diagnosis is made.

1.140 Clinical features of congenital rubella syndrome include (page 59):
   (a) Patent ductus arteriosus
   (b) Ventricular septal defect
   (c) Cataracts
   (d) Microcephaly
   (e) Deafness

1.141 Correct statements about the prevention of rubella include (page 59):
   (a) Human immunoglobulin can prevent teratogenic effects.
   (b) Human immunoglobulin has no effect on the symptoms of the illness.

(c) Vaccines prepared from human embryonic fibroblast cultures have more side effects than other live attenuated vaccines.
(d) The use of vaccine is contraindicated in pregnancy.
(e) Use of the vaccine during pregnancy has not revealed a risk of teratogenicity.

1.142 Correct statements about yellow fever include (page 60):
(a) It is caused by a flavivirus.
(b) It is common in Asia.
(c) Once infected, a mosquito remains so for its whole life.
(d) Monkeys form the sylvan reservoir.
(e) When the infection is mild it is indistinguishable from influenza.

1.143 Correct statements about the treatment and prevention of yellow fever include (page 60):
(a) It is an internationally notifiable disease.
(b) It is prevented by the 17-day chick embryo vaccine.
(c) It is prevented by the Dakar vaccine.
(d) Eradication of the breeding places of the mosquito will help reduce the prevalence of the disease.
(e) Treatment is supportive.

1.144 Correct statements about dengue include (page 61):
(a) It is transmitted by *Aëdes aegypti.*
(b) Humans are infectious in the first 3 days of the illness.
(c) Once infected, mosquitoes remain so for the rest of their lives.
(d) Backache.
(e) Biphasic fever.

1.145 Correct statements about Japanese encephalitis include (page 61):
(a) It is caused by a flavivirus.
(b) Mosquitoes are the vector.
(c) Humans are accidental hosts.
(d) Antibody detection in serum by IgM capture ELISA is a rapid diagnostic test.
(e) An inactivated mouse brain vaccine is effective.

1.146 Correct statements about the epidemiology of influenza include (page 62):
(a) The incidence increases during summer months.
(b) Influenza A is generally responsible for pandemics and epidemics.
(c) Influenza B often causes small or localized outbreaks, e.g. in camps and schools.
(d) Influenza C commonly produces disease in humans.
(e) Antigenic shift usually heralds the onset of a pandemic.

1.147 Correct statements about measles include (page 63):
(a) It is spread by droplet infection.

    (b) Koplik's spots occur before the onset of the rash.
    (c) It carries a high mortality in malnourished children.
    (d) It is a relatively mild disease in the healthy child.
    (e) Subacute sclerosing panencephalitis is a complication.

1.148 Human immunoglobulin in measles is indicated in (page 63):
    (a) Adults
    (b) The elderly
    (c) Previously unimmunized children below 3 years of age
    (d) Pregnant women
    (e) Debilitating disease

1.149 Correct statements about mumps include (pages 63–64):
    (a) It is spread by droplet infection.
    (b) Humans are the only known natural hosts.
    (c) Epididymo-orchitis is a recognized complication.
    (d) The diagnosis of mumps is on the basis of the clinical features.
    (e) Live attenuated mumps virus vaccine is contraindicated in children over the age of 1 year.

1.150 The rabies virus (pages 64–65):
    (a) is bullet shaped
    (b) penetrates nerve endings and travels in the axoplasm to the brain and spinal cord
    (c) causes hydrophobia
    (d) is common in Australia
    (e) is carried by bats.

1.151 Correct statements about rabies include (pages 64–65):
    (a) Almost all bites of rabid animals result in clinical disease.
    (b) The classical Negri bodies are detected in 90% of all patients with rabies.
    (c) Once the disease is established, therapy is symptomatic and death is inevitable.
    (d) Rabid animals can transmit the disease by licking abraded skin or mucosa.
    (e) Bites from rabid bats can cause the disease in humans.

1.152 Correct statements about the prevention of rabies include (page 65):
    (a) Vaccines of nervous-tissue origin are the vaccines of choice.
    (b) Human diploid cell strain vaccine is an experimental vaccine.
    (c) Duck embryo vaccine is a live attenuated virus vaccine.
    (d) Pre-exposure prophylaxis is given to all individuals in areas where rabies is prevalent.
    (e) Duck embryo vaccine should not be administered for post-exposure prophylaxis.

1.153 Correct statements about prion disease include (pages 66–67):
   (a) They result in spongiform encephalopathy.
   (b) Creutzfeldt–Jakob disease has occurred as result of the administration of human growth hormone.
   (c) Gerstmann–Straussler–Scheinker syndrome occurs in families.
   (d) These agents are considered to be orthodox viruses.
   (e) In the infected host there is no evidence of inflammatory cytokines or immune reactions.

1.154 Recognized clinical features of primary pulmonary histoplasmosis include (pages 68–69):
   (a) It is usually asymptomatic.
   (b) The only evidence of infection is conversion of a histoplasmin skin reaction from negative to positive.
   (c) The radiological features are similar to Ghon complex of tuberculosis.
   (d) Calcification in the spleen occurs in patients from areas of high endemicity.
   (e) It is confined to the Ohio and Mississippi Rivers.

1.155 Recognized clinical features of chronic pulmonary histoplasmosis include (pages 68–69):
   (a) It is usually seen in white males.
   (b) It is usually seen in those under the age of 50.
   (c) Pulmonary cavities.
   (d) Pulmonary infiltrates.
   (e) Fibrous streaking from the periphery to the hilum of the lung.

1.156 Recognized clinical features of disseminated histoplasmosis include (pages 68–69):
   (a) Lymphadenopathy
   (b) Hepatosplenomegaly
   (c) Weight loss
   (d) Addison's disease
   (e) Thrombocytopenia

1.157 In histoplasmosis (pages 68–69):
   (a) the histoplasmin skin test is usually negative
   (b) definitive diagnosis can be made by culturing the fungi
   (c) antibodies usually develop within 3 weeks of the onset of illness
   (d) antibodies are best detected by the complement fixation test
   (e) mild forms of primary pulmonary histoplasmosis do not require therapy

1.158 Clinical features of fulminant aspergillosis include (page 69):
   (a) Acute pneumonia
   (b) Meningitis
   (c) Lytic bone lesions

(d) Granulomatous lesions in the liver
(e) Endocarditis

1.159 Cryptococcus neoformans (pages 69–70):
(a) is a yeast-like fungus
(b) is spread by pigeon droppings
(c) enters the body by inhalation of spores
(d) elicits a granulomatous reaction in tissue
(e) causes pulmonary fibrosis

1.160 Correct statements about coccidioidomycosis include (pages 69–70):
(a) It is rare in the Americas.
(b) Epidemics occur following dust storms.
(c) The majority of the patients are asymptomatic.
(d) Infection is detected by the conversion of a skin test.
(e) In acute coccidioidomycosis complete recovery is rare.

1.161 Recognized clinical manifestations of rhinocerebral mucormycosis include (pages 70–71):
(a) It is mainly seen in diabetics with ketoacidosis.
(b) Nasal stuffiness
(c) Facial oedema
(d) Necrotic nasal turbinates
(e) Facial pain

1.162 Correct statements about chronic mucocutaneous candidiasis include (page 71):
(a) It usually occurs in children.
(b) It is associated with a T-cell defect.
(c) It presents with hyperkeratotic plaque-like lesions on the skin.
(d) It is associated with hypothyroidism.
(e) It is associated with hypoparathyroidism.

1.163 Recognized features of visceral leishmaniasis include (pages 71–72):
(a) It usually affects young people.
(b) Skin pigmentation.
(c) Spleen is enlarged.
(d) It is transmitted by the sandfly.
(e) Humans do not serve as reservoirs.

1.164 Correct statements about the diagnosis and treatment of visceral leishmaniasis include (pages 71–72):
(a) An intradermal leishmanin skin test is of value in diagnosis.
(b) Leishman–Donovan bodies may be demonstrated in buffy-coat preparations of blood.
(c) The organism can be cultured in Nicolle–Novy–Macneal culture medium.

(d) African kala-azar is relatively resistant to therapy.

(e) Pentavalent antimony compounds are the drugs of choice.

1.165 African trypanosomiasis (page 73):
(a) follows the bite of the tsetse fly
(b) is caused by *Trypanosoma brucei*
(c) of the Gambian variety is a chronic illness with symptom-free periods
(d) of the Rhodesian form causes death usually within a year
(e) death is often due to myocarditis in the Rhodesian sleeping illness

1.166 Correct statements about Chagas' disease include (pages 75–76):
(a) It is not a zoonotic disease.
(b) It is caused by *Trypanosoma cruzi*
(c) It is transmitted by the reduviid bug
(d) The heart is invariably spared.
(e) Vaccination can prevent the disease.

1.167 Correct statements about toxoplasmosis include (pages 76–77):
(a) Humans are a definitive host.
(b) It may be clinically indistinguishable from infectious mononucleosis.
(c) Asymptomatic lymphadenopathy is the commonest mode of presentation.
(d) The Sabin–Feldman dye test is used to diagnose it.
(e) Pyrimethamine and sulphadiazine are used in combination to treat severe disease.

1.168 Correct statements about *Pneumocystis carinii* infection include:
(a) It causes interstitial pneumonia in the immunocompromised patients.
(b) Physical signs in the chest are minimal or absent.
(c) Transbronchial biopsy is the favoured way to detect the organism.
(d) High-dose co-trimoxazole is used in treatment.
(e) Co-trimoxazole is useful in protecting high-risk patients from infection.

1.169 Correct statements about malaria include (pages 77–78):
(a) *Plasmodium vivax* preferentially invades senescent red blood cells.
(b) *Plasmodium falciparum* has exoerythrocytic schizogony.
(c) Those with blood Duffy-negative are highly susceptible to *P. vivax* malaria.
(d) Tumour necrosis factor-α blood levels correlate with the severity of the disease.
(e) Herpes labialis frequently occurs in established malaria.

1.170 The following associations are correct (pages 77–81):
(a) *P. vivax* – relapses
(b) *P. malariae* – nephrotic syndrome
(c) *P. falciparum* – cerebral malaria

    (d) *P. falciparum* – blackwater fever

    (e) Polymorphisms of ICAM-1 – cerebral malaria

1.171 Drugs used in the treatment of chloroquine-resistant malaria include (pages 80–81):

    (a) Mefloquine

    (b) Halofantrine

    (c) Artemisin

    (d) Proguanil

    (e) Quinine

1.172 Correct statements about tropical splenomegaly include (page 80):

    (a) It is seen in areas where malaria is hyperendemic.

    (b) It usually occurs before the age of 4.

    (c) Serum IgM levels are typically low.

    (d) It responds to antimalarial therapy.

    (e) Malarial parasites are detected in peripheral blood smears.

1.173 The following statements about malaria are correct (page 80):

    (a) Spleen rate is the percentage of children between 2 and 10 years with splenomegaly.

    (b) Spleen rate is used as a measure of the endemicity of malaria in a community.

    (c) Infant parasite rate is defined as the percentage of infants below 1 year of age in whom malarial parasites are demonstrable in peripheral blood smears.

    (d) Infant parasite rate is the most sensitive index of transmission of malaria to a locality.

    (e) Serological methods are widely used in the diagnosis.

1.174 Correct statements about amoebiasis include (pages 81–82):

    (a) Active homosexuals are susceptible.

    (b) Pus from an amoebic abscess has an 'anchovy sauce' appearance.

    (c) Liver abscess is associated with an elevated alkaline phosphatase.

    (d) The amoebic fluorescent antibody titre is usually positive in asymptomatic cyst passers.

    (e) Metronidazole is ineffective in amoebic liver abscess.

1.175 The following associations are correct (page 83):

    (a) Giardiasis – malabsorption

    (b) *Cryptosporidum parvum* – diarrhoea in those with AIDS

    (c) *Brugia malayi* – scrotal involvement is common.

    (d) Loa loa – calabar swellings

    (e) *Onchocerca volvulus* – ocular lesions

1.176 The following associations are correct (pages 84–91):

    (a) *Toxocara canis* – cutaneous larva migrans.

(b) *Necator americanus* – visceral larva migrans.
(c) Trichinosis – muscle cramps
(d) *Strongyloides stercoralis* – malabsorption
(e) *Trichuris trichura* – rectal prolapse.

1.177 Percutaneous spread of filariform larvae occurs with (Fig. 1.44):
(a) *Trichuris trichura*
(b) *Enterobius vermicularis*
(c) *Ascaris lumbricoides*
(d) Hookworm
(e) *Strongyloides stercoralis*

1.178 The following associations are correct (pages 91–94):
(a) *Schistosoma mansoni* – granulomatous hepatitis
(b) *S. haematobium* – obstructive uropathy
(c) *Clonorchis sinensis* – cholangiocarcinoma
(d) *Paragonimus westermani* – pulmonary involvement
(e) Schistosomiasis – Katayama fever

1.179 The following associations are correct (pages 94–95):
(a) Beef tapeworm – cysticercosis
(b) *Diphyllobothrium latum* – megaloblastic anaemia
(c) Hydatid disease – hepatic cysts
(d) *Trichomonas vaginalis* – vaginal discharge
(e) Gonococcus – Fitz-Hugh–Curtis syndrome

1.180 Causes of urethritis include (Table 1.43):
(a) *Chlamydiae trachomatis*
(b) *Ureaplasma urealyticum*
(c) Mycoplasma
(d) Varicella zoster
(e) Gonococcus

1.181 Causes of genital ulceration include (Table 1.44):
(a) Chancroid
(b) Herpes simplex
(c) Behçet's syndrome
(d) Granuloma inguinale
(e) Lymphogranuloma venereum

1.182 The following associations are correct (Table 1.45):
(a) 'Snail-track' ulcers – primary syphilis
(b) Chancre – secondary syphilis
(c) Tertiary syphilis – aortic regurgitation
(d) Secondary syphilis – tabes dorsalis
(e) Congenital syphilis – Hutchinson's teeth

1.183 The following statements about investigations for syphilis are correct (pages 101–103):
(a) *Treponema pallidum* grows in a culture dish.
(b) The VDRL is a specific test.
(c) The *Treponema pallidum* haemagglutination assay (TPHA) will differentiate between syphilis and yaws.
(d) The FTA-abs test remains positive for life, even after treatment.
(e) Dark-ground microscopy is the most sensitive and specific method for the identification of *Treponema pallidum*.

1.184 The following statements about the management of syphilis are correct (pages 102–103):
(a) Early syphilis should be treated with long-acting penicillin.
(b) Jarisch–Herxheimer reaction, a consequence of penicillin treatment, occurs in a small minority of patients with secondary syphilis.
(c) All patients treated for syphilis must be followed up at about 3 monthly intervals for the first 2 years following treatment.
(d) For neurosyphilis penicillin treatment should be given for a year.
(e) In pregnant patients who are allergic to penicillin, tetracycline is the drug of choice.

1.185 The following associations are correct (pages 103–104):
(a) Chancroid – *Chlamydia trachomatis*
(b) Lymphogranuloma venereum – *Calymmatobacterium granulomatis*
(c) Granuloma inguinale – *Haemophilus ducreyi*
(d) Bacterial vaginosis – *Gardnerella vaginalis*
(e) Anogenital warts – human papilloma virus

1.186 Correct statements about herpes simplex include (page 104):
(a) Asymptomatic infection is common
(b) Primary genital herpes is rarely accompanied by systemic symptoms.
(c) Recurrent attacks are generally more severe than the initial attack.
(d) Acyclovir therapy reduces the frequency of recurrent attacks.
(e) When active lesions are present, condoms effectively prevent sexual transmission.

1.187 Correct statements about herpes simplex during pregnancy include (page 104):
(a) Transplacental infection of the fetus does not occur if infection is acquired for the first time during pregnancy.
(b) The risk of transmitting infection to the baby from the birth canal is very low in the primary episode rather than in recurrent attacks.
(c) Acyclovir is licensed for use in pregnancy.
(d) Obstetric opinion is divided regarding whether caesarian section may be performed if the women has an attack during labour.
(e) It causes genital warts.

1.188 Correct statements about human papilloma virus include (page 104):
- (a) It causes anogential warts.
- (b) It causes laryngeal papillomas.
- (c) It is associated with cervical intraepithelial neoplasia in women.
- (d) Podophyllin extracts are used in treatment.
- (e) Up to one-third of patients have coexisting infections with other sexually transmitted diseases.

1.189 Human immunodeficiency virus (page 107):
- (a) is a DNA virus
- (b) replicates through an RNA intermediate
- (c) is a retrovirus
- (d) uses the enzyme reverse transcriptase for replication
- (e) can bind to receptors on CD4 lymphocytes

1.190 Correct statements about the diagnosis of HIV include (pages 107–113):
- (a) Detection of IgG antibody to envelope components (gp 120 and its subunits) is the most commonly used marker of this infection.
- (b) In babies born to HIV-infected women, the anti-HIV antibody is a reliable marker of active infection.
- (c) IgG antibody to p24 can be detected in late stages of the disease.
- (d) Viral p24 antigen is a useful marker in individuals who have been infected recently.
- (e) Recent law allows the physician to test for HIV without the patient's express consent.

1.191 AIDS occurs in the following population groups (pages 107–113):
- (a) Heterosexual men
- (b) Bisexual men
- (c) Haemophiliacs
- (d) Intravenous drug abusers
- (e) Children whose mothers have AIDS

1.192 Correct statements about the the natural history of HIV include (pages 107–113):
- (a) The majority of patients with HIV infection are asymptomatic for a substantial period of time.
- (b) Asymptomatic individuals are not infectious.
- (c) Older age is associated with a slower disease progression.
- (d) As HIV infection progresses the CD4 count increases.
- (e) Pregnancy exacerbates the rate of disease progression.

1.193 The following statements regarding HIV are correct (pages 107–113):
- (a) Zidovudine has a beneficial effect on HIV neurological disease.
- (b) There are reports of anterior uveitis presenting as acute red eye associated with rifabutin therapy for mycobacterial infections in HIV.
- (c) Resistant cases of aphthous ulcers in HIV may respond to thalidomide.

(d) Thrombocytopenic patients undergoing dental procedures may need therapy with human immunoglobulin.

(e) HIV nephropathy is less frequently seen in black male patients.

1.194 Mucocutaneous manifestations of HIV infection include (pages 107–113):
   (a) Psoriasis
   (b) Ichthyosis
   (c) Pityriasis versicolor
   (d) Oral hairy leucoplakia
   (e) Acne

1.195 The following associations in HIV infection are correct (pages 107–113):
   (a) Toxoplasmosis – multiple ring-enhancing lesions on CT head scan
   (b) CMV retinitis – pizza-pie appearance on fundus examination
   (c) CMV colitis – 'owl eye' cytoplasmic inclusion bodies on histology
   (d) Papovavirus – progressive multifocal leucoencephalopathy
   (e) Kaposi's sarcoma – *Mycobacterium tuberculosis*

1.196 Neoplasms known to occur in AIDS include (page 118):
   (a) Squamous carcinoma of the tongue
   (b) Burkitt's lymphoma
   (c) Primary brain lymphoma
   (d) Kaposi's sarcoma
   (e) Squamous carcinomas of the anal canal

1.197 Neurological manifestations of AIDS include (page 111):
   (a) Dementia
   (b) Peripheral neuropathy
   (c) Atypical aseptic meningitis
   (d) Subacute encephalitis
   (e) Progressive encephalopathy

1.198 Parasites causing infections in AIDS include (Table 1.47):
   (a) *Cryptococcus neoformans*
   (b) *Histoplasma capsulatum*
   (c) *Pneumocystis carinii*
   (d) Cryptosporidia
   (e) *Strongyloides stercoralis*

1.199 Fungi causing infections in AIDS include (Table 1.47):
   (a) *Isospora belli*
   (b) *Sarcocystis* sp.
   (c) *Candida* sp.
   (d) *Toxoplasma gondii*
   (e) *Mycobacterium kansasii*

1.200 The following statements are correct (page 115):
- (a) *Pneumocystis carinii* is not usually seen until patients are severely immunocompromised, with a CD4 count below 200.
- (b) Nebulized pentamidine, used in the long-term prophylaxis of *Pneumocystis carinii*, penetrates the upper lobes particularly efficiently.
- (c) The treatment of TB in the HIV-infected individual is curative.
- (d) Patients on ganciclovir therapy are more prone to infection with *Aspergillus fumigatus*.
- (e) *M. avium intracellulare* generally appears only in the later stages of HIV when patients are profoundly immunocompromised.

1.201 Correct statements about monitoring HIV infection include (page 119):
- (a) The absolute CD4 count, and the percentage of total lymphocytes that this represents, falls as HIV progresses.
- (b) The viral load is the best predictor of long-term prognosis.
- (c) HIV RNA is a marker of treatment efficacy.
- (d) CD4 count gives warning of the risk of immediate or short-term problems.
- (e) Serum β–2 microglobulin is a marker of lymphocyte activation.

1.202 Correct statements about HIV therapy include (pages 120–123):
- (a) Evidence from clinical trials has shown clear benefits from antiretrovirals used in combination rather than as monotherapy.
- (b) Several of the current combinations of drugs eradicate HIV.
- (c) Ritonavir is the only protease inhibitor which has no interactions with the cytochrome p450 system.
- (d) Non-nucleoside reverse transcriptase inhibitors (NNRTIs) bind and inhibit the reverse transcriptase of HIV-2.
- (e) The major toxicity with zidovudine is bone marrow toxicity.

1.203 Correct statements about HIV therapy include (pages 120–123):
- (a) Initiation of therapy with two NNRTIs plus a protease inhibitor produces a more substantial and longer-lasting reduction in viral load in a greater proportion of patients than that obtained with two NNRTIs alone.
- (b) Saquinavir is frequently chosen as initial therapy as it does not preclude the use of indinavir or ritonavir at later date, whereas the reverse does not apply.
- (c) Early data suggest that since the availability of zidovudine prophylaxis in pregnancy, the numbers of HIV-infected children born to HIV-positive mothers has fallen substantially.
- (d) Treatment of mothers with zidovudine monotherapy during pregnancy may have implications with regard to the possible emergence of azidovudine-resistant virus.
- (e) A combination of zidovudine and lamivudine is used in post-exposure prophylaxis.

1.204 A 40-year-old male with AIDS presents with a 20-day history of left frontal headache. The patient is afebrile and has no focal neurological signs, and mental status is normal. A CT head scan shows a 3 × 4 cm solitary mass in the left frontal region which enhances with intravenous contrast agent. There is no hydrocephalus, although there is significant oedema surrounding the lesion. The following management strategies are appropriate at this stage:

(a) Empirical treatment with pyrimethamine and sulphadiazine
(b) Serology for *Toxoplasma gondii*
(c) Magnetic resonance imaging (MRI) of the head to look for multiple lesions
(d) Lumbar puncture for the diagnosis of toxoplasmosis and primary lymphoma
(e) Brain biopsy

1.205 A 25-year-old promiscuous male present with purulent urethral discharge and burning micturition 4 days after unprotected sexual intercourse with a new female partner. Initial diagnostic tests will include:

(a) Urethral Gram stain
(b) Urinanalysis
(c) Culture for *N. gonorrhoeae*
(d) VDRL
(e) Complement fixation test for *C. burnetii*

1.206 A 41-year-old male of West Indian origin with a 15-year history of pulmonary fibrosis and sarcoidosis presents with a 3-week history of low-grade fever, haemoptysis and loss of weight. He has been on intermittent steroid therapy for the last 8 years but has been off steroids for 3 months. Clinical examination reveals diffuse inspiratory wheeze; chest X-ray shows lung fibrosis with bilateral apical lesions. A diagnosis of mycetoma due to aspergillosis is confirmed. The following statements are correct:

(a) The patient requires systemic amphotericin B to eradicate the mycetomas.
(b) About half the mycetomas regress spontaneously.
(c) The diagnosis is confirmed by microscopy and culture of the organism.
(d) In the absence of surgical removal, life-threatening haemoptysis may occur.
(e) High-dose intravenous penicillin is the drug of choice.

1.207 A 28-year-old male doctor from India presents with a 3-week history of fever and pain in the right upper quadrant. The patient lives in the UK and visits his family in Madras every year. On examination he is febrile and has tenderness in the right upper quadrant. The differential diagnosis includes:

(a) Hepatoma
(b) Echinococcal cyst

(c) Amoebic liver abscess
(d) Pyogenic liver abscess
(e) Metastatic adenocarcinoma

1.208 A 32-year-old male presents 4 months following cardiac transplantation with fever, non-productive cough and progressive shortness of breath. On examination he is febrile and has crackles at both bases. Chest X-ray shows diffuse interstitial changes. Correct statements about investigations for the diagnosis of cytomegalovirus include:
(a) CMV IgG titres identify latent infection.
(b) CMV IgM titres identify primary infection.
(c) PCR provides a sensitive method of detecting CMV in blood.
(d) Open lung biopsy is required for diagnosis.
(e) The virus can be identified by the presence of characteristic intranuclear 'owl eye' inclusions.

Cell and Molecular Biology, genetic Disorders and Immunology

2.1 The cell membrane (page 125):
  (a) consists of a bilayer of amphipathic lipid molecules
  (b) contains phospholipids
  (c) contains cholesterol
  (d) contains glycolipids
  (e) is a dynamic fluid compartment

2.2 Functions of the cell membrane include (page 126):
  (a) Selective ion transport
  (b) Modulation of cell function through receptor sites
  (c) Cell recognition and communication.
  (d) Endocytosis
  (e) DNA replication

2.3 Correct statements about G proteins include (page 126):
  (a) When stimulated, G protein exchanges GDP for GTP.
  (b) The separation of the α subunit from the β and γ subunits brings about the biological effects within the cell.
  (c) The heterotrimeric G protein-coupled receptors span the cell membrane seven times.
  (d) G protein is the guanosine analogue of ATP.
  (e) G proteins are absent in the acetylcholine receptor.

2.4 The endoplasmic reticulum (page 127):
  (a) is a network of channels throughout the cytoplasm from the nucleus to the cell membrane
  (b) is involved in the processing of secretory proteins
  (c) contains enzyme systems that hydroxylate hydrophobic compounds
  (d) transports lysosomal enzymes to lysosomes
  (e) is involved in the modification and packaging of secretory proteins

2.5 The mitochondria contains enzymes responsible for (page 127):
  (a) cell digestion, such as acid hydrolases
  (b) oxidative phosphorylation
  (c) the citric acid cycle
  (d) the electron-transport chain
  (e) ATP synthesis

2.6 The following statements about the cytoplasm are correct (page 127):
   (a) The endoplasmic reticulum is involved in the processing of secretory proteins.
   (b) Proteins of the oncogene family *Bcl*-2 are found in the outer membrane of the mitochondria.
   (c) The ubiquitin–proteosome pathway is capable of degrading most cell proteins.
   (d) The Golgi apparatus acts as a focal point for the complex intracellular traffic that takes place between all of the subcellular components.
   (e) Translation of protein occurs in the cytoplasm.

2.7 Correct statements about cell cytoskeleton include (page 127):
   (a) Colchicine disrupts microtubule assembly.
   (b) The anticancer drug paclitaxel causes cell death by binding to microtubules.
   (c) Cell movement is mediated by the anchorage of actin filaments to the plasma membrane.
   (d) Actin-binding proteins modulate the behaviour of microfilaments.
   (e) Vinblastine disrupts microtubule assembly.

2.8 The nucleus contains (page 128):
   (a) Golgi apparatus
   (b) Mitochondria
   (c) Lysosomes
   (d) Endoplasmic reticulum
   (e) DNA

2.9 Correct statements about the cell cycle include (Fig 2.3, page 128):
   (a) During the G1 phase the cell synthesizes RNA, proteins, lipids and polysaccharides.
   (b) During the S phase the genome is replicated.
   (c) G2 is an inactive phase.
   (d) The cell cycle starts with the inactive phase.
   (e) The G1 phase is followed by the G2 phase.

2.10 Correct statements about calcium include (page 128):
   (a) Calcium enters the cell by voltage-gated calcium channels.
   (b) Most of the calcium is bound by the endoplasmic reticulum.
   (c) Calbindin binds and transports calcium ions across membranes.
   (d) Calcineurin inactivates calcium channels.
   (e) Calmodulin, by binding calcium, activates many calmodulin-dependent kinases.

2.11 The following statements are correct (page 128):
   (a) The cell cycle is modified by the cyclin family of proteins.
   (b) Interferons activate the JAK–STAT pathway.
   (c) Transmembrane integrins link the extracellular matrix to

microfilaments at focal areas where cells also attach to their basal laminae.
(d) Charcot–Marie–Tooth disease is a consequence of mutant connexons.
(e) Cadherins mediate cell-to-cell adhesion.

2.12 Correct statements about unifactorial genetic disorders include (pages 141–148):
(a) They are due to a combination of environmental and genetic factors.
(b) There is no clear pattern of inheritance.
(c) There is a low risk to relatives.
(d) They are usually due to single gene defects.
(e) These disorders are numerous, although each individual disorder is rare.

2.13 Each strand of DNA contains (page 129):
(a) Deoxyribose phosphate backbone
(b) Adenine
(c) Guanine
(d) Thymine
(e) Cytosine

2.14 The following statements about DNA are correct (page 129):
(a) Two strands of DNA are held together by oxygen bonds between the two bases.
(b) Thymine always pairs with adenine.
(c) DNA in a cell is coiled around histone proteins to form nucleosomes.
(d) Chromosomes are seen during metaphase.
(e) The two strands of DNA twist to form a single helix.

2.15 Correct statements about codons include (page 129):
(a) Three adjacent nucleotides code for a particular amino acid.
(b) Some amino acids are coded by more than one codon.
(c) Codons are used as signals for initiating polypeptide chain synthesis.
(d) Codons are used as signals for terminating polypeptide chain synthesis.
(e) 'Nonsense' codons code for arginine.

2.16 Correct statements about genes include (page 129):
(a) A gene is a portion of DNA that codes for a single polypeptide sequence.
(b) Structural genes are responsible for synthesis of specific proteins.
(c) Control genes are thought to modify the action of structural genes.
(d) Exons are coding sequences.
(e) Introns are intervening sequences that are non-coding.

2.17 Correct statements about messenger RNA include (page 131–132):
(a) It carries genetic information from the nucleus to the cytoplasm.
(b) Translation begins when the triplet AUG (methionine) is encountered.
(c) It is found mainly in the nucleolus and cytoplasm.

(d) The poly A tail is translated.
(e) Before it leaves the nucleus, the exons are excised and introns are spliced together.

2.18 The following associations of DNA-binding proteins causing human pathology are correct (Table 2.1):
(a) Zinc finger – steroid receptors
(b) Helix–turn–helix – cAMP response element-binding protein
(c) Leucine zipper – *cFos* cell replication oncogene
(d) Zinc finger – *WT-1* oncogene product (Wilms' tumour)
(e) Helix–loop–helix – *Myc* oncogene

2.19 Correct statements about regulators of gene expression include (page 135):
(a) RNA polymerases bind to the promoter regions.
(b) Operator regions act as repressors by binding to DNA sequences within the promoter site.
(c) Operator regions act as positive regulators.
(d) The promoter region is normally a considerable distance from the site of transcription initiation.
(e) The enhancer region is normally adjacent to the site of transcription initiation.

2.20 The following statements are correct (page 136):
(a) The euchromatin are condensed regions that consist of supercoiled DNA around histones.
(b) The supercoiling of DNA around histones gives tighter control of specific gene expression.
(c) Exons enable the production of alternative proteins for one gene.
(d) In eukaryocytes, genomic RNA is associated with nuclear proteins called histones.
(e) Most of human DNA is highly repetitive, consisting of long arrays of tandem repeats.

2.21 Pulsed field gel electrophoresis (page 137):
(a) is a technique used for long-range mapping of the genome
(b) is used to separate very long pieces of DNA
(c) can be used for identification of gene deletions
(d) is the same as PCR
(e) is used to detect gene rearrangements

2.22 The following statements are correct (page 138):
(a) Restriction endonucleases are bacterial enzymes that recognize their own individually specific DNA sequence and cleave double-stranded DNA at these sites.
(b) Southern blotting is a technique for detection of a specific DNA gene using a specific radiolabelled DNA probe.

(c) A fundamental property of DNA is that when the two strands are separated by heating they will reassociate and stick together again because of their complementary base sequences.
(d) Bacterial plasmids consist of a circular ring of DNA.
(e) Gene sequencing can be used for the identification of many single-gene disorders.

2.23 The following statements regarding the DNA probe are correct (page 137):
(a) The presence or position of a particular gene can be identified using a gene probe.
(b) The gene probe consists of DNA with a base sequence that is complementary to that of the gene.
(c) A probe is a piece of single-stranded DNA radiolabelled with ^{32}P.
(d) Complementary DNA (cDNA) probes can be synthesized from the messenger RNA of the gene under study using reverse transcriptase.
(e) DNA probes can be cloned by incorporating the DNA fragment into a bacterial plasmid.

2.24 The following associations are correct (page 137):
(a) DNA fragments – Northern blotting
(b) RNA fragments – Southern blotting
(c) Proteins – Western blotting
(d) Nucleotide sequence – dideoxy sequencing
(e) Protein amplification – PCR

2.25 The following statements about DNA cloning are correct (page 138):
(a) Plasmids are self-replicating episomal circular DNA molecules found in bacteria which carry antibody resistance genes.
(b) Yeast artificial chromosomes are derived from centromeric and telomeric DNA sequences found in the yeast.
(c) A cosmid is a hybrid between a plasmid and a bacteriophage.
(d) Several hundred kilobases of DNA can be inserted into a bacteriophage.
(e) A DNA fragment of interest is inserted into the vector DNA sequence using an enzyme ligase.

2.26 Correct statements about the polymerase chain reaction (PCR) include (page 138):
(a) Small amounts of DNA can be amplified enormously using this technique.
(b) It allows rapid analysis of DNA without the need for radioactive probes or autoradiography.
(c) The DNA is heated to allow primers to anneal to their complementary sequence.
(d) It can be used for prenatal diagnosis of cystic fibrosis.
(e) DNA polymerase is used to extend primers in opposite directions using the target DNA as a template.

2.27 X-linked disorders include (Table 2.8):
  (a) Rare forms of diabetes mellitus
  (b) Pompé's disease
  (c) Retinitis pigmentosa
  (d) Duchenne muscular dystrophy
  (e) Haemophilia B

2.28 Molecular biological techniques in genetics are useful in (pages 129–157):
  (a) the investigation of gene structure
  (b) prenatal diagnosis of disease
  (c) carrier detection of genetic disease
  (d) the biosynthesis of insulin
  (e) diagnosis of Huntington's chorea

2.29 The following statements about chromosomes are correct (pages 139–140):
  (a) Human gametes contain 46 chromosomes.
  (b) Chromosomes contain one linear molecule of DNA that is wound around histone proteins into smaller units called nucleosomes.
  (c) Primary male sexual characteristics are determined by the *SRY* gene.
  (d) The short arm of the chromosome is called q.
  (e) Chromosomes are numbered from the smallest (No 1) to the largest (No 46).

2.30 The following statements about chromosomes are correct (page 140):
  (a) Lyonization is a process whereby one of the two X chromosomes in the cells of females become transcriptionally inactive, so the cell has only one dose of X-linked genes.
  (b) Replication of linear chromosomes starts at coding sites at the two extreme ends.
  (c) Stem cells have longer telomeres than their terminally differentiated daughters.
  (d) Cells from patients with progeria have extremely long telomeres.
  (e) The mitochondria of cells have their own chromosomes.

2.31 Correct statements about chromosomal disorders include (page 141, Table 2.2):
  (a) Over half of spontaneous abortions have chromosomal abnormalities.
  (b) At least one-fifth of all live births have chromosomal abnormalities.
  (c) Autosomal aneuploidy is usually more severe than the sex-chromosome aneuploidies.
  (d) Abnormalities of the sex chromosome are three times as common as abnormalities of the autosome.
  (e) Congenital malformations are more prevalent than single-gene disorders.

2.32 Non-disjunction (page 141–142):
  (a) is an abnormality of nuclear division

(b) is characterized by the failure of chromosomes to separate during nuclear division
(c) can occur with autosomes
(d) cannot occur with sex chromosomes
(e) occurring during mitosis can result in mosaicism

2.33 The following associations are correct (pages 141–143):
(a) Prader–Willi syndrome – deletion of a part of the long arm of chromosome 15.
(b) Anirida–Wilms – duplication of a part of the short arm of chromosome 11.
(c) DiGeorge syndrome – microdeletion in the long arm of chromosome 22.
(d) Charcot–Marie–Tooth disease – small duplication of a region of chromosome 17.
(e) Tumourigenesis – chromosome translocations in somatic cells.

2.34 Reciprocal translocation (page 142):
(a) occurs when any two homologous chromosomes lying together break simultaneously and a portion of one joins up with a portion of the other
(b) results in the cell having 47 chromosomes
(c) causes physical deformities in carriers of this balanced translocation
(d) can involve more than two chromosomes
(e) involves an end-to-end reversal of a segment within a chromosome.

2.35 Robertsonian translocation (page 142):
(a) occurs when two acrocentric chromosomes join and the short arm is lost
(b) results in the cell having 45 chromosomes
(c) is an unbalanced translocation
(d) of the 14/21 chromosome in a woman results in a 1 in 8 risk of delivering a baby with Down's syndrome
(e) of the 14/21 chromosome in an individual results in a 50% risk of producing a carrier like themselves.

2.36 Abnormalities of sex chromosomes include (page 142, Table 2.4):
(a) Down's syndrome
(b) Patau's syndrome
(c) Leber's optic atrophy
(d) Myoclonic epilepsy with ragged red fibres
(e) Klinefelter's syndrome

2.37 Mitochondrial chromosomes (page 142):
(a) contain double-stranded DNA
(b) are transmitted only by mothers
(c) have a different genetic code from nuclear DNA

(d) abnormalities result in mitochondrial myopathies

(e) code for components of mitochondrial respiratory chain and oxidative phosphorylation

2.38 Mutations (page 144):
(a) are changes in the DNA
(b) are random
(c) cannot be inherited
(d) can be due to gene invasion
(e) can be due to gene fusions

2.39 The following associations are correct (page 144):
(a) Point mutation within the globin gene – sickle cell disease
(b) Termination mutations – haemoglobin Constant Spring
(c) Deletions in the dystrophin gene – Duchennes muscular dystrophy
(d) Frame shift mutations – thalassaemia
(e) Insertion/deletion polymorphism in the angiotensin-converting enzyme (ACE) gene – cardiac disease

2.40 Substitution (page 144):
(a) involves the substitution of one base or one triplet for another
(b) of valine for glutamic acid occurs in Hb S disease
(c) of amino acids has resulted in over 300 haemoglobin variants
(d) of a single amino acid can result in glucose-6-phosphate dehydrogenase deficiency
(e) can result in a splicing mutation.

2.41 Correct statements about autosomal dominant disorders include (page 145):
(a) Cystic fibrosis is the commonest autosomal dominant disorder in the UK.
(b) These disorders manifest themselves only when an individual is homozygous for the disease allele.
(c) Incomplete penetrance may occur with patients having the dominant disorder but not having the clinical manifestations.
(d) About half the offspring will carry the disease allele.
(e) The overall incidence is 7 per 1000 live births.

2.42 Examples of autosomal dominant disorders include (Table 2.5):
(a) Cystic fibrosis
(b) Oculocutaneous albinism
(c) Haemochromatosis
(d) Infantile polycystic kidney disease
(e) Wilson's disease

2.43 Examples of autosomal recessive disorders include (Table 2.6):
(a) Marfan's syndrome

    (b) Huntington's chorea
    (c) Neurofibromatosis
    (d) Adult polycystic kidney disease
    (e) Dystrophia myotonica

2.44 Examples of polygenic inheritance include (Table 2.9):
    (a) Congenital pyloric stenosis
    (b) Hypertension
    (c) Rheumatoid arthritis
    (d) Epilepsy
    (e) Ischaemic heart disease

2.45 X-linked dominant disorders include (page 146):
    (a) Vitamin D-resistant rickets
    (b) Colour blindness
    (c) Haemophilia
    (d) Duchenne muscular dystrophy
    (e) Becker's muscular dystrophy

2.46 Characteristics of autosomal recessive disorders include (page 146):
    (a) The affected individual is homozygous for the gene.
    (b) The parents are unaffected healthy carriers.
    (c) The parents are also homozygous.
    (d) There is usually no family history.
    (e) Consanguinity increases the risk of a recessive disorder.

2.47 Characteristics of X-linked recessive disorders include (page 147):
    (a) In the male, X-linked recessive genes only manifest when the gene is homozygous.
    (b) These conditions usually affect females.
    (c) They are transmitted by healthy male carriers.
    (d) The male offspring of a male with the disorder will not have the disease as long as his wife is not a carrier.
    (e) All female offspring of an affected male will be carriers.

2.48 The following associations are correct (page 147):
    (a) Y-linked single gene disorder – vitamin D-resistant rickets.
    (b) Triplet repeat mutations – myotonic dystrophy
    (c) Anticipation – offspring of patients with myotonic dystrophy
    (d) Imprinting – fetal recognition of chromosomes inherited from mother or father
    (e) Triplet repeat expansion – Huntington's disease

2.49 The following statements are correct (pages 148–150):
    (a) Linkage can be important in the detection of diseases in which no marker is known.

(b) Restriction fragment length polymorphism (RFLP) is DNA fragments of identical sizes.
(c) RFLP can be used as markers of genetic disorders.
(d) The lod score is a measure of the statistical significance of the observed co-segregation of the disease gene and the marker DNA sequence.
(e) Positional cloning is used to isolate genes whose protein products are not known, but whose existence can be inferred from a disease phenotype.

2.50 Oncogenes (page 151):
(a) are genes that are present in normal cells
(b) in cancer cells become altered in expression or structure
(c) share genes that share some homology with genes of oncogenic viruses
(d) can be activated by viruses
(e) can be activated by structural point mutations

2.51 The following associations are correct (page 152):
(a) *Abl* gene – chronic lymphatic leukaemia
(b) N-*myc* – neuroblastoma
(c) N-*myc* – small cell carcinoma of the lung
(d) L-*myc* – Small cell carcinoma of the lung
(e) Fusion gene – chronic myeloid leukemia

2.52 The following tumours have a familial predisposition (Table 2.10):
(a) Retinoblastoma
(b) Wilms' tumour
(c) Mycetoma
(d) Eumycetoma
(e) Granuloma

2.53 The following statements about the *p53* gene include (page 152):
(a) It has been found in almost all human tumours.
(b) It is a nuclear phosphoprotein that affects apoptosis.
(c) In colorectal carcinomas the mutant *p53* is shorter lived than the normal allele.
(d) Mutation of a single copy of the gene is not sufficient to promote tumour formation because a heterodimer of mutated and normal *p53* would still be functioning normally.
(e) It is a DNA-binding protein.

2.54 The following statements are correct (pages 152–153):
(a) The transcription factor dimer E2F-DP1 prevents the progression from the G1 to the S phase.
(b) Proteins WAF-1/p21, p16 and p17 inhibit the activation of the retinoblastoma gene by cyclin D-related proteins.
(c) The retinoblastoma gene normally stops the cell cycle.

(d) The human papilloma virus binds to the retinoblastoma gene.
(e) The SV40 virus large T antigen binds both retinoblastoma and *p53* gene.

2.55 Apoptosis (page 153):
(a) is mediated by the enzyme CASPASE
(b) is cell death where the organelles remain intact
(c) Requires energy (ATP)
(d) is associated with an inflammatory response
(e) is due to overexpression of *Bcl*-2

2.56 The following statements are correct (pages 153, 154, 157, 160):
(a) The *Knudson multi-hit hypothesis* proposes that an inherited mutation in one gene allele may be insufficient to cause a tumour but will cause a significant susceptibility to the development of a particular cancer.
(b) The Hardy–Weinerg equilibrium states that in the absence of mutation, non-random mating, selection and genetic drift, the genetic constitution of the population remains the same from one generation to the next.
(c) Gene therapy entails placing a normal copy of a gene into the cells of patient who has a defective copy of that gene.
(d) In cystic fibrosis it is sufficient to introduce one functional normal allele of the relevant gene in order to overcome the genetic deficiency.
(e) The proteome is the protein expression characteristic of normal and diseased cells.

2.57 The aims of genetic counselling include (page 154):
(a) Establishing an accurate diagnosis
(b) Estimation of risk in future pregnancies of developing or transmitting a disorder
(c) Information on prognosis and follow-up
(d) Prenatal diagnosis
(e) Carrier detection

2.58 The following associations are correct (page 155):
(a) β-Thalassaemia – Mediterranean population
(b) Sickle cell disease – African origin
(c) Tay–Sachs disease – Ashkenazi Jews
(d) Cystic fibrosis – Caucasian populations
(e) Thalassaemia – Asian population

2.59 Anticipation is seen in the following genetically inherited diseases (Table 2.12):
(a) Cystic fibrosis
(b) Friedreich's ataxia
(c) Spinocerebellar ataxia
(d) Spinobulbar muscular atrophy
(e) Machado–Joseph ataxia

2.60 Amniocentesis (Information box 2.4):
  (a) is performed in the first trimester
  (b) is an outpatient procedure
  (c) is preceded by ultrasound to localize the placenta
  (d) involves the aspiration of approximately 200 ml of amniotic fluid
  (e) involves the aspiration of amniotic fluid via the transabdominal route

2.61 The supernatant of centrifuged amniotic fluid is used for chemical analysis
  to detect (page 155):
  (a) Adrenogenital syndrome – 17-hydroxyprogesterone
  (b) Mucopolysaccharidases – Glycosaminoglycosis
  (c) Neural tube defects – α-fetoprotein
  (d) Cystic fibrosis – alkaline phosphatase
  (e) Discoloration of fluid – impending death of fetus

2.62 The following statements about Down's syndrome are correct (page 156):
  (a) The sole measurement of the urinary metabolite of hCG, β-core, is
      reported to detect as many Down's cases as do current serum
      biochemical trimester tests.
  (b) First-trimester maternal serum screening for trisomy 21 using
      pregnancy-associated plasma protein-A (PAP-A) is under evaluation.
  (c) Ultrasound detection of a thickened oedematous flap of skin at the base
      of the neck – *nuchal translucency* – is reported to detect as many as
      80% of Down's fetuses during the first trimester.
  (d) Over half of the patients will require surgery for congenital defects.
  (e) Over half of the patients will develop Alzheimer-like neuronal
      degeneration after the age of 40.

2.63 The following associations about methods available for prenatal diagnosis
  are correct (Information box 2.4):
  (a) Ultrasonography – neural tube defects
  (b) Amniocentesis – measurement of acetyl cholinesterase
  (c) Fetoscopy – fetal sampling
  (d) Chorionic villous sampling – DNA analysis
  (e) Chorionic villous sampling – chromosomal analysis

2.64 Immunological competence (pages 160–175):
  (a) resulting from stimulation with a foreign substance is innate immunity
  (b) due to natural immunity is the last line of defence
  (c) due to acquired immunity produces a specific response to an antigen
  (d) due to acquired immunity retains its 'memory' for future contact with
      that particular antigen
  (e) resulting from the genetic constitution is the first line of defence

2.65 Natural immunity is provided by (pages 170–185):
  (a) Mechanical barriers
  (b) Humoral immunity

(c) Extracellular fluids
(d) Phagocytic cells
(e) Cell-mediated immunity

2.66 Mechanical barriers and secretions include (pages 170–185):
(a) Intact skin
(b) Mucosa
(c) Sweat
(d) Tears
(e) Normal microbial flora

2.67 The following associations are correct (pages 170–185):
(a) β-Lysin – Gram-positive bacteria
(b) C-reactive protein – complement activation
(c) Interferons – antiviral activity
(d) Gastric acid – antibacterial activity
(e) Lysosyme – Gram-positive bacteria

2.68 Lymphoid tissue in man is present in (page 172):
(a) Brain
(b) Lymph nodes
(c) Bone marrow
(d) Thymus
(e) Spleen

2.69 Mucosally associated lymphoid tissue is present in (page 172):
(a) Gut
(b) Pharynx
(c) Bronchus
(d) Breast
(e) Lacrimal glands

2.70 Correct statements about lymphoid tissue include (page 172):
(a) The resting cortex contains B lymphocytes.
(b) The resting paracortex contains T lymphocytes.
(c) The resting medulla contains connective tissue.
(d) Plasma cells live for months.
(e) Following antigenic stimulation the medulla is packed with plasma cells.

2.71 The afferent limb of the immune response (pages 160–185):
(a) recognizes the antigen
(b) processes the antigen
(c) sets in motion a series of cellular mechanisms against the antigen
(d) induces the antigen
(e) sets in motion a series of humoral mechanisms against the antigen

2.72 Lymphocytes (pages 167–172):
   (a) such as long-living T and B cells carry immunological memory
   (b) of B-cell type constitute 20% of the total lymphocytes
   (c) of the null-cell type constitute 75% of the total lymphocytes
   (d) of the T and B-cell type communicate by direct contact
   (e) of the T and B-cell type communicate by soluble factors

2.73 T lymphocytes (pages 167–172):
   (a) arise in the bone marrow
   (b) are transformed into immunocompetent cells in the thymus
   (c) can be activated to form 'blast cells' by specific antigens
   (d) can be activated to form 'blast cells' by non-specific mitogens such as phytohaemagglutinin
   (e) are transformed into antibody-producing cells when activated

2.74 Subsets of the T lymphocytes include (pages 170–171):
   (a) T receptor
   (b) Helper cells
   (c) Cytotoxic cells
   (d) Suppressor cells
   (e) Delayed hypersensitivity

2.75 CD4 T cells (pages 170–171):
   (a) include helper cells
   (b) include cytotoxic cells
   (c) recognize antigen with MHC class I molecules
   (d) contain receptor for HTLV-3
   (e) comprise 50–60% of peripheral T cells

2.76 The T-cell receptor (pages 170–171):
   (a) consists of CD8 cells
   (b) consists of α and β chains
   (c) has two constant regions
   (d) has variable N-terminal ends
   (e) has several hypervariable regions

2.77 Correct statements about T cells include (pages 170–171):
   (a) T cells secrete antibodies.
   (b) T-helper and B-cell interaction is essential for an optimal humoral response to most antigens.
   (c) T-cell mediated immunity can be transferred by giving T-cells to a genetically compatible individual.
   (d) T-cell interaction with antigen releases non-specific factors called lymphokines which amplify the immunological response.
   (e) T lymphocytes live for months or years.

2.78 Null cells (pages 170–171):
- (a) possess the phenotype markers of both T and B cells
- (b) possess Fc receptors for IgG
- (c) originate in the fetal liver
- (d) of the natural killer type lyse tumour cells
- (e) which are identical to killer cells have cytotoxic properties against target cells coated by antibody

2.79 Neutrophils (page 161):
- (a) are polymorphonuclear granulocytes
- (b) live for 6–20 hours
- (c) constitute approximately 60% of the total number of leucocytes
- (d) bear high-affinity surface receptors for IgE
- (e) are cells of acute inflammation

2.80 The following statements about neutrophil function are correct (page 162):
- (a) Up-regulation of adhesion molecules, L-selectin and integrins on neutrophils decreases the 'stickiness' of the phagocyte.
- (b) Decrease in the E-selectin and ICAM-1 on the blood vessel endothelial cells causes the cells to become 'sticky'.
- (c) The main chemoattractants in vivo are the complement activation products C51 and C31 and the macrophage-derived cytokine leukotriene B4.
- (d) Neutrophils are useful against intracellular organisms such as mycobacteria.
- (e) Opsonization is more effective if the particle is first coated with specific antibody and complement, because neutrophils have receptors for both the *Fc* portion of antibody molecules (FcR) and complement components (CR), which bind strongly to the coated particle.

2.81 Mast cells (page 164):
- (a) are present in the skin and mucosal surfaces
- (b) are involved in immediate hypersensitivity reactions
- (c) bear receptors to complement components C3 and C5
- (d) of the T type contain tyrosine
- (e) of the TC type contain trypsin and chymotrypsin.

2.82 Basophils (page 164):
- (a) are seen in the secretions of patients with allergic rhinitis
- (b) are seen in increased numbers in the circulation of non-allergenic individuals
- (c) lack receptors to complement components
- (d) are involved in delayed hypersensitivity reactions
- (e) bear high-affinity Ig E receptors

2.83 Eosinophils (page 163):
- (a) bear high-affinity receptors for IgE

(b) are seen in the circulation in allergic diseases
(c) are seen in the circulation in helminth infections
(d) are seen in the secretions of patients with allergic rhinitis
(e) are more potent phagocytes than neutrophils

2.84 The primary activities of eosinophils include (page 163):
(a) Secretion of IgG
(b) Synthesis of mast cells
(c) Engulfment and digestion of antigen–antibody complexes
(d) Release of histamine
(e) Release of granule proteins

2.85 The eosinophil granule proteins include (page 164):
(a) IgG
(b) Major basic protein
(c) Eosinophilic cation protein
(d) Eosinophil-derived neurotoxin
(e) Eosinophil peroxidase

2.86 Types of immunological response include (pages 160–185):
(a) Antigen production
(b) Humoral antibody production
(c) Immune tolerance
(d) Cell-mediated response
(e) Anaphylaxis.

2.87 The antigenicity of substance (pages 160–185):
(a) is its ability to induce an immune response
(b) is determined by its size
(c) is determined by its foreignness
(d) is determined by the complexity of the material
(e) is determined by the type of immune response

2.88 The following statements about antigens are correct (pages 160–185):
(a) They are substances that do not elicit immune responses in vertebrates.
(b) Each microorganism bears a single antigen on its surface specific to it.
(c) Epitopes are specific areas of the antigen against which antibodies are directed.
(d) Each antigen consists of a number of epitopes.
(e) Antisera produced against microorganisms consist of a number of different antibodies, each being specific for the epitope against which it has been raised.

2.89 The non-covalent forces between antigen and antibody are mediated by (pages 160–185):
(a) Hydrogen bonding
(b) Hydrostatic bonding

(c) Van der Waals' forces
(d) Hydrophobic forces
(e) Eosinophils

2.90 The following statements about antibody specificity are correct
(pages 160–185):
(a) Each antibody is specific for a particular epitope.
(b) Epitopes may be present on more than one antigen.
(c) Antibodies raised against one antigen can react with another antigen that contains the same epitope.
(d) Cross-reactivity means antisera raised against certain organisms will react with those of others.
(e) Cross-reactivity is due to sharing of epitopes.

2.91 The following statements about antibody production are correct
(pages 160–185):
(a) Macrophages trap the antigen.
(b) The degraded antigen is carried on the surface of the macrophage as small peptides.
(c) The macrophage presents the degraded antigen to T and B-cell lymphocytes.
(d) Receptive lymphocytes undergo 'blast formation', producing a clone of cells.
(e) It occurs in neutrophils.

2.92 The following statements about antibody response are correct
(pages 160–185):
(a) On initial exposure to the antigen the circulating antibody appears within 3 hours.
(b) The primary antibody response is mounted by IgG.
(c) The primary response results in the generation of 'memory' T and B cells.
(d) Subsequent exposure to the same antigen results in the generation of IgM antibodies.
(e) During the secondary antigenic challenge antibodies appear more quickly and reach a higher titre.

2.93 The following statements about lymphocytes are correct (pages 160–185):
(a) Plasma cells arise from T lymphocytes.
(b) Plasma cells do not synthesize antibodies.
(c) T helper cells synthesize antibodies.
(d) T suppressor cells regulate antibody synthesis.
(e) B cells give rise to helper cells.

2.94 Macrophage factors involved in antibody synthesis include (pages 160–185):
(a) Helper factor
(b) Suppressor factor
(c) Genetically restricted factor

(d) Interleukin-1
(e) Interleukin-6

2.95 The following statements are correct (pages 160–185):
(a) Serum proteins are T-dependent antigens.
(b) Erythrocytes are T-dependent antigens.
(c) *Escherichia coli* are T-independent antigens.
(d) Pneumococcal polysaccharides are T-independent antigens.
(e) T-dependent antigens require cooperation between T and B cells to synthesize antibodies.

2.96 Immunoglobulins (pages 160–185):
(a) consist of four carbohydrate chains
(b) have two identical heavy chains
(c) have two identical light chains
(d) heavy chains are linked by a hydrogen bond
(e) are encoded by genes located on three chromosomes

2.97 Five types of heavy chains in immunoglobulins include (pages 160–185):
(a) κ Chain
(b) λ Chain
(c) α Chain
(d) γ Chain
(e) μ Chain

2.98 The following associations between immunoglobulin classes and their heavy chains are correct (pages 160–185):
(a) IgA and δ Chain
(b) IgG and γ Chain
(c) IgD and α Chain
(d) IgM and μ Chain
(e) IgE and ε Chain

2.99 The following statements about immunoglobulin molecules are correct (pages 160–185):
(a) Papain splits the immunoglobulin into three regions.
(b) The Fab fragment combines with the antigen.
(c) The variable region of the Fab fragment is unique for each antibody.
(d) The constant region determines the class of immunoglobulin.
(e) The constant region determines the cytophilic activities of immunoglobulin.

2.100 The following associations between the constant region and its activities are correct (pages 160–185):
(a) CH1 – binds the C4b fragment of complement
(b) CH2 – control of C1q complement fixation
(c) CH2 – catabolic rate of the whole molecule

(d) Interaction between CH2 and CH3 – binding to staphylococcal protein A

(e) CH3 – binding to the Fc receptor of macrophages and monocytes

2.101 The following statements about immunoglobulins are correct (pages 160–185):
(a) Immunoglobulin A play a primary role in mucosal immunity.
(b) Immunoglobulin D is the major antibody produced during secondary immune response.
(c) IgE plays a primary role in the defence against helminthic infection.
(d) IgG can fix complement via the classical pathway.
(e) IgM can fix complement via the classical pathway.

2.102 Complement (page 164):
(a) is a series of at least 20 serum glycoproteins
(b) binds to antigen–antibody complexes in a specific sequence
(c) contributes to humoral immunity by opsonization
(d) contributes to humoral immunity by phagocytosis
(e) contributes to humoral immunity by complement fixation

2.103 The classical pathway is triggered by (pages 164–165):
(a) antigen–antibody complex
(b) IgM antibody alone
(c) mannan-binding protein
(d) IgE
(e) Cobra venom

2.104 Correct statements about the complement pathway include (pages 164–165):
(a) The Fc site on the antibody is a binding site for the first component of the complement.
(b) C1a inactivates the C42 complex.
(c) In structure the first component of the complement resembles a bunch of tulips.
(d) Bystander lysis is a process by which non-target cells are destroyed.
(e) C8 causes cells to be leaky.

2.105 The following associations regarding the biologically antigenic active molecules generated during the complement cascade are correct (pages 164–165):
(a) C3a – liberation of histamine by mast cells
(b) C3b – engulfment of antigenic particles by phagocytes
(c) C5a – chemotaxis for neutrophils
(d) C5a – mast cell degranulation
(e) C5,6,7 – chemotaxis for neutrophils

2.106 Activators of the alternative pathway include (page 165):
(a) Yeast cell walls
(b) IgG
(c) IgA
(d) Endotoxin found in the cell wall of Gram-negative bacteria
(e) C3 nephritic factor

2.107 Modulation of the alternative complement cascade is achieved by (page 165):
(a) C1a esterase inhibitor
(b) Anaphylatoxin inactivator
(c) Factor H
(d) C3b inactivator
(e) C2

2.108 Actions of complement include (page 165):
(a) Recruitment of cells and proteins to inflammatory sites
(b) Cell-mediated immunity
(c) Destruction of pathogens and tumour cells
(d) Removal of immune complexes
(e) Immunomodulation of B-cell responses to specific antigen through binding to complement receptors on the B-cell surface

2.109 Cellular immunity is involved in (pages 170–185):
(a) Anaphylaxis
(b) Complement activation
(c) Immunity against viruses
(d) Immunity against parasites
(e) Immunity against bacteria resistant to phagocytosis

2.110 Antigen presentation (in cellular immunity) (pages 170–185):
(a) to T cells is by eosinophils
(b) results in the T cells releasing a factor that induces the antigen-presenting cells to generate interleukin 1
(c) Interleukin-1 production activates the T cell to produce interleukin-2.
(d) Interleukin-2 drives the antigenically activated cells to proliferate.
(e) with class II molecules are recognized by T-helper cells.

2.111 In cell-mediated cytotoxicity the binding of Tc cells and NK cells to their targets results from (pages 170–185):
(a) antibody combining with antigen-specific receptors
(b) antigen-specific receptors on the Tc cells
(c) determinants recognized by NK cells
(d) antibody receptors on K cells
(e) Fc receptors on K cells

2.112 The following statements are correct (page 166):
  (a) Natural killer cells have the morphology of lymphocytes.
  (b) The measurement of C-reactive protein in the serum is used to monitor disease activity.
  (c) Serum amyloid P protein is helpful in the diagnosis of secondary amyloidosis.
  (d) Heat-shock proteins act as molecular chaperones, preserving the cell's protein structures.
  (e) Acute-phase reactants are proteins that are synthesized to tumours.

2.113 Statements about the following cytokines are correct (page 166):
  (a) IFN-γ is used to improve phagocyte function in patients with chronic granulomatous disease.
  (b) Nuclear factor-κB is a pivotal transcription factor in chronic inflammatory diseases.
  (c) Chemokines are primarily associated with chemoattractant function.
  (d) Tumour necrosis factor plays a key role in inflammation.
  (e) Granulocyte–colony-stimulating factor is used in the treatment of neutropenia.

2.114 The following statements are correct (page 167):
  (a) Clusters of differentiation (CD) molecules are typically absent on the cell surface of leucocytes in normal people.
  (b) B lymphocytes differentiate to become plasma cells.
  (c) The plasma cell is terminally differentiated.
  (d) B cells produce antibody.
  (e) B lymphocytes can be differentiated by the presence of CD19 and CD20 molecules.

2.115 Correct statements about antibody molecules (immunoglobulins) include (page 168):
  (a) They are glycoproteins.
  (b) The Fc portion is antigen specific.
  (c) The variable 'V' domain is the part that binds to cell surface immunoglobulin receptors.
  (d) Antigen binding occurs on the constant 'C' domain.
  (e) The type of light chain determines the antibody isotypes.

2.116 The following statements about antibody production are correct (page 169):
  (a) The primary immune response is always of the IgG isotype.
  (b) The IgG response requires additional T-cell help.
  (c) The secondary response is the production of IgM antibodies.
  (d) Memory B cells remain in the body for many years.
  (e) Memory B cells react rapidly to re-challenge to the same antigen by producing IgM.

2.117 Major functions of antibody include (page 169):
   (a) Elimination of infective organisms
   (b) Antitoxin activity
   (c) Sensitization cells for antibody-dependent cell cytotoxicity (ADCC)
   (d) Acting as antigen receptor on T cells
   (e) Presenting the antigen to helper T cells

2.118 The following statements about immunoglobulins are correct (page 169):
   (a) If antigen-specific IgM is present in the newborn infant, it is a good marker for intrauterine infection.
   (b) Patients lacking IgG suffer recurrent, even life-threatening, bacterial infections.
   (c) IgA is found in mucous membrane secretions.
   (d) IgD levels are low in conditions with B-cell activation.
   (e) The main physiological role of IgG is anti-nematode activity.

2.119 Correct statements about T cells include (page 170–171):
   (a) T cells are characterized by the absence of CD3 surface molecules.
   (b) CD4+ lymphocytes recognize antigen only when presented with MHC class I molecules.
   (c) T-helper 2 (Th2) cells produce cytokines that favour IgE responses.
   (d) Cytotoxic/suppressor cells can down regulate immune responses.
   (e) The role of natural killer cells is to eliminate tumour and virus-infected cells.

2.120 The HLA system (page 172):
   (a) is located on the long arm of chromosome 6
   (b) consists of a series of closely linked genetic loci
   (c) is situated on the major histocompatibility complex
   (d) class I series is expressed on all nucleated cells
   (e) class II series is expressed predominantly on B lymphocytes

2.121 The following statements regarding genetic linkage and HLA are correct (page 172):
   (a) Crossing over cannot occur within the HLA region.
   (b) There is no interracial variation in HLA antigens.
   (c) All genes in the major histocompatibility complex tend to be inherited together.
   (d) The term halotype is used to indicate the particular set of HLA genes an individual carries on each chromosome 6.
   (e) The genes at a given locus are inherited as co-dominants.

2.122 The following statements about the products of HLA genes are correct (page 173):
   (a) The HLA genes code for cell-surface glycoproteins.
   (b) Class I antigens are expressed on all cell types.
   (c) Class I antigens are distinguished serologically by the microlymphocytotoxic test.

(d) Class II antigens are expressed on B cells.

(e) HLA-D antigens are recognized by mixed lymphocyte culture.

2.123 Correct statements about the immunoregulatory function of HLA molecules include (page 174):

(a) T cells use HLA antigens as recognition molecules.

(b) Helper T cells are identified by monoclonal antibody CD8.

(c) Cytotoxic T cells are identified by monoclonal antibody CD4.

(d) Helper T cells usually recognize class II antigens.

(e) Cytotoxic T cells generally recognize class I antigens

2.124 The following statements are correct (page 175):

(a) When tolerance fails or is incomplete, autoimmunity can result.

(b) Tissue typing for organ grafting requires HLA typing only for HLA A and B, but not for C and DR antigens.

(c) Requirements for matching in bone marrow transplantation are much less stringent than for organ transplantation.

(d) HAL-DR4 is present in over three-quarters of patients with systemic lupus erythematosus due to hydralazine.

(e) Autosomal genes control the acetylator status.

2.125 The following associations between immune defects and opportunist organisms are correct (Table 2.22):

(a) Lytic complement pathway defects – meningococcus.

(b) Cell-mediated immunodeficiency – *Listeria monocytogenes*

(c) Antibody deficiency – *Campylobacter* spp.

(d) Opsonin defects – pneumococcus

(e) Neutropenia and defective neutrophil function – *Staphylococcus aureus*

2.126 HLA B27 is associated with (Table 2.21):

(a) Juvenile rheumatoid arthritis

(b) Reiter's syndrome

(c) Psoriatic arthropathy

(d) Ankylosing spondylitis

(e) Acute anterior uveitis

2.127 HLA B8 and HLA DR3 are associated with (Table 2.21):

(a) Autoimmune chronic active hepatitis

(b) Dermatitis herpetiformis

(c) Idiopathic membranous glomerulonephritis

(d) Myasthenia gravis with thymoma

(e) Sjögren's syndrome

2.128 The following associations are correct (Table 2.21):

(a) HLA A3 – haemochromatosis

(b) HLA B5 – Behçet's syndrome

(c) HLA DR4 – rheumatoid arthritis

(d) HLA BW 47 – congenital adrenal hyperplasia
(e) HLA DR5 – Hashimoto's thyroiditis

2.129 Interferon has been used in the treatment of:
(a) Chronic hepatitis B
(b) Leprosy
(c) AIDS-related Kaposi's tumour
(d) Hairy-cell leukaemia
(e) Multiple myeloma

2.130 The following associations between complement deficiencies and various diseases are correct (page 179):
(a) C1 esterase inhibitor – hereditary angio-oedema
(b) C1q – discoid lupus erythematosus
(c) Mannan-binding protein – recurrent viral infections in children
(d) C3 – partial lipodystrophy
(e) C5-9 – recurrent infections with *Neisseria* spp.

2.131 Cell-mediated immunity is impaired in (Table 2.23):
(a) Purine nucleoside phosphorylase deficiency
(b) Ataxia telangiectasia
(c) Wiskott–Aldrich syndrome
(d) Job's syndrome
(e) Chronic granulomatous disease

2.132 Defective phagocyte function occurs in (Table 2.23):
(a) Chediak–Higashi syndrome
(b) Myeloperoxidase deficiency
(c) DiGeorge syndrome
(d) Nezelof syndrome
(e) Chronic granulomatous disease

2.133 Mechanisms of CD4 loss/dysfunction in HIV infection include (Table 2.24):
(a) Direct cytophatic effects of HIV
(b) Lysis of infected cells by HIV-specific cytotoxic cells
(c) Immunosuppressive effects of soluble HIV proteins on uninfected cells
(d) Molecular mimicry between gp 120/160 and MHC class I
(e) Tc-mediated lysis of uninfected cells CD4+T cells that have bound gp120 to the CD4 molecule

2.134 The following statements about defects in the function of neutrophils include (page 178):
(a) In leucocyte adhesion defect, bone marrow transplantation is contraindicated.
(b) Shwachman's syndrome may resemble cystic fibrosis.
(c) In chronic granulomatous disease the production of superoxide is normal.

(d) The Chediak–Higashi syndrome is characterized by giant granules in myeloid cells and large granular lymphocytes.
(e) In chronic granulomatous disease the regular interferon-γ can reduce the frequency of infections.

2.135 Impaired neutrophil function is associated with (page 179):
(a) Corticosteroids
(b) Influenza
(c) Diabetes mellitus
(d) Hypophosphatamia
(e) Hodgkin's disease

2.136 The following associations are correct (page 180):
(a) X-linked hypogammaglobulinemia – *btk* gene
(b) Common variable immunodeficiency – late-onset antibody deficiency
(c) IgA deficiency – gluten-sensitive enteropathy
(d) Isolated IgG_2 subclass deficiency – increased infection with capsulated organisms
(e) DiGeorge anomaly – abnormal thymic development

2.137 The following associations are correct (page 182):
(a) Wiskott–Aldrich syndrome – thrombocythaemia.
(b) Ataxia telangiectasia – high IgA levels
(c) Tacrolimus – impaired T-cell mechanism
(d) Protein – calorie malnutrition – *Pneumocystis carinii* pneumonia
(e) Ataxia telangiectasia – Oncogene nibrin.

2.138 Correct statements about type I hypersensitivity reaction include (page 182):
(a) An allergic reaction is produced within 30 minutes of exposure to the allergen.
(b) Atopy is diagnosed on skin-prick testing.
(c) Type I reaction can be transferred passively.
(d) Prausnitz–Küstner reaction is a wheal and flare reaction.
(e) It is mediated by antibodies of the IgE class.

2.139 Histamine is (page 183):
(a) present as a preformed mediator
(b) present in mast cells
(c) present in basophils
(d) a vasoconstrictor
(e) a bronchodilator

2.140 Arachidonic acid is metabolized to produce (page 184):
(a) Membrane lipids
(b) Prostaglandins
(c) Leukotrienes

(d) Platelet-activating factor
(e) Aspirin

2.141 The main actions of arachidonic metabolites include (page 184):
(a) Inflammatory cell mucosal infiltration
(b) Bronchoconstriction
(c) Bronchial mucosal oedema
(d) Mucus hypersecretion
(e) Hypertension

2.142 Organ-specific autoimmune diseases include (Table 2.27):
(a) Systemic lupus erythematosus
(b) Scleroderma
(c) Overlap syndrome
(d) Rheumatoid arthritis
(e) Addison's disease

2.143 Type II hypersensitivity reaction (page 183):
(a) is where antibodies are directed to the cell surface
(b) can lead to autoimmune haemolytic reaction
(c) can result in insulin-resistant diabetes
(d) is mediated by antibodies of the IgE class
(e) is mediated by antibodies of the IgD class

2.144 Correct statements about type III hypersensitivity reaction include (page 183):
(a) Immune complexes are deposited in the tissues.
(b) In serum sickness reaction the immune complexes are insoluble.
(c) In Arthus reaction the immune complexes are soluble.
(d) Causes erythema nodosum.
(e) Causes pulmonary aspergillosis.

2.145 Type IV reaction (page 183):
(a) takes less than 12 hours to develop
(b) can be transferred from one animal to another by serum
(c) is mediated by delayed hypersensitivity cells
(d) by B cytotoxic cells
(e) can be transferred from one animal to another by certain types of lymphocytes

2.146 Type V reaction is (page 183):
(a) the stimulating antibody reaction
(b) mediated by antibodies of the IgG class
(c) important in the pathogenesis of neonatal hyperthyroidism
(d) mediated by antibodies of the IgE class
(e) mediated by killer lymphocytes

2.147 Type VI reactions are involved in (page 183):
- (a) Hashimoto's thyroiditis
- (b) Graft-versus-host disease
- (c) Autoimmune diseases
- (d) Tumour rejection
- (e) Defence against helminthic reactions

2.148 Conventional therapy for controlling a genetic defect includes (page 157):
- (a) Anticonvulsant therapy for tuberous sclerosis
- (b) Avoiding fava beans in G-6PD deficiency
- (c) Avoiding barbiturates in porphyria
- (d) Dietary phenylalanine restriction in phenylketonuria
- (e) Factor VIII replacement in haemophilia A

2.149 The following associations are correct (page 186):
- (a) Indirect immunofluorescence – detects organ-specific antibodies
- (b) Particle agglutination – detection of rheumatoid factors
- (c) ELISA – detection of autoantibodies
- (d) Purified protein derivative (PPD) – lymphocyte function
- (e) Concanavalin A – activates B lymphocytes

Nutrition

3.1 The following associations between food and disease are correct (page 189):
    (a) Saturated fat – ischaemic heart disease
    (b) Aflatoxin – cancer
    (c) Vitamin A deficiency – tumours
    (d) High fat content – cancers
    (e) Nitrates – cancer

3.2 The following statements are correct (pages 189–190):
    (a) Energy balance is the difference between energy intake and energy expenditure.
    (b) Refined carbohydrates contribute to obesity.
    (c) Pectins and gums in food slow down monosaccharide absorption.
    (d) Low growth rates in utero are associated with high death rates from cardiovascular disease in adult life.
    (e) In the UK the reference nutrient intake (RNI) is being replaced by recommended daily amounts (RDA) to provide more help in interpreting dietary surveys.

3.3 Daily energy expenditure is a sum of (page 191, Fig 3.2):
    (a) Total calorie intake
    (b) Basal metabolic rate
    (c) Thermic effect of food eaten
    (d) Occupational activities
    (e) Non-occupational activities

3.4 The following statements are correct (page 191):
    (a) Total energy expenditure is measured using a double-labelled water method.
    (b) The basal metabolic rate is calculated by measuring oxygen consumption.
    (c) The basal metabolic rate is higher than resting metabolic rate.
    (d) There is a 10-fold increase in muscle energy demands during exercise.
    (e) In developing countries carbohydrate intake constitutes less than 25% of the average daily requirement.

3.5 Protein (page 192):
    (a) The total amount of nitrogen excreted in the urine represents the balance between protein breakdown and synthesis.
    (b) In order to maintain nitrogen balance, at least 40–50 g of protein are needed.
    (c) In developing countries adequate protein intake is achieved mainly from vegetable proteins.
    (d) Urinary urea forms 80–90% of total urinary nitrogen.
    (e) Protein breakdown provides more energy per gram than fat.

3.6 Correct statements include (page 192):
  (a) Most proteins from vegetables are deficient in at least one indispensable amino acid.
  (b) A diminished concentration of homocysteine in the plasma is an independent risk factor for vascular disease.
  (c) Homocysteine is derived from methionine in the diet.
  (d) Homocysteine is an amino acid that lacks sulphur.
  (e) There are at least 20 essential amino acids.

3.7 Essential fatty acids include (pages 192–193):
  (a) Eicosapentaenoic acid
  (b) α-Linolenic acid
  (c) Docosahexanoic acid
  (d) Linolenic acid
  (e) Arachidonic acid

3.8 Dietary fat has been implicated in the causation of the following cancers (page 193):
  (a) Leukaemia
  (b) Squamous cell carcinoma
  (c) Breast
  (d) Colon
  (e) Prostate

3.9 Current recommendations of fat intake for the UK are (page 193):
  (a) Saturated fatty acids should provide at least one-fifth of the dietary energy.
  (b) *Cis*-monounsaturated fatty acids should provide approximately 12% of the dietary energy.
  (c) *Cis*-polyunsaturated fatty acids should provide about 6% of the dietary energy.
  (d) Total fat intake should be no more than 35% of the total dietary energy.
  (e) The daily *trans* fatty acid intake should exceed 10% of the daily dietary energy.

3.10 Correct statements about cholesterol include (page 193):
  (a) Its absorption is decreased by olestra.
  (b) Egg white is rich in cholesterol.
  (c) It is virtually absent from plants.
  (d) It is synthesized by the body.
  (e) The average intake in the UK is less than 100 mg/day.

3.11 Correct statements about non-starch polysaccharides (NSP) include (page 193):
  (a) Dietary fibre is largely NSP.
  (b) Cellulose is digested by gut enzymes.
  (c) Non-specific polysaccharides are broken down by colonic bacteria.

(d) The breakdown of NSP in the colon produces gas.

(e) Unprocessed plant food lacks NSP.

3.12 The daily consumption of non-starch polysaccharides can be increased by the consumption of (page 193):

(a) Sugar

(b) Bread

(c) Potatoes

(d) Fruits

(e) Vegetables

3.13 Causes of protein–energy malnutrition include (Table 3.5):

(a) Postoperative sepsis

(b) Anorexia

(c) Dementia

(d) Physical trauma

(e) Renal failure

3.14 Factors leading to malnutrition include (page 194):

(a) Anorexia

(b) Increased catabolism in the septic patient

(c) Cachexia factor in cancer patients

(d) Malabsorption in patients with GI disease

(e) Uncontrolled insulin-dependent diabetes mellitus

3.15 Correct statements about the pathogenesis of starvation include (page 194):

(a) In the first 24 hours following low dietary intake, the body relies on glycogenolysis for energy.

(b) Central nervous system changes from ketone bodies to glucose as the main source of energy.

(c) Lipolysis occurs only when the serum insulin levels are high.

(d) Insulin/glucose ratios are high.

(e) Glucocorticoids stimulate the ubiquitin–proteasome pathway.

3.16 Insulin promotes (page 195):

(a) lipolysis

(b) gluconeogenesis

(c) glycogen synthesis

(d) protein synthesis

(e) synthesis of glucagon

3.17 Glucagon increases (page 195):

(a) glycogenolysis

(b) gluconeogenesis

(c) ketone body formation

(d) lipolysis

(e) muscle glycogen

3.18 Tumour necrosis factor (page 195):
    (a) stimulates lipoprotein lipase
    (b) is a catecholamine
    (c) is a cytokine
    (d) is the same as cachexia factor in cancer patients
    (e) does not affect metabolism

3.19 Causes of weight loss include (page 195):
    (a) Hypothyroidism
    (b) Malignancy
    (c) Anorexia
    (d) Insulin-dependent diabetes mellitus
    (e) Tuberculosis

3.20 Hallmarks of protein–energy malnutrition include (Table 3.6):
    (a) Weight gain
    (b) Increased triceps skinfold thickness
    (c) Increased mid-arm muscle circumference
    (d) Reduced serum albumin
    (e) Raised serum transferrin.

3.21 Kwashiorkor (page 196):
    (a) occurs in breastfed children
    (b) occurs with a very low protein and high carbohydrate diet
    (c) patients have oedema
    (d) patients have a high plasma insulin
    (e) is rarely associated with low serum albumin

3.22 Features of marasmus include (page 196):
    (a) Muscle wasting
    (b) Oedema
    (c) Apathy and lethargy
    (d) Diarrhoea
    (e) Increased body fat

3.23 Large increases in energy during refeeding in malnutrition can lead to (page 197):
    (a) Stroke
    (b) Heart failure
    (c) Circulatory collapse
    (d) Death
    (e) Increased appetite

3.24 Problems faced during the treatment of malnutrition include (page 197):
    (a) Anorexia
    (b) Hypothermia
    (c) Hypoglycaemia

(d) Diarrhoea

(e) Accompanying infection.

3.25 Conditions associated with malnutrition include (pages 196–197):

(a) Diarrhoea

(b) Vitamin deficiency

(c) Iron deficiency

(d) Selenium deficiency

(e) Folic acid deficiency

3.26 Severe protein–energy malnutrition can result in (pages 196–197):

(a) Death

(b) Impaired physical growth

(c) Intellectual impairment

(d) Behavioural abnormalities

(e) Cancer

3.27 The following statements are correct (page 198):

(a) The richest food source of vitamin A is the liver.

(b) Between a quarter and a third of dietary vitamin A in the UK is derived from retinoids.

(c) β-Carotene is cleaved in the intestinal mucosa by carotene dioxygenase.

(d) α-Carotene is the main carotenoid found in carrots.

(e) Retinol is added to margarine in the UK.

3.28 Correct statements about the metabolism of vitamin A include (page 198):

(a) Retinol is transported in the plasma bound to γ-globulin.

(b) Retinaldehyde is found in both the rods and the cones of the retina.

(c) Retinoic acid is involved in the control of cell differentiation.

(d) Retinyl phosphate is a cofactor in the synthesis of most glycoproteins containing mannose.

(e) Retinol is formed by the oxidation of retinaldehyde.

3.29 Clinical features of vitamin A deficiency include (page 198):

(a) Rickets

(b) Osteomalacia

(c) Follicular hyperkeratosis

(d) Xerophthalmia

(e) Coagulation defects

3.30 Clinical features of niacin deficiency include (page 203):

(a) Beriberi

(b) Wernicke–Korsakoff syndrome

(c) Pellagra

(d) Peripheral neuropathy

(e) Scurvy

3.31 The following causes of vitamin deficiency are correct (Table 3.9):
  (a) In vegans – vitamin B_{12}
  (b) Ileal disease – vitamin B_{12}
  (c) Alcohol dependency – thiamine
  (d) Small bowel disease – folate
  (e) Intestinal bacterial overgrowth – vitamin B_{12}

3.32 Correct statements about vitamin A include (page 198):
  (a) The best guide to diagnosis of deficiency is a response to replacement therapy.
  (b) It is destroyed by cooking.
  (c) In excess it is teratogenic.
  (d) It is a precursor of β-carotene.
  (e) In excess it can cause liver damage.

3.33 Vitamin K (page 200):
  (a) is present in many plant foods
  (b) can be synthesized by intestinal bacteria
  (c) deficiency is most commonly seen in biliary obstruction
  (d) is water soluble
  (e) deficiency will increase prothrombin time

3.34 The following statements are correct (page 200):
  (a) Vitamin K is a cofactor necessary for the production of proteins involved in the formation of bone.
  (b) Vitamin K is a cofactor for the post-translational carboxylation of specific protein-bound glutamate residues in γ-carboxyglutamate.
  (c) Oral therapy with vitamin K is used in primary biliary cirrhosis.
  (d) Oral anticoagulants synergize the action of vitamin K.
  (e) Vitamin K is absorbed in the upper small gut.

3.35 Vitamin E (page 201):
  (a) occurs mainly in vegetable oils
  (b) in large doses prevents the subsequent risk of non-fatal myocardial infarction
  (c) can prevent ataxia in children with abetalipoproteinaemia
  (d) requirements depend on the intake of polyunsaturated fatty acids
  (e) deficiency leads to haemolytic anaemia in premature infants

3.36 Thiamin (page 201):
  (a) is a cofactor involved in the oxidative decarboxylation of acetyl CoA in mitochondria
  (b) is fat soluble
  (c) deficiency results in an accumulation of lactate and pyruvate
  (d) deficiency can occur when the only food is undermilled or parboiled rice
  (e) deficiency occurs in severe prolonged hyperemesis gravidarum

3.37 Recognized features of beriberi include (page 202):
   (a) Dry beriberi and wet beriberi commonly occur together.
   (b) Dry beriberi presents with a polyneuropathy.
   (c) In wet beriberi pedal oedema is rare.
   (d) High-output cardiac failure occurs in wet beriberi.
   (e) In infantile beriberi the mother shows no signs of thiamin deficiency.

3.38 Correct statements about the diagnosis and treatment of beriberi include (pages 202–203):
   (a) A rapid disappearance of oedema after thiamine is diagnostic.
   (b) The diagnosis is confirmed by measurement of transketolase activity in red cells.
   (c) In wet beriberi the response to thiamine occurs in hours.
   (d) In dry beriberi the response to thiamine is often slow to occur.
   (e) Infantile beriberi is treated by giving thiamine to the mother.

3.39 Features of Wernicke–Korsakoff syndrome include (page 202):
   (a) Dementia
   (b) Ataxia
   (c) Ophthalmoplegia
   (d) Nystagmus
   (e) Occurs in alcoholics

3.40 Riboflavin (page 203):
   (a) is widely distributed throughout all plant and animal cells
   (b) is destroyed appreciably by cooking
   (c) is not destroyed by sunlight
   (d) deficiency causes angular stomatitis
   (e) deficiency causes seborrhoeic dermatitis

3.41 Niacin (page 203):
   (a) is necessary in the hexose monophosphate shunt
   (b) is necessary for fatty acid synthesis
   (c) is lost by removing bran from cereals
   (d) deficiency causes pellagra
   (e) can be synthesized in humans from tryptophan

3.42 Pellagra may occur in (pages 203–204):
   (a) people who virtually only eat maize
   (b) those on isoniazid therapy
   (c) Hartnup disease
   (d) carcinoid syndrome
   (e) phaeochromocytoma

3.43 Recognized features of pellagra include (page 204):
   (a) Casal's necklace
   (b) Constipation

(c) Diarrhoea
(d) Dementia
(e) Dermatitis

3.44 The following drugs interact with pyridoxal phosphate to produce vitamin B$_6$ deficiency (page 204):
(a) Vitamin A
(b) Isoniazid
(c) Hydralazine
(d) Penicillamine
(e) Biotin

3.45 Vitamin C (page 204):
(a) has been shown to be useful in the common cold in clinical trials
(b) is involved in the hydroxylation of proline to hydroxyproline
(c) is necessary for the formation of collagen
(d) can be synthesized from glucose by humans.
(e) is easily leached out of vegetables

3.46 Recognized clinical features of vitamin C deficiency include (Table 3.11):
(a) 'Corkscrew' hair
(b) Perifollicular haemorrhages
(c) Swollen, spongy gums
(d) Anaemia
(e) Impaired wound healing

3.47 The following statements are correct (page 205):
(a) Iron deficiency is particularly prevalent in women of reproductive age.
(b) Iron deficiency is seen in South African Bantu men who cook in iron pots.
(c) Cobalt deficiency causes anaemia.
(d) Chromium deficiency causes glucose intolerance.
(e) Manganese deficiency causes growth retardation.

3.48 Correct statements about Menkes' kinky hair syndrome include (page 205):
(a) It is due to an excess of copper.
(b) It is a sex-linked abnormality.
(c) Infants with this abnormality develop growth failure
(d) Mental retardation develops in affected infants.
(e) Anaemia also occurs.

3.49 Recognized features of acrodermatitis enteropathica include (page 206):
(a) Malabsorption of zinc
(b) Growth retardation
(c) Hair loss
(d) Candidiasis
(e) Bacterial infection

3.50 Iodine (page 206):
  (a) excess causes endemic goitre
  (b) excess results in cretinism
  (c) is added to salt in developed countries
  (d) exists in foods as inorganic iodines which are efficiently absorbed
  (e) deficiency tends to occur in mountainous areas

3.51 Correct statements include (page 206):
  (a) Fluoridation of water increases the prevalence of dental caries.
  (b) Excessive fluoride intake results in the discoloration of tooth enamel.
  (c) Keshan disease is a selenium-responsive cardiomyopathy.
  (d) Increased calcium is required in pregnancy and lactation.
  (e) Calcium deficiency is usually due to vitamin D deficiency.

3.52 Theories postulated to explain ageing include (page 207):
  (a) Programmed ageing
  (b) Genomic instability theory
  (c) Free radical theory
  (d) Random genetic error theory
  (e) Alzheimer's theory

3.53 Factors that cause nutritional problems in the elderly include (page 207):
  (a) Dental problems
  (b) Lack of cooking skills
  (c) Depression
  (d) Lack of motivation
  (e) Lack of exposure to sunlight

3.54 Conditions in which obesity is an associated feature include (Table 3.14):
  (a) Laurence–Moon–Biedl syndrome
  (b) Hyperthyroidism
  (c) Cushing's syndrome
  (d) Stein–Levanthal syndrome
  (e) Anorexia nervosa

3.55 Correct statements regarding the mechanisms of obesity include (page 208):
  (a) Studies in twins have suggested that genetic influences have no role in the pathogenesis of obesity.
  (b) Obese people eat more than they admit to eating.
  (c) In obesity no single abnormality involving appetite control has been identified.
  (d) Obese patients need to expend more energy during physical activity as they have a larger mass to move.
  (e) Obese people tend to have a defect in thermogenesis in their brown adipose tissue.

3.56 The following statements are correct (page 208):
  (a) In massively obese subjects leptin mRNA in subcutaneous adipose tissue is lower than in controls.
  (b) β_{-3} Adrenergic receptors are the principal receptors mediating catecholamine-stimulated lipolysis in brown and white fat tissue.
  (c) Recent experimental evidence suggests that leptin stimulates the release of neuropeptide Y.
  (d) The *ob* gene produces a protein called leptin.
  (e) The main satiety centre is the paraventricular nucleus and the ventromedial wall of the hypothalamus.

3.57 Conditions associated with obesity include (Table 3.14):
  (a) Menstrual abnormalities
  (b) Osteoarthritis
  (c) Hypertension
  (d) Coronary artery disease
  (e) Stroke

3.58 Correct statements about diet in obesity include (page 210):
  (a) The common diets allow an intake of 1000 kcal per day.
  (b) The aim of any dietary regimen is to lose approximately 1 kg/day.
  (c) Weight loss is initially greater owing to the breakdown of protein and glycogen.
  (d) Alcohol consumption should be encouraged as it burns the fat.
  (e) A permanent change in eating habits is not required once the patient loses weight.

3.59 Correct statements about obesity include (page 210):
  (a) Weight cannot be lost by exercise alone.
  (b) Most obese people oscillate in weight.
  (c) Drugs are a substitute for strict dieting.
  (d) Obesity is associated with increased mortality.
  (e) A large cuff must be used in obese patients to obtain accurate blood pressure recordings.

3.60 Surgical procedures still used in the treatment of obesity include (page 210):
  (a) Vagotomy
  (b) Jejunoileal bypass
  (c) Wiring the jaws to prevent eating
  (d) Gastric plication
  (e) Gastric balloon

3.61 Enteral feedings in malnourished patients can be given by (page 211):
  (a) mouth
  (b) fine-bore nasogastric tube
  (c) intravenously

    (d) percutaneous endoscopic gastrostomy
    (e) needle catheter jejunostomy

3.62 Complications of central venous catheter placement include (page 212):
    (a) Thrombosis
    (b) Pneumothorax
    (c) Embolism
    (d) Catheter-related sepsis
    (e) Hypertension

3.63 Complications of peripheral parenteral nutrition include (pages 212–213):
    (a) Hyperglycaemia
    (b) Electrolyte disturbances
    (c) Hypercalcaemia
    (d) Liver dysfunction
    (e) Thrombophlebitis

3.64 The following associations regarding food allergies are correct (page 213):
    (a) Diarrhoea – strawberries
    (b) Asthma – eggs
    (c) Rhinitis – milk
    (d) Migraine – cheese
    (e) Urticaria – shellfish

3.65 Correct statements about alcohol include (page 214):
    (a) In general the effects of a given intake of alcohol seem to be worse in women.
    (b) The long-term effects of alcohol depend on the type of beverage.
    (c) Hangovers depend on congeners such as isoamyl alcohol.
    (d) Heavy sporadic drinkers are at greater risk than heavy persistent drinkers.
    (e) The amount of alcohol that produces damage varies from individual to individual.

3.66 Correct statements about the metabolism of ethanol include (page 214):
    (a) It is converted into acetaldehyde in the cytoplasm of the liver cell.
    (b) Acetaldehyde is converted to acetate mainly in the liver mitochondria.
    (c) Acetate is oxidized by peripheral tissues to carbon dioxide, fatty acids and water.
    (d) Alcohol dehydrogenase is found in the gastric mucosa.
    (e) A pint of beer provides 250 kcal.

3.67 Correct statements about alcohol consumption in pregnancy include (page 214):
    (a) Pregnant women are permitted to consume small quantities.
    (b) Even small amounts can cause small babies.

(c) Fetal alcohol syndrome occurs in fetuses of alcohol-dependency syndrome.
(d) Fetal alcohol syndrome is characterized by mental retardation.
(e) Fetal alcohol syndrome is characterized by growth impairment.

3.68 Neurological manifestations of excessive alcohol consumption include (Table 3.18):
(a) Epilepsy
(b) Wernicke–Korsakoff syndrome
(c) Myopathy
(d) Polyneuropathy
(e) Multiple sclerosis

3.69 Cardiovascular manifestations of excessive alcohol consumption include (Table 3.18):
(a) Hypertension
(b) Myocardial infarction
(c) Cardiomyopathy
(d) Beriberi
(e) Cardiac arrhythmias

3.70 Metabolic manifestations of excessive alcohol consumption include (Table 3.18):
(a) Cushing's syndrome
(b) Gout
(c) Hyperlipidaemia
(d) Hyperglycaemia
(e) Obesity

3.71 Gastrointestinal manifestations of excessive alcohol consumption include (Table 3.18):
(a) Acute gastritis
(b) Carcinoma of the oesophagus
(c) Carcinoma of the rectum
(d) Pancreatitis
(e) Cirrhosis

3.72 Haemopoietic manifestations of excessive alcohol consumption include (Table 3.18):
(a) Leucopenia
(b) Thrombocytopenia
(c) Macrocytosis
(d) Osteomalacia
(e) Osteoporosis

3.73 The following associations between foodstuffs and dietary sources of fatty acids are correct (Information box 3.1):
(a) Animal fat – saturated fatty acids
(b) Vegetable oils – n-6 fatty acids
(c) Fish oils – n-3 fatty acids
(d) Vegetable foods – n-3 fatty acids
(e) Margarine – *trans* fatty acids

3.74 Factors in the WHO programme for the prevention of protein–energy malnutrition include (Information box 3.3):
(a) Growth monitoring
(b) Oral rehydration
(c) Breastfeeding supplemented by food after six months
(d) Immunization against infectious diseases
(e) Family planning

3.75 The main complications of nasogastric feeding include (Practical box 3.1):
(a) Aspiration into the bronchus
(b) Blockage of the tube
(c) Diarrhoea
(d) Hyperglycaemia
(e) Hyperkalaemia

Gastroenterology

4.1 Correct statements about hiccups include (page 218):
  (a) Hiccups are voluntary diaphragmatic contractions with closure of the glottis.
  (b) Chlorpromazine is used to treat continuous hiccups
  (c) Diazepam may be effective in the treatment of hiccups.
  (d) Hiccups are a feature of chronic renal failure.
  (e) If untreated, hiccups can become continuous.

4.2 Causes of vomiting include (Table 4.1):
  (a) Urinary tract infection
  (b) Uraemia
  (c) Raised intracranial pressure
  (d) Severe pain
  (e) Hypercalcaemia

4.3 Early morning vomiting is seen in (Table 4.1):
  (a) Pyloric stenosis
  (b) Uraemia
  (c) Alcoholism
  (d) Pregnancy
  (e) Motion sickness

4.4 The following statements regarding altered bowel habit are correct (page 218):
  (a) Diarrhoea implies the frequent passage of small amounts of stool.
  (b) Diarrhoea implies the passing of increased amounts of loose stool.
  (c) Stools in steatorrhoea float because of increased air content.
  (d) Patients with steatorrhoea may pass only one motion a day.
  (e) Watery stools of large volume are due to organic disease.

4.5 Weight loss is a feature of (page 219):
  (a) Insulin-dependent diabetes mellitus
  (b) Hypothyroidism
  (c) Malabsorption
  (d) Anorexia nervosa
  (e) Tuberculosis

4.6 The following statements regarding sigmoidoscopy are correct (page 220):
  (a) Over two-thirds of colonic neoplasms are within the range of flexible sigmoidoscopy.
  (b) Most patients require colonic irrigation before the procedure.
  (c) Contact bleeding during the procedure is a recognized feature of normal mucosa.

(d) Air insufflation during the procedure often reproduces the pain of irritable bowel syndrome.

(e) Sigmoidoscopy should be a part of the routine examination in all cases of diarrhoea.

4.7 The following statements regarding barium contrast studies are correct (page 221):

(a) Swallowing bread with barium is useful in the investigation of undiagnosed dysphagia.

(b) A single-contrast barium meal is the recommended procedure to examine the stomach.

(c) The barium enema allows examination of the colon from the lowest part of the rectum to the caecum.

(d) Small-bowel follow-through is the only way of demonstrating the gross anatomy of the small intestine.

(e) In small bowel enema a tube is passed through the duodenum and a large volume of dilute barium is passed.

4.8 Causes of aphthous ulcers include (page 223):

(a) Behçet's disease

(b) Coeliac disease

(c) Crohn's disease

(d) Ulcerative colitis

(e) Idiopathic

4.9 The following statements about leucoplakia are correct (pages 224–225):

(a) It consists of white patches in the mouth which are easily removed.

(b) It is a premalignant condition.

(c) Leucoplakia can be caused by smoking.

(d) A biopsy should always be taken.

(e) Treatment with isotretinoin reduces disease progression.

4.10 Correct statements about oral hairy leucoplakia include (page 225):

(a) It is rarer in HIV-infected homosexual men than in any other high-risk group.

(b) It is associated with Epstein–Barr virus.

(c) Hairy leucoplakia on the side of the tongue is pathognomonic of AIDS.

(d) Hairy leucoplakia in AIDS indicates a good prognosis.

(e) It is due to Kaposi's sarcoma.

4.11 Causes of dry mouth include (page 225):

(a) Ptyalism

(b) Sjögren's syndrome

(c) Tricyclic antidepressants

(d) Diuretics

(e) Anxiety

4.12 Correct statements about the pathogenesis of gastro-oesophageal reflux disease include (page 227):
(a) The resting lower oesophageal sphincter (LOS) tone is high.
(b) The LOS tone fails to decrease when lying flat.
(c) There is increased oesophageal mucosal resistance to acid.
(d) A large hiatus hernia can impair the 'pinchcock' mechanism of the diaphragm.
(e) Delayed gastric emptying has been implicated.

4.13 Causes of dysphagia include (Table 4.2):
(a) Bulbar palsy
(b) Myasthenia gravis
(c) Scleroderma
(d) Goitre
(e) Enlarged left atrium

4.14 Investigations for oesophageal disorders include (Table 4.2):
(a) Manometry
(b) Bernstein test
(c) pH monitoring
(d) Mediastinoscopy
(e) Barium swallow

4.15 Recognized features of achalasia include (page 229):
(a) Weight gain
(b) Aspiration pneumonia
(c) Severe retrosternal chest pain
(d) Aperistalsis of the body of the oesophagus
(e) Failure of relaxation of the lower oesophageal sphincter

4.16 The following statements are correct (page 230):
(a) In systemic sclerosis most patients show increased peristalsis of the oesophagus on manometry.
(b) Diffuse oesophageal spasm produces retrosternal chest pain which is relieved by nitrates.
(c) Chagas' disease produces a picture similar to achalasia.
(d) 'Nutcracker' oesophagus is characterized by high-amplitude peristalsis within the oesophagus.
(e) Oesophageal stricture is a recognized feature of systemic sclerosis.

4.17 Causes of oesophageal infection include (page 231):
(a) *Streptococcus milleri*
(b) *Streptococcus viridans*
(c) *Candida* spp.
(d) Herpes simplex
(e) Cytomegalovirus

4.18 Factors associated with increased gastro-oesophageal reflux include
(Table 4.3):
(a) Pregnancy
(b) Diffuse oesophageal spasm
(c) Cholinergic drugs
(d) Calcium channel blockers
(e) Obesity

4.19 The following statements are correct (page 229):
(a) Cisapride is a dopamine antagonist.
(b) Metoclopramide is devoid of dopaminergic activity.
(c) Omeprazole inhibits the hydrogen–potassium proton pump.
(d) Ranitidine is a H_2 receptor agonist.
(e) Cisapride increases oesophageal peristalsis.

4.20 The following statements are correct (page 229):
(a) The major complication of reflux is peptic stricture.
(b) There is no increased incidence of carcinoma in hiatus hernia per se.
(c) Long-standing acid reflux causes columnization of the oesophageal mucosa.
(d) Barrett's oesophagus is premalignant.
(e) Peptic stricture usually occurs in patients below the age of 20.

4.21 Predisposing factors for carcinoma of the oesophagus include (page 232):
(a) Plummer–Vinson syndrome
(b) Achalasia
(c) Barrett's oesophagus
(d) Tylosis
(e) Long-standing dysphagia

4.22 The following statements about the structure of the stomach and
duodenum are correct (page 234):
(a) The parietal cells secrete hydrochloric acid.
(b) The chief cells secrete pepsinogen.
(c) There are two major forms of gastrin: G17 and G34.
(d) The duodenal mucosa contains Brunner's glands.
(e) The Brunner's glands secrete alkaline mucus.

4.23 Major gastric functions include (page 234):
(a) Emulsification of fat
(b) Secretion of intrinsic factor
(c) Acid secretion
(d) Reservoir for food
(e) Conservation of water

4.24 Correct statements about NSAIDs and the GI tract include (page 235):
(a) NSAIDs stimulate cyclooxygenase.

(b) NSAIDs more specific for COX II have less effect on the gastric mucosa.
(c) Rectal administration of NSAIDs prevents upper GI tract effects.
(d) H_2 receptor blockers may be effective in preventing duodenal ulcers due to NSAIDs.
(e) NSAIDs deplete mucosal prostaglandins.

4.25 The possible pathogenetic factors of *H. pylori* infection result in (page 236):
(a) An increase in fasting and meal-stimulated gastritis.
(b) An increase in somatostatin (D cells) in the antrum.
(c) A decrease in pepsinogen I secretion.
(d) An alteration in the mucous protective layer.
(e) A cytotoxin layer.

4.26 Factors influencing gastric acid secretion include (Fig 4.9):
(a) Passage of food into the duodenum
(b) Gastric distension by food
(c) Gastrocolic reflex
(d) The thought of food
(e) The smell of food

4.27 Ménétrièr's disease (page 237):
(a) is a common condition
(b) is characterized by thinning of the gastric mucosal folds
(c) is characterized histologically by hyperplasia of the mucin-producing cells
(d) may be complicated by hypoalbuminaemia
(e) is treated with cisapride

4.28 *Helicobacter pylori* (page 235):
(a) is an intracellular pathogen
(b) colonizes the epithelial cells
(c) is a urease-producing bacterium
(d) displays intrafamilial clustering
(e) can be eradicated using triple therapy comprising bismuth, amoxycillin and metronidazole

4.29 Correct statements about the clinicopathological features of *H. pylori* infection include (page 236):
(a) Cag A-positive strains are not associated with gastroduodenal disease.
(b) *H. pylori*-positive healthy volunteers have an increased sensitivity to gastrin.
(c) The earlier the *H. pylori* is acquired the greater the risk of atrophy and metaplasia.
(d) Over 90% of patients with gastric B-cell lymphomas have *H. pylori.*
(e) *H. pylori* is present in a greater proportion of patients with non-ulcer dyspepsia than in asymptomatic controls.

4.30 The following statements about the diagnosis of *H. pylori* are correct (page 236):
(a) The urea breath test with ^{13}C is a quick and easy way of detecting the presence of *H. pylori* and is used as a screening test.
(b) IgG titres are useful for confirming eradication.
(c) The rapid urease test cannot be performed with gastric biopsies.
(d) The urea breath test with $^{13}CO_2$ requires a mass spectrometer.
(e) *H. pylori* can be detected histologically using Giemsa-stained sections of gastric mucosa.

4.31 Factors thought to be involved in the causation of peptic ulceration include (page 238):
(a) Alcohol
(b) Steroids
(c) Genetic susceptibility
(d) Non-secretors of blood groups substances in saliva
(e) Blood group O

4.32 The following statements regarding peptic ulcer are true (page 238):
(a) Epigastric pain is a characteristic feature of the disease.
(b) The pain of duodenal ulcer classically occurs at night.
(c) The symptoms of a duodenal ulcer are periodic, with relapses and remissions.
(d) Back pain may suggest a penetrating posterior duodenal ulcer.
(e) Epigastric tenderness is a reliable discriminating sign of peptic ulcer.

4.33 The following statements about the treatment of duodenal ulcer are correct (page 238):
(a) Bed rest and special diet are the mainstay of treatment.
(b) The effectiveness of treatment should be assessed by follow-up X-ray or endoscopy.
(c) H_2 receptor antagonists are usually the first choice of therapy.
(d) Omeprazole produces healing rates of 100% after 4 weeks of treatment.
(e) Antacids are prescribed for severe cases of ulcer disease.

4.34 The following statements about the treatment of gastric ulcer are correct (page 238):
(a) Follow-up endoscopy is necessary after therapy.
(b) Fifty per cent of patients with gastric ulceration will have a recurrence within 2 years if untreated.
(c) Spicy foods should be avoided.
(d) Omeprazole is not useful in the treatment of gastric ulcers.
(e) Misoprostol should be avoided in the elderly.

4.35 Indications for surgical therapy of peptic ulcer include (pages 239–241):
(a) Malignant gastric ulcer
(b) Gastric outflow obstruction

(c) Recurrent haemorrhage
(d) Perforated gastric ulcer which is oversown
(e) Duodenal ulcer

4.36 The following statements about partial gastrectomy in the treatment of peptic ulcer are true (page 240):
(a) The aim is to remove the antral area, which secretes gastrin.
(b) Polya gastrectomy is now the commonest operation for patients with a gastric ulcer.
(c) In Billroth I partial gastrectomy the lower part of the stomach is removed and the stomach remnant is connected to the duodenum.
(d) In Billroth II the stomach remnant is connected to the first loop of the duodenum and the duodenum is closed.
(e) Partial gastrectomy has a lower operative mortality than vagotomy.

4.37 Complications of surgery for peptic ulcer include (page 240):
(a) Recurrent ulcer
(b) Megaloblastic anaemia
(c) Dumping syndrome
(d) Bilious vomiting
(e) Osteomalacia

4.38 Anaemia following peptic ulcer surgery is due to (page 240):
(a) Haemolysis
(b) Sequestration in the spleen
(c) Iron deficiency
(d) Folic acid deficiency
(e) Vitamin B_{12} deficiency

4.39 The following statements about gastric carcinoma are correct (page 241):
(a) It is the sixth most common fatal cancer in the UK.
(b) There is no link between *H. pylori* infection and gastric cancer.
(c) There is a higher incidence of gastric cancer in men.
(d) Benign gastric ulcers have not been shown to develop into gastric cancer.
(e) Most gastric cancers, such as colonic carcinomas, arise from pre-existing adenomas.

4.40 Recognized clinical features of gastric cancer include (page 242):
(a) Virchow's node
(b) Weight gain due to increased appetite
(c) Dermatomyositis
(d) Acanthosis nigricans
(e) Epigastric pain which is easily distinguishable from the pain of peptic ulcer disease

4.41 The following statements about the prognosis of gastric carcinoma are correct (page 242):
(a) The prognosis is excellent
(b) Early diagnosis means longer survival.
(c) Mass screening techniques in Japan have improved survival.
(d) Early surgery means complete cure.
(e) Early gastric cancer has a 5-year survival of 90% outside Japan.

4.42 The differential diagnosis of perforated peptic ulcer includes (Information box 4.3, page 240):
(a) Myocardial infarction
(b) Pancreatitis
(c) Bronchitis
(d) Cholecystitis
(e) Pyloric stenosis

4.43 The following statements regarding melaena are correct (page 243):
(a) The black colour is due to free iron.
(b) At least 50 ml of blood are required to produce melaena.
(c) Melaena is the vomiting of blood.
(d) It can occur with bleeding from any lesion in areas proximal to and including the caecum.
(e) The colour of blood appearing per rectum is dependent not only on the site of bleeding but also on the time of transit in the gut.

4.44 Causes of upper GI haemorrhage include (Fig 4.16):
(a) Chronic peptic ulceration
(b) Cigarette smoking
(c) Pseudoxanthoma elasticum
(d) Alcohol
(e) Low-dose corticosteroids

4.45 Factors that affect the management of upper GI haemorrhage include (page 244):
(a) Age of the patient
(b) Amount of blood lost
(c) Continuing visible blood loss
(d) Signs of chronic liver disease on examination
(e) Presence of the classic features of shock

4.46 The following factors are associated with increased mortality from acute upper GI haemorrhage (page 245):
(a) Age above 80 years
(b) Melaena rather than haematemesis
(c) Continuing visible blood loss
(d) Recurrent haemorrhage
(e) Proton-pump inhibitors

4.47 The following statements regarding the treatment of acute upper GI haemorrhage are correct (page 245):
  (a) H_2 receptor antagonists affect the mortality rate of GI haemorrhage.
  (b) Surgery is the treatment of choice in acute gastric ulceration.
  (c) Omeprazole should be tried before surgery in chronic gastric ulcers.
  (d) Surgical repair of a Mallory–Weiss tear is required in most cases.
  (e) Surgery is the treatment of choice in chronic duodenal ulcer.

4.48 Causes of lower GI bleeding include (Fig. 4.17):
  (a) Meckel's diverticulum
  (b) Angiodysplasia
  (c) Ischaemic colitis
  (d) Haemorrhoids
  (e) Carcinoma of the colon

4.49 Neuroreceptors present in the nerve supply to the gut include (page 246):
  (a) α-Adrenergic receptors
  (b) Nicotinic receptors
  (c) Muscarinic receptors
  (d) β-Adrenergic receptors
  (e) Peptidergic receptors

4.50 Functions of the small intestine include (Table 4.4):
  (a) Immunologic defence against antigens
  (b) Structural defence against antigens
  (c) Hormone production
  (d) Transit of nutrients
  (e) Absorption

4.51 The following statements regarding absorption are correct (page 247):
  (a) Simple diffusion requires energy.
  (b) An energy-dependent sodium pump is required for simple diffusion.
  (c) Amino acids are transported into the cell by a number of different carrier systems.
  (d) Fructose absorption occurs by facilitated diffusion.
  (e) Monosaccharides are transported into cells largely by active transport.

4.52 The following statements regarding fat digestion are correct (page 248):
  (a) Dietary fat consists mainly of cholesterol with some triglycerides.
  (b) Emulsification of fat occurs in the stomach.
  (c) Hydrolysis of triglycerides occurs in the duodenum.
  (d) Bile salts are absorbed in the jejunum.
  (e) Micelles have a hydrophobic centre of monoglycerides, fatty acids and cholesterol.

4.53 Common presenting features of small bowel disease include (page 250):
  (a) Weight gain

(b) Steatorrhoea
(c) Abdominal pain
(d) Tenesmus
(e) Anaemia due to vitamin B_{12} deficiency

4.54 The following statements regarding tests for small bowel disease are correct (page 252):
(a) The glucose tolerance test is useful in assessing sugar absorption in the proximal small bowel.
(b) A smear of jejunal juice is helpful in the diagnosis of *Giardia intestinalis.*
(c) The ^{14}C-glycocholic acid breath test is used to detect bacterial overgrowth.
(d) The Schilling test is performed to look for folate deficiency.
(e) Small bowel follow-through will show gross dilatation in pseudo-obstruction.

4.55 Causes of malabsorption include (Table 4.6):
(a) *Giardia* infestation
(b) Bacterial overgrowth
(c) Neomycin therapy
(d) Abetalipoproteinaemia
(e) Obstructive jaundice

4.56 The following statements about coeliac disease are correct (page 254):
(a) The jejunal mucosa shows subtotal villous atrophy.
(b) It is associated with dermatitis herpetiformis.
(c) It is rare in black Africans.
(d) The inheritance is autosomal dominant.
(e) It is associated with splenic atrophy.

4.57 Coeliac disease is associated with the following conditions (page 254):
(a) Atopy
(b) Small intestinal lymphoma
(c) Fibrosing alveolitis
(d) Non-insulin dependent diabetes
(e) Chronic liver disease

4.58 The following statements about the investigation of coeliac disease are correct (page 255):
(a) In the presence of endomysial antibodies and a typical clinical picture a confirmatory jejunal biopsy may not always be required to make a diagnosis.
(b) Anti-reticulin antibodies are the investigation of first choice.
(c) Folate deficiency is almost invariably present.
(d) The jejunal biopsy shows flattened mucosa.
(e) A blood film may show Howell–Jolly bodies.

4.59 The following occur in ileal resection (page 257):
   (a) Bile salts and fatty acids enter the colon and interfere with water and electrolyte absorption, causing diarrhoea.
   (b) Increased bile salt synthesis cannot compensate for loss of bile salts resulting in steatorrhoea.
   (c) Renal oxalate stones caused by increased oxalate absorption.
   (d) There is high serum B_{12}
   (e) Macrocytosis.

4.60 Recognized features of Whipple's disease include (page 257):
   (a) Usually affects females
   (b) Peripheral lymphadenopathy
   (c) Arthritis
   (d) On electron microscopy bacilli can be seen within macrophages
   (e) Dramatic improvement with antibiotic therapy

4.61 Recognized clinical features of carcinoid syndrome include (page 261):
   (a) Pulmonary stenosis
   (b) Tricuspid incompetence
   (c) Flushing
   (d) Abdominal pain
   (e) Watery diarrhoea

4.62 The following statements about carcinoid tumours are correct (page 261):
   (a) They originate from enterochromaffin cells.
   (b) They are clinically silent until metastases are present.
   (c) Benign tumours are easily discriminated from malignant tumours by histology.
   (d) Carcinoid syndrome occurs in the majority of patients with the tumour.
   (e) Octreotide is contraindicated in these patients.

4.63 The following statements about the epidemiology of inflammatory bowel disease are correct (page 261):
   (a) Crohn's disease is more prevalent than ulcerative colitis.
   (b) Crohn's disease is common before the age of 10.
   (c) Non-Jews are more prone to inflammatory bowel disease than Jews.
   (d) There is an increased risk of ulcerative colitis among smokers.
   (e) HLA-B27 is increased in patients with associated ankylosing spondylitis.

4.64 Predisposing factors for small bowel tumours include (page 261):
   (a) Coeliac disease
   (b) Ulcerative colitis
   (c) Crohn's disease
   (d) Immunoproliferative small intestinal disease
   (e) Carcinoid syndrome

4.65 The following pathological associations are correct (pages 262–263):
(a) Crohn's disease – 'backwash ileitis'
(b) Ulcerative colitis – 'skip lesions'
(c) Crohn's disease – cobblestone appearance of mucosa
(d) Ulcerative colitis – inflammation of all layers of the bowel
(e) Crohn's disease – granulomas

4.66 Indicators of severe ulcerative colitis include (Table 4.9):
(a) Low ESR
(b) Anaemia
(c) Hypoalbuminaemia
(d) Fever
(e) Bradycardia

4.67 Extraintestinal manifestations of inflammatory bowel disease include (Table 4.10):
(a) Pyoderma gangrenosum
(b) Erythema nodosum
(c) Sacroiliitis
(d) Uveitis
(e) Kidney stones

4.68 Hepatic manifestations of inflammatory bowel disease include (Table 4.10):
(a) Fatty change
(b) Pericholangitis
(c) Sclerosing cholangitis
(d) Cirrhosis
(e) Chronic active hepatitis

4.69 Complications of inflammatory bowel disease include (page 267):
(a) Septicaemia
(b) Toxic megacolon
(c) Perforation
(d) Haemorrhage
(e) Carcinoma

4.70 The following statements regarding the prognosis of Crohn's disease are correct (page 268):
(a) These patients have recurrent lapses.
(b) All patients have a significant relapse over a 20-year period.
(c) Mortality is twice that of the normal population.
(d) Crohn's disease in childhood causes growth retardation.
(e) Most deaths are associated with surgery.

4.71 The following statements regarding the prognosis of ulcerative colitis are correct (page 268):
(a) The course is variable.

(b) In proctitis the prognosis is poor.
(c) The overall mortality is not altered even when treated promptly.
(d) Overall the mortality is not greater than that of normal population.
(e) Pregnancy increases both maternal and fetal mortality.

4.72 The following statements regarding the anatomy of the colon are correct (page 268):
(a) It starts at the caecum.
(b) The mucosa is lined with epithelial cells with crypts and villi.
(c) The blood supply is from the superior and inferior mesenteric vessels.
(d) The rectum is about 12 cm long.
(e) The anal canal has an internal and an external sphincter.

4.73 The following statements regarding the physiology of the colon are correct (page 269):
(a) The main role of the colon is the secretion of fluids and electrolytes.
(b) Approximately 2 l of fluid pass the ileocaecal value each day.
(c) The absorption of fluid takes place mainly on the right side of the colon.
(d) When the rectum contains approximately 100 ml of faeces the urge to defaecate is experienced.
(e) The rectum is emptied by the relaxation of the internal anal sphincter.

4.74 Diverticula (page 269):
(a) are found in over half of patients over the age of 50
(b) are most frequently found in the sigmoid colon
(c) are associated with a high-fibre diet
(d) are commoner in the eastern hemisphere
(e) can be present over the whole colon

4.75 Complications of diverticular disease include (page 270):
(a) Bowel perforation
(b) Abscess formation
(c) Fistula formation
(d) Generalized peritonitis
(e) Diverticulosis

4.76 Causes of constipation include (Table 4.12)
(a) Opiates
(b) Hypercalcaemia
(c) Hyperthyroidism
(d) Hirschsprung's disease
(e) Aluminium antacids

4.77 Causes of megacolon include (page 271):
(a) Chagas' disease
(b) Hirschsprung's disease

(c) Chronic constipation
(d) Dermatitis herpetiformis
(e) Malabsorption

4.78 Causes of faecal incontinence include (Table 4.14):
(a) Spina bifida
(b) Multiple sclerosis
(c) Rectal carcinoma
(d) Faecal impaction
(e) Dementia

4.79 Correct statements about familial adenomatous polyposis include (page 273):
(a) It is inherited as an autosomal recessive trait.
(b) Constant endoscopic surveilliance is necessary as all patients will eventually develop cancer if followed long enough.
(c) The NSAID sulindac has been shown to decrease the number and size of polyps.
(d) The duodenum is spared.
(e) Congenital hypertrophy of the retinal pigment epithelium is seen in two-thirds of patients.

4.80 The following statements about the epidemiology of colorectal carcinoma are correct (page 273):
(a) Adenocarcinomas are the second most common tumour in the UK.
(b) The risk of developing this carcinoma is substantially increased among NSAID users.
(c) It is rare in Asia.
(d) The incidence increases with age.
(e) There is no correlation between the consumption of meat and animal fat and colon cancer.

4.81 The following statements about colorectal carcinoma are correct (page 273):
(a) Most colorectal cancers develop as a result of a stepwise progression from normal mucosa to adenomatous polyp to invasive cancer.
(b) There is a 1.7-times increased lifetime risk of developing colorectal cancer if one first-degree relative is affected.
(c) About 90% of colorectal cancers occurs in individuals who do not have a strong family history of the disease.
(d) Over half the tumours are in the rectosigmoid area.
(e) The primary tumour can be removed surgically in over 90% of cases.

4.82 The following associations regarding laxatives are correct (Table 4.13):
(a) Stimulant laxative – ispaghula husk
(b) Osmotic laxative – senna
(c) Bulking agent – lactulose

(d) Stimulant laxative – dioctyl sodium sulphosuccinate
(e) Bulking agent – bisacodyl

4.83 The following associations are correct (page 276):
(a) Osmotic diarrhoea – lactulose
(b) Secretory diarrhoea – cholera
(c) Inflammatory diarrhoea – shigellosis
(d) Abnormal motility – irritable bowel syndrome
(e) Inflammatory diarrhoea – ulcerative colitis

4.84 Recognized causes of chronic diarrhoea include (Table 4.17, page 278):
(a) Faecal impaction in the elderly
(b) Thyrotoxicosis
(c) Diabetic neuropathy
(d) Fungal infections
(e) Rotavirus

4.85 GI problems seen in patients with AIDS include (Table 4.18, page 279):
(a) *Cryptosporidium* diarrhoea
(b) Hairy leucoplakia
(c) Herpes oesophagitis
(d) Candidiasis
(e) Kaposi's sarcoma

4.86 Recognized clinical features of irritable bowel syndrome include (page 281):
(a) Nocturnal diarrhoea
(b) Ribbon-like stools
(c) Constipation
(d) Marked weight loss
(e) Left iliac fossa pain

4.87 Conditions which can mimic acute abdomen include (page 281):
(a) Diabetic ketoacidosis
(b) Myocardial infarction
(c) Porphyria
(d) Lead poisoning
(e) Pneumonia

4.88 Causes of intestinal obstruction include (Table 4.20, page 283):
(a) Volvulus of the sigmoid colon
(b) Adhesions
(c) Gall stones
(d) Crohn's disease
(e) Diverticular disease

4.89 Causes of bacterial peritonitis include (Table 4.21):
(a) Ascites due to liver disease

(b) Chronic peritoneal dialysis
(c) Tuberculosis
(d) Perforation of gastric ulcer
(e) Mesothelioma

4.90 Neoplastic colorectal polyps are seen in (Table 4.15, page 279):
(a) Peutz–Jegher's syndrome
(b) Juvenile polyposis
(c) Carcinoid syndrome
(d) Cronkhite–Canada syndrome
(e) Familial adenomatous polyposis

4.91 A 38-year-old man presents with a 3-year history of difficulty in swallowing, recurrent cough at night and loss of weight. A barium swallow shows a moderately dilated oesophagus with a smooth, tapering distal 'beak'. The following statements are correct (page 230):
(a) The diagnosis is clinical and therefore an upper GI endoscopy is not indicated.
(b) Botulinum toxin into the lower oesophageal sphincter may be helpful.
(c) Endoscopic dilatation of the lower oesophageal sphincter using a pneumatic bag is appropriate therapy.
(d) Oesophageal manometry will reveal aperistalsis of the oesophagus as well as failure of relaxation of the lower oesophageal sphincter.
(e) In older patients nifedipine is contraindicated.

4.92 A 55-year-old woman with atrial fibrillation present with sudden onset of severe abdominal pain and haematochezia. On examination she has mild tenderness on deep palpation. Abdominal radiography shows ileus of the small bowel with thumbprinting (submucosal oedema). The following diagnostic procedures are appropriate (page 271):
(a) Small bowel barium studies
(b) Mesenteric angiography
(c) Upper GI endoscopy
(d) Sigmoidoscopy
(e) Barium enema

4.93 A 85-year-old man presents with fever, vomiting, acute lower abdominal pain and blood in the stools. Lower GI barium studies reveal a localized area of 'sawtooth' irregularity in the colon. The following statements are correct (page 271):
(a) The barium studies confirm colonic carcinoma.
(b) The next step is ultrasound of the liver for metastases.
(c) Serum carcinoembyronic antigen should be done.
(d) The patient has portal hypertension.
(e) The barium studies exclude ischaemic colitis.

4.94 A 45-year-old man is seen in A and E with a 1-day history of black tarry stools. He is asymptomatic. His blood pressure is 100/60 mmHg, with a resting pulse rate 105 beats per minute. The following statements are correct (page 243):
- (a) These clinical features exclude peptic ulcers.
- (b) The patient requires emergency surgery.
- (c) A postural fall in blood pressure indicates significant loss of blood volume of at least 10%.
- (d) This patient has rectal carcinoma.
- (e) These clinical features confirm a perforated colonic ulcer.

4.95 Upper GI endoscopy is contraindicated in the following situations:
- (a) A 55-year-old man with a history of peptic ulcer and clinical features of distended rigid abdomen, rebound tenderness and absent bowel sounds
- (b) A 35-year-old man with HIV and difficulty in swallowing, with a pain
- (c) An 80-year-old man with ischaemic heart disease and a non-healing gastric peptic ulcer after 6 weeks of antacid therapy
- (d) A 41-year-old alcoholic with hepatic failure and variceal bleeding
- (e) A 32-year-old with recently diagnosed familial adenomatous polyposis.

4.96 A 58-year-old man presents with fever, pain in the left lower quadrant and constipation. Clinical examination shows a temperature of 38.8°C and tenderness on palpation. Complete blood count shows a WBC of 16 000. The following statements are correct (page 270):
- (a) The patient requires emergency flexible sigmoidoscopy.
- (b) Broad-spectrum intravenous antibiotics are appropriate treatment.
- (c) A surgical opinion should be sought.
- (d) Spiral CT may help to differentiate this condition from malignant disease.
- (e) Ultrasound is more sensitive than CT in making the diagnosis.

Liver, Biliary Tract and Pancreatic Diseases

5.1 Correct statements about the epidemiology of hepatobiliary diseases include (pages 287–316):
(a) Hepatitis B virus is the major cause of liver disease in the western world.
(b) Alcohol is the major cause of liver disease in the rest of the world.
(c) Hepatitis B vaccine has almost eradicated the disease in the western world.
(d) Liver transplantation is of value in chronic liver disease.
(e) Liver transplantation is of little value in acute liver disease.

5.2 The following statements regarding the anatomy of the liver are correct (page 287):
(a) It is the largest organ in the body.
(b) Its upper border lies between the right fifth and sixth ribs.
(c) Riedel's lobe is an extension of the lateral portion of the right lobe.
(d) The right lobe contains the quadrate and caudate lobes.
(e) It is located in the right lumbar region.

5.3 The following statements regarding the blood supply of the liver are correct (pages 287–288):
(a) The hepatic artery supplies a quarter of its total blood flow.
(b) The hepatic artery is a branch of the coeliac axis.
(c) The portal venous system supplies about half of its total oxygen supply.
(d) Both the hepatic artery and the portal vein enter the liver via the porta hepatis.
(e) Blood is supplied via the portal tracts into the sinusoids in the parenchyma of the liver.

5.4 The following statements about the parenchyma of the liver are correct (page 288):
(a) Each polyhedral lobule contains a central vein and peripheral portal triads.
(b) The portal triad is in the middle of each acinus.
(c) The cells near the central veins are more resistant to hypoxic damage than the cells near the portal triads.
(d) The space of Disse lies between the sinusoids and the hepatocytes.
(e) The sinusoids contains fluid that drains to the lymphatics in the portal tracts.

5.5 The following statements about the biliary system are correct (page 288):
(a) The common hepatic duct is a combination of cystic duct and the hepatic duct.
(b) The common bile duct is about 8 mm wide.

(c) The gall bladder dilutes hepatic bile with its own secretion.
(d) The sphincter of Oddi prevents bile entering the duodenum in the fasting state.
(e) The common bile duct and pancreatic duct open into the second part of the duodenum.

5.6 Causes of hypoalbuminaemia include (page 289):
(a) Fulminant hepatic failure
(b) Trauma with sepsis
(c) Nephrotic syndrome
(d) Protein-losing enteropathy
(e) Chronic liver disease

5.7 The liver synthesizes (page 289):
(a) Coagulation factor VIII
(b) γ-Globulins
(c) Albumin
(d) Transferrin
(e) Caeruloplasmin

5.8 Sources for gluconeogenesis include (page 289):
(a) Lactate
(b) Amino acids from muscles
(c) Glycerol from lipolysis of fat stores
(d) Ketone bodies
(e) Fatty acids

5.9 The following statements about lipid metabolism are correct (page 289):
(a) The liver synthesizes very low-density lipoproteins.
(b) The liver synthesizes high-density lipoproteins.
(c) Low-density lipoproteins are degraded by the liver.
(d) The kidney is one of the major sites of HDL metabolism.
(e) Diet is the main source of cholesterol.

5.10 The following statements about the secretion of bile are correct (pages 289–290):
(a) A bile salt-dependent process contributes about 230 mL per day.
(b) A bile salt-independent process contributes about 230 mL per day.
(c) Canalicular multispecific organic anion transporter mediates transport of a broad range of compounds, including bilirubin diglucuronide.
(d) Cystic fibrosis transmembrane conductance regulator controls chloride secretion.
(e) The secretion of bicarbonate-rich solution is stimulated by somatostatin.

5.11 Bile acids (page 289):
(a) are synthesized from dietary triglycerides

(b) are reabsorbed in the colon
(c) the entire pool recycles through the enterohepatic circulation six to eight times a day
(d) main function is lipid solubilization
(e) are conjugated with glycine to increase their solubility

5.12 Bilirubin (pages 290–291):
(a) is produced mainly from the catabolism of myoglobin, cytochromes and catalases
(b) is formed by the reduction of biliverdin
(c) is conjugated with glucuronic acid in the endoplasmic reticulum
(d) is reabsorbed in the small intestine to form the enterohepatic circulation
(e) remains elevated in the blood for a short time after cholestasis is resolved because the conjugated form binds strongly to serum albumin

5.13 The liver catabolizes (page 291):
(a) Insulin
(b) Growth hormone
(c) Parathormone
(d) Oestrogens
(e) Glucocorticoids

5.14 The reticuloendothelial system of the liver (page 292):
(a) acts as a 'sieve' for bacteria carried to it from the gastrointestinal system
(b) contains Kupffer's cells, which are phagocytic
(c) contains lymphoid cells in the portal tract
(d) degrades the phagocytosed antigens with the production of antibody
(e) is thought to play a role in tissue repair

5.15 Routine liver function tests sent for biochemical examination include serum (page 292):
(a) Prothrombin time
(b) Proteins
(c) Aminotransferases
(d) Alkaline phosphatase
(e) γ-Glutamyl transpeptidase

5.16 High levels of aspartate aminotransferase are seen in (page 293):
(a) Cardiac infarction
(b) Muscle injury
(c) Congestive cardiac failure
(d) Liver cell necrosis
(e) Pulmonary infarctions

5.17 The following statements about aminotransferases are correct (page 293):
(a) Aminotransferases were previously known as transaminases.

(b) Aspartate aminotransferase is a mitochondrial enzyme.
(c) Alanine aminotransferase is a cytosolic enzyme.
(d) Alanine aminotransferase is more specific for the liver than aspartate aminotransferase.
(e) Aminotransferases leak into the blood with liver cell damage.

5.18 Aspartate aminotransferase is present in (page 293):
   (a) Lung
   (b) Brain
   (c) Kidney
   (d) Muscle
   (e) Heart

5.19 Alkaline phosphatase is present in (page 293):
   (a) Heart
   (b) Bone
   (c) Intestine
   (d) Placenta
   (e) Lung

5.20 Serum alkaline phosphatase is raised in (page 293):
   (a) Myocardial infarction
   (b) Metastatic liver disease
   (c) Extrahepatic cholestasis
   (d) Intrahepatic cholestasis
   (e) Primary biliary cirrhosis

5.21 γ-Glutamyl transpeptidase (page 293):
   (a) has a similar pathway of excretion to serum alkaline phosphatase
   (b) is a microsomal enzyme
   (c) when raised is a good guide to alcohol intake
   (d) can be induced by phenytoin
   (e) when mildly elevated indicates liver disease

5.22 Recognized clinical features of chronic liver disease include (page 293):
   (a) Hypergammaglobulinaemia
   (b) Burr cells
   (c) Hypoalbuminaemia
   (d) β–γ fusion on plasma protein electrophoresis
   (e) Prolonged prothrombin time

5.23 The following haematological associations in liver disease are correct (page 292–295):
   (a) Acute viral hepatitis – aplastic anaemia
   (b) Alcohol – macrocytosis
   (c) Hypersplenism – pancytopenia

(d) Acute liver failure – haemolysis
(e) Bleeding–microcytic hypochromic blood picture

5.24 The following statements about liver function tests are correct (page 294):
(a) Antimitochondrial antibody is found in most patients with primary biliary cirrhosis.
(b) High concentrations of α-fetoprotein in adults indicate hepatocellular carcinoma.
(c) Prothrombin time is a crude indicator of liver disease.
(d) A second recirculation peak of the bromsulphthalein test occurs in Gilbert's syndrome.
(e) High titres of nucleic, actin, liver/kidney microsomal antibodies are found in chronic active hepatitis.

5.25 Correct statements about imaging techniques in hepatobiliary or pancreatic disease include (page 294):
(a) Most gall stones are visible on a plain abdominal X-ray.
(b) Ultrasound is usually the first investigation of choice in hepatobiliary disease.
(c) CT can detect calcification not seen on plain X-rays.
(d) Cholecystography is the investigation of choice in jaundiced patients with suspected gall bladder disease.
(e) Ultrasound detects space-occupying lesions in the liver of less than 1 cm in diameter.

5.26 The following statements about scintiscanning are correct (page 295):
(a) With a technetium colloid scan there is no hepatic uptake in alcoholic hepatitis.
(b) With a technetium colloid scan most of the uptake is the spleen and bone marrow in advanced cirrhosis.
(c) The ^{99m}Tc-HIDA scan is useful in acute cholecystitis.
(d) The ^{99m}Tc-HIDA scan is useful in neonatal hepatitis due to biliary atresia.
(e) When technetium colloid is injected intravenously it is taken up by the reticuloendothelial cells of the liver and spleen.

5.27 Endoscopic retrograde cholangiopancreatography is used to (page 296):
(a) diagnose acute haemorrhagic pancreatitis
(b) remove common bile duct stones
(c) remove stones from the gall bladder
(d) introduce biliary stents in extrahepatic cholestasis
(e) diagnose acute hepatitis

5.28 Correct statements about percutaneous transhepatic cholangiography include (page 296):
(a) A large-bore needle is used.

(b) It outlines the biliary tree in jaundiced patients with dilated intrahepatic ducts on ultrasound.
(c) Prophylactic antibiotics should be given before the procedure.
(d) Bleeding is one the main complications.
(e) It is safe in patients with platelet count $<80 \times 10^9$ L^{-1}.

5.29 Usual contraindications to needle liver biopsy include (Table 15.2):
(a) Prothrombin prolonged by more than 3 s
(b) Platelet count $<80 \times 10^9$ L^{-1}
(c) Ascites
(d) Extrahepatic cholestasis
(e) Uncooperative patient

5.30 Indications for liver biopsy include (Table 15.2):
(a) In most cases of jaundice
(b) In most cases of acute hepatitis
(c) Unexplained hepatomegaly
(d) Pyrexia of unknown origin
(e) Cirrhosis

5.31 Complications of liver biopsy include (page 296):
(a) Pleurisy
(b) Intraperitoneal bleeding
(c) Perihepatitis
(d) Haemobilia
(e) Transient septicaemia

5.32 Recognized symptoms of chronic liver disease include (page 297):
(a) Abdominal distension
(b) Haematemesis
(c) Pruritus
(d) Amenorrhoea
(e) Drowsiness

5.33 Spider naevi (page 297):
(a) are found in acute liver disease
(b) are telangiectasia
(c) consist of a central arteriole with radiating small vessels
(d) are found below the nipple line
(e) are found in pregnancy

5.34 Palmar erythema is seen in (page 297):
(a) Chronic liver disease
(b) Pregnancy
(c) Rheumatoid arthritis
(d) Thyrotoxicosis
(e) Severe acute liver disease

5.35 Recognized signs of chronic liver disease include (page 297):
  (a) Gynaecomastia
  (b) Testicular atrophy
  (c) Clubbing
  (d) Dupuytren's contracture
  (e) Xanthomas

5.36 Recognized features of decompensated cirrhosis include (page 298):
  (a) Fetor hepaticus
  (b) Flapping tremor of the outstretched hands
  (c) Drowsiness
  (d) Ascites
  (e) Stupor

5.37 Jaundice (page 298):
  (a) is a yellow coloration of skin and mucous membranes
  (b) is detectable when the serum bilirubin exceeds 30–60 mmol/L^{-1}
  (c) with pale stools indicates excessive breakdown of red cells
  (d) with dark-coloured urine is 'acholuric jaundice'
  (e) is usually mild in haemolytic jaundice

5.38 Recognized causes of haemolytic jaundice include (page 298):
  (a) Gilbert's syndrome
  (b) Crigler–Najjar syndrome
  (c) Dubin–Johnson syndrome
  (d) Rotor syndrome
  (e) Sickle cell disease

5.39 Causes of conjugated hyperbilirubinaemia include (page 298):
  (a) Gilbert's syndrome
  (b) Rotor syndrome
  (c) Crigler–Najjar syndrome type I
  (d) Crigler–Najjar syndrome type II
  (e) Dubin–Johnson syndrome

5.40 Causes of cholestatic jaundice include (page 299):
  (a) Common bile duct stones
  (b) Carcinoma of the head of the pancreas
  (c) Sclerosing cholangitis
  (d) Viral hepatitis
  (e) Pregnancy

5.41 The following associations in liver disease are correct (page 300):
  (a) Recent consumption of shellfish – suggests hepatitis B
  (b) Tattoos – increase the chance of hepatitis A
  (c) Blood transfusion – hepatitis C

(d) Recurrent jaundice in family members – Gilbert's syndrome
(e) Sewage workers – leptospirosis

5.42 The following clinical associations in hepatobiliary disease are correct (page 301):
(a) Knobbly irregular liver – viral hepatitis
(b) Splenomegaly – portal hypertension
(c) Ascites – cirrhosis
(d) Palpable gall bladder – carcinoma of the pancreas
(e) Smooth tender liver – metastases

5.43 Causes of hepatomegaly include (Table 5.3):
(a) Leukaemia
(b) Lymphoma
(c) Heart failure
(d) Amyloid
(e) Early cirrhosis

5.44 The following statements are correct (pages 300–301):
(a) In early hepatitis serum AST tends to be high.
(b) In early hepatitis there is only a small rise in alkaline phosphatase.
(c) Serum alkaline phosphatase is high with extrahepatic obstruction.
(d) Abnormal mononuclear cells in blood are a feature of toxoplasmosis.
(e) Abnormal mononuclear cells in blood are a feature of infectious mononucleosis.

5.45 Infective agents causing acute liver damage include (Fig 5.12):
(a) *Toxoplasma gondii*
(b) *Leptospira icterohaemorrhagiae*
(c) Yellow fever virus
(d) Cytomegalovirus
(e) Epstein–Barr virus

5.46 Causes of acute parenchymal liver damage include (Fig 5.12):
(a) Aflatoxin
(b) *Amanita phalloides*
(c) Carbon tetrachloride
(d) Halothane
(e) Paracetamol

5.47 The following statements are correct (pages 302–309):
(a) In hepatitis A the damage is due to the virus itself.
(b) In hepatitis B the damage is due to an immunological reaction to the virus.
(c) Most hepatitis C infections are asymptomatic.
(d) Hepatitis E usually progresses to chronic liver disease.
(e) HGV almost always causes either acute or chronic hepatitis.

5.48 Hepatitis A (pages 302–303):
  (a) is the commonest type of viral hepatitis
  (b) is spread by the faeco-oral route
  (c) has a carrier state
  (d) occurs worldwide
  (e) is more frequent in lower socioeconomic classes

5.49 Hepatitis A virus (page 303):
  (a) is excreted in faeces for about 2 weeks before the onset of the illness
  (b) disease is maximally infectious just before the onset of jaundice
  (c) is a RNA virus
  (d) is transmitted vertically
  (e) causes liver cancer

5.50 Biochemical changes in hepatitis A virus infection include (page 303):
  (a) A raised serum AST, which precedes the jaundice.
  (b) Serum alkaline phosphatase is usually less than 300 IU L^{-1}.
  (c) Serum bilirubin is normal in the prodromal stage.
  (d) AST may remain elevated for up to 6 months after the jaundice has subsided.
  (e) Urinary urobilinogen is increased in the prodromal period.

5.51 Haematological changes in hepatitis A virus infections include (pages 303–304):
  (a) Leucopenia with relative lymphocytosis
  (b) Aplastic anaemia
  (c) Coombs'-positive haemolytic anaemia
  (d) Prolonged prothrombin time
  (e) Raised ESR

5.52 The following statements about investigations in hepatitis A virus infection are correct (page 304):
  (a) Anti-HAV IgG antibodies are common in the general population over the age of 50.
  (b) Anti-HAV IgM indicates an acute infection.
  (c) Older patients should have an ultrasound of the abdomen to exclude bile duct obstruction.
  (d) Liver biopsy is essential to make a tissue diagnosis.
  (e) Patients ought to have an ERCP once the jaundice has subsided.

5.53 The following statements about course and prognosis in hepatitis A virus infection are correct (page 304):
  (a) Most patients make a complete recovery.
  (b) Mortality is high in young adults.
  (c) Death is due to fulminant necrosis.

(d) About a quarter of the patients develop chronic liver disease.
(e) Immunoglobulins against hepatitis A virus shorten the course of the illness.

5.54 The following statements about the treatment of hepatitis A are correct (page 304):
(a) There is no specific treatment.
(b) Admission to hospital is usually necessary.
(c) Low-fat diet shortens the durations of symptoms.
(d) Prolonged bed rest is helpful.
(e) Corticosteroids shorten the course of the illness.

5.55 The followings statements about preventing hepatitis A are correct (page 304):
(a) The virus is killed by boiling water for 10 minutes.
(b) The virus is destroyed by chlorination.
(c) Normal immunoglobulin provides protection for about 3 months.
(d) The most effective prophylactic measure is good hygiene and improved sanitation.
(e) Immunoglobulins provide protection in those without antibodies travelling to endemic areas.

5.56 The following associations are correct (Table 5.4):
(a) Hepatitis A – RNA virus
(b) Hepatitis B – DNA virus
(c) Hepatitis C – RNA virus
(d) Hepatitis D – DNA virus
(e) Hepatitis E – RNA virus

5.57 The faecal route of transmission is a feature of (Table 5.4):
(a) Hepatitis A
(b) Hepatitis B
(c) Hepatitis C
(d) Hepatitis D
(e) Hepatitis E (non-A, non-B)

5.58 The salivary route of transmission is a feature of (Table 5.4):
(a) Hepatitis A
(b) Hepatitis B
(c) Hepatitis C
(d) Hepatitis D
(e) Hepatitis E

5.59 The sexual route of transmission is a feature of (Table 5.4):
(a) Hepatitis A
(b) Hepatitis B
(c) Hepatitis C

(d) Hepatitis D
(e) Hepatitis E

5.60 Vertical transmission is a feature of (Table 5.4):
   (a) Hepatitis A
   (b) Hepatitis B
   (c) Hepatitis C
   (d) Hepatitis D
   (e) Hepatitis E

5.61 A carrier state is a feature of (Table 5.4):
   (a) Hepatitis A
   (b) Hepatitis B
   (c) Hepatitis C
   (d) Hepatitis D
   (e) Hepatitis E

5.62 Chronic liver disease is a recognized complication of (Table 5.4):
   (a) Hepatitis A
   (b) Hepatitis B
   (c) Hepatitis C
   (d) Hepatitis D
   (e) Hepatitis E

5.63 Liver cancer is a recognized complication of (Table 5.4):
   (a) Hepatitis A
   (b) Hepatitis B
   (c) Hepatitis C
   (d) Hepatitis D
   (e) Hepatitis E

5.64 Long incubation is a feature of (Table 5.4):
   (a) Hepatitis A
   (b) Hepatitis B
   (c) Hepatitis C
   (d) Hepatitis D
   (e) Hepatitis E

5.65 Transmission through blood products occurs with (Table 5.4):
   (a) Hepatitis A
   (b) Hepatitis B
   (c) Hepatitis C
   (d) Hepatitis D
   (e) Hepatitis E

5.66 Passive immunization is available for (Table 5.4):
   (a) Hepatitis A

(b) Hepatitis B
(c) Hepatitis C
(d) Hepatitis D
(e) Hepatitis E

5.67 Recognized routes of transmission of hepatitis B include (page 305):
(a) Transmission of infective blood
(b) Contaminated needles used by drug addicts
(c) Contaminated needles used by tattooists
(d) Sexual contact
(e) From mother to child during parturition

5.68 The inner core of the hepatitis B virus contains (page 305):
(a) HBsAg
(b) e antigen
(c) HBcAg
(d) DNA polymerase
(e) Single-stranded DNA

5.69 The following statements about the hepatitis B virus are correct (page 304):
(a) The whole virus is called the Dane particle.
(b) The virus replicates in the bloodstream.
(c) The outer surface coat is produced by multiplication in the cytoplasm.
(d) The inner core is formed by the liver cell nucleus.
(e) The core antigen has further antigenic determinants known as a, d, y, w and r.

5.70 The following statements about the hepatitis D virus are correct (page 307):
(a) It requires hepatitis B for its propagation.
(b) It can cause severe hepatitis in HBV carriers.
(c) When chronic is associated with a poor prognosis.
(d) Transmission is by the faeco-oral route.
(e) HBV vaccine is used for immunization.

5.71 Recognized clinical features of hepatitis B include (pages 305–306):
(a) Urticaria
(b) Polyarthritis
(c) Osteoarthroses
(d) Glomerulonephritis
(e) Arteritis

5.72 The time course of serological changes in hepatitis B includes (Fig 5.16):
(a) HBeAg rises early and usually declines rapidly.
(b) Anti-HBs appears late.
(c) Anti-HBc is the last antibody to appear.
(d) Anti-HBe appears before anti-HBc.
(e) HBsAg appears from about 6 weeks to 3 months after an acute infection.

5.73 Correct statements about serological changes in hepatitis B include (page 306):
(a) HBcAg is not usually seen in the blood.
(b) HBeAg correlates with increased severity and infectivity of the disease.
(c) High titres of IgM anti-HBc suggest continuing viral replication.
(d) The appearance of anti-HBe relates to a decreased infectivity.
(e) Anti-HBs indicates immunity.

5.74 Measures to prevent hepatitis B include (page 306):
(a) Avoid sharing needles.
(b) Avoid multiple homosexual partners.
(c) Counselling HBsAg-positive patients.
(d) Counselling e-antigen-positive patients.
(e) Avoid accidental needle punctures in hospitals.

5.75 Passive immunization for hepatitis B (page 306):
(a) consists of serum globulin containing a high titre of anti-HBs
(b) is given to sexual partners of patients with acute hepatitis B
(c) is given to babies born to hepatitis B-positive mothers
(d) is given to patients acutely exposed to body fluids in a laboratory
(e) is given to hospital staff acutely punctured by an infected needle

5.76 High-risk groups for hepatitis B include (page 306):
(a) Haemophiliacs
(b) Patients on haemodialysis
(c) Staff in institutions for the mentally handicapped
(d) Patients in institutions for the mentally handicapped
(e) Sexual contacts of HBsAg carriers

5.77 Vaccines for hepatitis B are prepared (page 307):
(a) from immune serum globulin containing a high titre of anti-HBs
(b) from plasma of carriers of hepatitis B
(c) by inserting a plasmid containing the gene of HBsAg into a yeast
(d) by inactivating all known viruses in the plasma containing HBsAg
(e) from hepatitis B immunoglobulin

5.78 The following statements about hepatitis B carriers are correct (page 307):
(a) Following acute hepatitis about half the patients will become carriers.
(b) Adults are more likely to remain carriers than children.
(c) Asymptomatic patients with no history of acute hepatitis may be chronic carriers.
(d) Carriers with HBeAg viral DNA are highly infective.
(e) Carriers with DNA polymerase in the serum are highly infective.

5.79 High-risk groups for chronic hepatitis B carrier state include (page 307):
(a) Hodgkins's disease patients
(b) Down's syndrome patients

(c) Patients on immunosuppressive therapy
(d) Patients on long-term dialysis
(e) Patients in long-term mental institutions

5.80 Correct statements regarding the prognosis of hepatitis B carriers include (page 307):
(a) Most remain HBsAg positive.
(b) Those who develop HBe antibodies are not highly infective.
(c) Some may carry the virus for years without developing chronic liver disease.
(d) Those with the e antigen are more likely to develop chronic hepatitis.
(e) Those with the e antigen are more likely to develop hepatocellular carcinoma.

5.81 Recognized manifestations of hepatitis C virus include (page 308):
(a) Agranulocytosis
(b) Cirrhosis
(c) Arthritis
(d) Aplastic anaemia
(e) Diffuse neurological manifestations

5.82 Causes of fulminant hepatic failure include (Table 5.7):
(a) Isoniazid
(b) Monoamine oxidase inhibitor
(c) Halothane anaesthesia
(d) Paracetamol overdose
(e) Carbon tetrachloride poisoning

5.83 Correct statements about investigations in fulminant hepatic failure include (page 309):
(a) Prothrombin time is the most useful index of severity.
(b) AST falls with progressive liver damage.
(c) Serum albumin increases.
(d) EEG is useful in grading encephalopathy.
(e) A very high prothrombin time indicates a good prognosis.

5.84 Viruses known to cause hepatitis include (page 310):
(a) Rotavirus
(b) Epstein–Barr virus
(c) Herpes simplex
(d) Yellow fever virus
(e) Cytomegalovirus

5.85 Recognized pathological features of chronic hepatitis include (page 310):
(a) Interface hepatitis
(b) Chronic inflammatory cell infiltrates are usually present in the portal tracts

(c) Lobular change
(d) Both necrosis and apoptosis
(e) Bridging fibrosis

5.86 The following statements about the chronic hepatitis B infection are correct (page 311):
(a) Viral persistence in patients with a very poor cell-mediated response leads to a healthy carrier state.
(b) When the viral genome becomes integrated into the host DBA, the level of HBV in the serum is low and the patient is HBe-negative and Hbe antibody-positive.
(c) The inactivation of p-53 induced apoptosis by protein X has been implicated in carcinogenesis.
(d) HGsAg may be seen as 'ground glass' appearance in the cytoplasm on haematoxylin and eosin staining.
(e) Chronic hepatitis occurs mainly in women.

5.87 Correct statements about the management and prognosis of hepatitis B include (page 311):
(a) Patients with normal aminotransferases should be treated.
(b) The main aim of treatment is the disappearance of HBeAg and HBV DNA from the serum.
(c) In patients in whom HBeAg disappears, remission is usually sustained.
(d) α-Interferon is the best available agent.
(e) Spontaneous seroconversion occurs in about a third of patients per year.

5.88 Correct statements about chronic hepatitis C include (page 308):
(a) Patients are usually symptomatic.
(b) Severe chronic hepatitis and cirrhosis can be present with only minimal elevation of aminotransferases.
(c) The diagnosis is made by finding HCV antibody in the serum.
(d) The presence of cirrhosis is a contraindication for treatment.
(e) Patients with decompensated cirrhosis should be considered for transplantation.

5.89 Recognized features of chronic persistent hepatitis include (page 310):
(a) Patients are usually male.
(b) It is usually asymptomatic.
(c) HBeAg is usually positive.
(d) Piecemeal necrosis is a prominent feature.
(e) Majority of the patients develop cirrhosis.

5.90 Correct statements about autoimmune hepatitis include (page 313):
(a) Patients may be asymptomatic.
(b) It is not associated with other autoimmune disorders.

    (c) Pancytopenia is present even before portal hypertension and
       splenomegaly.
    (d) Type II autoimmune hepatitis occurs most frequently in men.
    (e) Steroid and azathioprine induce remission in about 80% of cases.

5.91 Recognized features of autoimmune hepatitis include (page 313):
    (a) Glomerulonephritis
    (b) Fibrosing alveolitis
    (c) Migratory polyarthritis
    (d) Anti-liver/kidney microsomal (LKM-1) antibodies
    (e) Pleurisy

5.92 The following statements about the pathogenesis of cirrhosis are correct
(page 314):
    (a) Fibrosis is initiated by activation of the stellate cells.
    (b) $TGF_{\beta 1}$ is the most potent fibrinogenic mediator.
    (c) In the space of Disse the normal matrix is replaced by collagen and
       fibronectin.
    (d) Subendothelial fibrosis leads to loss of the endothelial fenestrations.
    (e) Activated stellate cells have an abundance of retinoid droplets.

5.93 Recognized features of cirrhosis include (page 314):
    (a) Necrosis of liver cells
    (b) Fibrosis
    (c) Nodule formation
    (d) Distortion of architecture
    (e) Deranged liver blood flow

5.94 Common causes of cirrhosis include (Table 5.10):
    (a) Haemochromatosis
    (b) Alcohol
    (c) Hepatitis C
    (d) Hepatitis B
    (e) Wilson's disease

5.95 Causes of cirrhosis include (Table 5.10):
    (a) Methotrexate
    (b) Budd–Chiari syndrome
    (c) Galactosaemia
    (d) α_{-1}-Antitrypsin deficiency
    (e) Cystic fibrosis

5.96 Features of micronodular cirrhosis include (page 314):
    (a) Nodules which are usually less than 3 mm in size
    (b) Nodules consisting of necrosed hepatocytes
    (c) Nodules surrounded by fibrous septa

    (d) Uniform involvement of all lobes

    (e) History of excessive alcohol consumption

5.97 Features of macronodular cirrhosis include (page 314):

    (a) Nodules of varying size

    (b) Normal lobules within larger nodules

    (c) Antecedent hepatitis B infection

    (d) Wilson's disease

    (e) Galactosaemia

5.98 Poor prognostic factors of cirrhosis include (Table 5.11):

    (a) Low serum albumin

    (b) Low serum sodium

    (c) Prolonged prothrombin time

    (d) Neuropsychiatric symptoms

    (e) Small liver

5.99 Indications for liver transplantation include (page 316):

    (a) Fulminant hepatic failure

    (b) Alcoholic liver disease

    (c) Primary biliary cirrhosis

    (d) Chronic hepatitis B

    (e) Cholangiocarcinoma

5.100 Recognized complications of cirrhosis include (Table 5.12):

    (a) Upper gastrointestinal haemorrhage

    (b) Ascites

    (c) Portosystemic encephalopathy

    (d) Renal failure

    (e) Primary liver cell carcinoma

5.101 Causes of portal hypertension include (Table 5.13):

    (a) Portal vein thrombosis

    (b) Schistosomiasis

    (c) Myelosclerosis

    (d) Constrictive pericarditis

    (e) Budd–Chiari syndrome

5.102 Clinical features of portal hypertension include (page 318):

    (a) Hepatomegaly

    (b) Splenomegaly

    (c) Haematemesis

    (d) Ascites

    (e) Hypersplenism

5.103 Correct statements about the management of acute variceal haemorrhage include (page 319):
(a) Acute variceal sclerotherapy arrests bleeding in less than 40% of cases.
(b) Transjugular intrahepatic portocaval shunt is used where bleeding cannot be stopped after two sessions of sclerotherapy 24 hours apart.
(c) Vasopressin infusion is safe in patients with ischaemic heart disease.
(d) Octreotide is as effective as balloon tamponade.
(e) Balloon tamponade is used mainly to control bleeding if sclerotherapy has failed or is unavailable.

5.104 Prophylactic measures for acute variceal haemorrhage include (page 320):
(a) Sengstaken–Blackmore tube
(b) Vasopressin
(c) Long-term injection sclerotherapy
(d) Portosystemic shunting
(e) Oral propranolol

5.105 Mechanisms of ascites in cirrhosis include (page 320):
(a) Excessive urinary sodium excretion
(b) Portal hypertension
(c) High serum albumin
(d) Low peripheral vascular resistance
(e) Activated renin–angiotensin–aldosterone system

5.106 Causes of ascites include (Table 5.14):
(a) Left ventricular failure
(b) Constrictive pericarditis
(c) Malignancy
(d) Tuberculosis
(e) Budd–Chiari syndrome

5.107 Causes of haemorrhagic ascites include (Table 5.14):
(a) Nephrotic syndrome
(b) Cirrhosis
(c) Acute pancreatitis
(d) Malignancy
(e) Ruptured ectopic pregnancy

5.108 Correct statements about the management of ascites in cirrhosis include (page 321):
(a) Dietary sodium restriction is unnecessary.
(b) Bed rest alone may lead to diuresis.
(c) The aim of diuretic therapy is to produce a net loss of 3 L of fluid.
(d) Paracentesis should always be followed up by plasma expander.
(e) Peritoneo-venous shunt is used in most patients.

5.109 Correct statements about spontaneous bacterial peritonitis include (page 322):
(a) It should be suspected in any patient with ascites with evidence of clinical deterioration.
(b) It can be caused by *E. coli.*
(c) A third-generation cephalosporin provides adequate cover pending culture results.
(d) A raised neutrophil count alone is sufficient evidence to instigate treatment.
(e) It is an indication for liver transplantation.

5.110 Portosystemic encephalopathy (page 322):
(a) is a neuropsychiatric syndrome secondary to chronic liver disease
(b) may be seen in patients following a portocaval shunt
(c) is irreversible
(d) is associated with increased aromatic amino acids in the blood
(e) is associated with increased reduced branch-chain amino acids in the blood

5.111 Suggested causative factors in portosystemic encephalopathy include (page 322):
(a) Accumulation of octapamine
(b) Ammonia
(c) Mercaptans
(d) Free fatty acids
(e) Activation of GABA inhibitory neurotransmitter system

5.112 Precipitating factors for portosystemic encephalopathy include (Table 5.15):
(a) High dietary protein
(b) Electrolyte imbalance
(c) Infection
(d) Narcotics
(e) Gastrointestinal haemorrhage

5.113 Recognized features of portosystemic encephalopathy include (page 323):
(a) Fetor hepaticus
(b) Asterixis
(c) Constructional apraxia
(d) Prolonged trail-making test
(e) Convulsions

5.114 Correct statements about portosystemic encephalopathy include (page 323):
(a) Abnormal routine liver function tests are useful in excluding it.
(b) EEG changes occur before coma supervenes.
(c) Visual evoked responses detect subclinical encephalopathy.

(d) Blood ammonia is useful in differentiating from other causes of coma.
(e) Diagnosis is clinical.

5.115 The immediate management of portosystemic encephalopathy includes (page 323):
(a) High-protein diet
(b) Sedation
(c) Enemas
(d) Oral neomycin
(e) Increased diuretic therapy

5.116 Correct statements about hepatorenal syndrome include (page 323):
(a) Low urinary sodium excretion
(b) Intact renal tubular function
(c) Normal kidney histology
(d) Liver transplantation is the best option
(e) Increase or initiate diuretic therapy

5.117 Recognized features of primary biliary cirrhosis include (page 324):
(a) Predominantly affects men
(b) Progressive destruction of bile ducts
(c) Antimitochondrial antibodies
(d) Increased IgM synthesis
(e) Raised serum cholesterol

5.118 The following statements regarding primary biliary cirrhosis are correct (page 324):
(a) The antigen M2 is specific.
(b) The finding of M4 and M8 antigens in patients with M2 is associated with more progressive disease.
(c) The presence of a high titre of antimitochondrial antibody indicates a more severe prognosis.
(d) Antibodies to bile ductules are specific to PBC.
(e) The E2 component of the pyruvate dehydrogenase complex is the major M2 antigen.

5.119 Clinical features of primary biliary cirrhosis include (page 324):
(a) Asymptomatic patients with raised alkaline phosphatase
(b) Pruritus
(c) Pigmentation of skin
(d) Xanthelasma
(e) Hepatosplenomegaly

5.120 Recognized associations in primary biliary cirrhosis include (page 324):
(a) Cardiomyopathy
(b) Keratoconjunctivitis sicca
(c) Renal tubular acidosis

(d) Membranous glomerulonephritis
(e) Emphysema of the lung

5.121 Correct statements about the therapy of primary biliary cirrhosis include (page 325):
(a) Penicillamine is useful.
(b) Corticosteroids have no benefit.
(c) Rifampicin has been shown to be of benefit in pruritus.
(d) Ursodeoxycholate is curative.
(e) Liver transplantation should be offered before the onset of jaundice in mild cases.

5.122 Causes of hepatic granulomas include:
(a) Sarcoidosis
(b) Tuberculosis
(c) Adverse effect of phenylbutazone therapy
(d) Brucellosis
(e) Schistosomiasis

5.123 Hereditary haemochromatosis is (page 325):
(a) a mutation on the short arm of chromosome 6
(b) an autosomal dominant disease
(c) associated with HLA-A3
(d) associated with excessive alcohol in most cases
(e) associated with dietary intakes of iron and chelating agents

5.124 Organs involved in hereditary haemochromatosis include (page 325):
(a) Lungs
(b) Heart
(c) Skin
(d) Endocrine glands
(e) Gonads

5.125 Histological features of the liver in hereditary haemochromatosis include (page 325):
(a) Pigmentation
(b) Fibrosis
(c) Iron deposition in the periportal hepatocytes late in the disease
(d) Cirrhosis
(e) Fatty change

5.126 Clinical features of hereditary haemochromatosis include (page 325):
(a) It is more common in women
(b) Most individuals present in the fifth decade
(c) Skin pigmentation
(d) Diabetes mellitus
(e) Hepatomegaly

5.127 Clinical features of hereditary haemochromatosis include (page 326):
  (a) Loss of libido
  (b) Gonadal atrophy
  (c) Deficiency of pituitary hormones
  (d) Cardiac failure
  (e) Chondrocalcinosis

5.128 Homozygotes in hereditary haemochromatosis show (page 326):
  (a) Elevated serum iron
  (b) Reduced total iron-binding capacity
  (c) Complete transferrin saturation
  (d) Elevated serum ferritin
  (e) Normal liver biochemistry

5.129 Venesection in hereditary haemochromatosis (page 326):
  (a) prolongs life.
  (b) abolishes the risk of malignancy
  (c) may reverse tissue damage
  (d) removes excess iron
  (e) requires monitoring of serum ferritin

5.130 Venesection in hereditary haemochromatosis usually improves (page 326):
  (a) Diabetes
  (b) Testicular atrophy
  (c) Chondrocalcinosis
  (d) Skin pigmentation
  (e) Hepatomegaly

5.131 Correct statements about screening in hereditary haemochromatosis include (page 326):
  (a) It must be done in all first-degree family members.
  (b) It is used to detect asymptomatic disease.
  (c) Serum ferritin is the investigation of choice.
  (d) Liver biopsy is a must.
  (e) Genetic markers are now available.

5.132 Recognized features of Wilson's disease include (pages 326–327):
  (a) Autosomal dominant inheritance
  (b) Common in consanguinity
  (c) Children usually present with hepatic problems
  (d) Young adults have more neurological problems
  (e) Characterized by failure to excrete copper

5.133 The following statements about copper metabolism are correct (pages 326–327):
  (a) Dietary copper is absorbed from the stomach.
  (b) Dietary copper is absorbed from the upper small intestine.

(c) It is transported loosely bound to albumin.
(d) It is incorporated into caeruloplasmin in the liver.
(e) Copper is normally excreted in the bile.

5.134 Correct statements about the Kayser–Fleischer ring include (page 327):
(a) It is due to copper deposition in the Descemet's membrane in the cornea.
(b) It appears as a greenish brown pigment at the corneoscleral junction just within the cornea.
(c) It may be absent in young children with Wilson's disease.
(d) It may be seen in cryptogenic cirrhosis.
(e) Slit-lamp examination is often required for identification.

5.135 Biochemical features of Wilson's disease include (page 327):
(a) Low serum copper
(b) Normal serum copper
(c) Low serum caeruloplasmin
(d) Increased hepatic copper
(e) Increased 24-hour urinary copper

5.136 The following statements regarding the management of Wilson's disease are correct (page 327):
(a) All siblings should be screened.
(b) All children should be screened.
(c) Asymptomatic homozygous relatives should be treated.
(d) Long-term pencillamine leads to biochemical but not clinical improvement.
(e) Urinary copper levels should be monitored during penicillamine therapy.

5.137 Death in Wilson's disease is from (page 327):
(a) Myocardial infarction
(b) Cardiomyopathy
(c) Bleeding varices
(d) Liver failure
(e) Intercurrent infection

5.138 Features of α_1-antitrypsin deficiency include (page 327):
(a) Inheritance is autosomal recessive
(b) Periodic acid–Schiff-positive diastase-resistant globules in the hepatocytes
(c) Pulmonary emphysema
(d) It responds to penicillamine
(e) Liver transplantation is contraindicated

5.139 Pathological features of alcoholic liver disease include (page 328):
(a) Collagen deposition around the central hepatic veins
(b) Polymorphonuclear infiltration in zone 3

(c) Mallory bodies in the hepatocytes
(d) Bridging fibrosis between portal tracts and terminal hepatic veins
(e) Fat deposition

5.140 Causes of Budd–Chiari syndrome include (page 329):
(a) Polycythaemia vera
(b) Oral contraceptive pill
(c) Leukaemia
(d) Congenital venous webs
(e) Alcoholic liver disease

5.141 Features of Budd–Chiari syndrome include (page 330):
(a) Enlarged caudate lobe
(b) A negative hepatojugular reflux
(c) Splenomegaly
(d) Mild jaundice
(e) Ascites

5.142 The following associations are correct (pages 331–332):
(a) Liver abscess – *Streptococcus milleri*
(b) Amoebic abscess – *Echinococcus granulosus*
(c) Hydatid disease – Casoni skin test
(d) Amoebic liver disease – ELISA
(e) Schistosomiasis – praziquantel therapy

5.143 Causes of jaundice in pregnancy include (page 332):
(a) Viral hepatitis
(b) Hyperemesis gravidarum
(c) HELLP syndrome
(d) Recurrent intrahepatic cholestasis
(e) Acute fatty liver

5.144 The following associations are correct (page 334):
(a) Reye's syndrome – aflatoxin
(b) Hepatocellular carcinoma – oral contraceptives
(c) Cholangiosarcoma – *Clonorchis sinensis*
(d) Veno-occlusive disease – bush tea
(e) Pelioses hepatitis – oral contraceptives

5.145 The following associations about drug-induced liver damage are correct (Table 5.14):
(a) Tetracyclines – microvesicular fat deposition
(b) Amiodarone – 'Alcoholic' hepatitis-like picture
(c) Methyldopa – chronic active hepatitis
(d) Chlorpromazine – cholestasis
(e) Acute hepatitis – isoniazid

5.146 Risk factors for cholesterol gall stones include (Table 5.15):
    (a) Males rather than females
    (b) Nulliparity
    (c) Ileal disease
    (d) Acromegaly treated with octreotide
    (e) Obesity

5.147 Correct statements about the management of gall stones include (page 328):
    (a) Laparoscopic cholecystectomy is the operation of choice.
    (b) In open cholecystectomies an increased mortality occurs in the obese.
    (c) Cholesterol gall stones can be dissolved by bile acids.
    (d) They can be removed endoscopically with a Dormia basket.
    (e) Shock-wave lithotripsy is becoming the treatment of choice.

5.148 Investigations used in the assesment of pancreatic disease include (Table 5.18):
    (a) Faecal fat
    (b) Glucose tolerance test measuring insulin and glucose
    (c) Duodenal enzymes after the Lundh meal
    (d) CT scan
    (e) ERCP

5.149 Causes of pancreatitis include (Table 5.19):
    (a) Gall stones
    (b) Alcohol
    (c) ERCP
    (d) Hyperlipidaemia
    (e) Mumps

5.150 Complications of pancreatitis include (Table 5.20):
    (a) Pseudocyst
    (b) Portal vein thrombosis
    (c) Disseminated intravascular coagulation
    (d) Paralytic ileus
    (e) Respiratory failure

5.151 Factors that indicate a poor prognosis in acute pancreatitis include (Table 5.19):
    (a) Elevated serum calcium
    (b) Hyperglycaemia
    (c) Leucocytosis
    (d) Elevated blood urea
    (e) Hypoxia

5.152 The following associations are correct (page 346):
    (a) Grey–Turner's sign – pancreatic carcinoma
    (b) Cullen's sign – acute pancreatitis

(c) Courvoiser's sign – pancreatic carcinoma
(d) Thrombophlebitis – pancreatic carcinoma
(e) Defective chloride channel in the cell membrane – cystic fibrosis

5.153 The following statements about Zollinger–Ellison syndrome are correct (page 352):
(a) They arise mainly from the G cells in the pancreas.
(b) Peptic ulcers occur.
(c) Diarrhoea is a common feature.
(d) Serum gastrin levels are low.
(e) Omeprazole should be avoided.

5.154 Endocrine tumours known to affect the gut include (page 352):
(a) Vipomas
(b) Glucogonoma
(c) Enteroglucogonoma
(d) Somatostatinoma
(e) Medullary carcinoma thyroid

5.155 A 58-year-old man was diagnosed as having haemochromatosis. His 24-year-old son is asymptomatic, has no physical signs of the condition and his liver function tests are normal. To screen the son for haemochromatosis the following investigations are appropriate:
(a) Serum iron
(b) Serum transferrin saturation
(c) Serum ferritin level
(d) Serum amylase
(e) Fasting blood sugar

5.156 A 38-year-old woman has jaundice and generalized itching. She is found to have adenocarcinoma of the pancreas with multiple liver metastases. Liver function tests show a bilirubin 14 mg/dL urine bilirubin positive, alanine transaminase 98 mg/dL, aspartate transaminase 79 mg/dL, serum alkaline phosphatase 800 u/L. She is treated palliatively with stent placement at the site of obstruction. Ten days after the stent placement she feels much better, with no itching and normal urine colour. The jaundice, however, persisted. Liver function tests now show a bilirubin 7 mg/dL, urine bilirubin negative, alanine transaminase 49 mg/dL, aspartate transaminase 35 mg/dL, serum alkaline phosphatase 420 u/L. Further management at this stage includes:
(a) Obtain an ultrasound to determine the site of the stent.
(b) Insert a new stent as the old one is blocked.
(c) Obtain a surgical opinion for urgent choledochoenterostomy.
(d) Insert a needle into the biliary tree for percutaneous drainage.
(e) Continue observation.

5.157 A 26-year-old woman returns from a visit to Bangladesh and presents in A and E with malaise of 10 days duration, dark urine for several days and pain in the right hypochondrium for 5 days. The patient is not on any medications. Her physical examination reveals icterus and mild tender hepatomegaly. Her ALT 1000, AST 800, alkaline phosphatase 200 uL, bilirubin 10 mg/DL, PT 13 s, haematocrit 40 and white blood cell count of 9000/μL. The following statements are correct:

(a) Liver biopsy is mandatory.

(b) An ultrasound of the liver is the next test to rule out dilated hepatic ducts.

(c) The patient is in immediate danger of fulminant hepatic failure and will require liver transplantation.

(d) The patient has Gilberts' syndrome.

(e) The patient has viral hepatitis.

5.158 A 42-year-old man with portal hypertension and ascites secondary to alcoholic cirrhosis presents with fever and pain in the abdomen. On examination his temperature is 38.2°C, pulse 110 bpm and blood pressure 110/60 mmHg. The abdomen is grossly distended and there is bilateral pitting leg oedema. His bilirubin is 13 mg/dL, haemoglobin 11.8 g/dL, white blood cell count of 15 000 μl, platelet count of 100,000 μl, prothrombin time 17 s and serum albumin 2.6 g/dL. Ascitic fluid examination reveals albumin 0.8 g/dL, white blood cell count of 700 μl, polymorphonuclear leucocyte count of 85%. Gram stain of ascitic fluid revealed no organisms. The following statements are true:

(a) The patient has bacterial peritonitis.

(b) Empiric antibiotics should not be started until the culture and sensitivity report are received.

(c) Further paracentesis should be done only under ultrasound guidance.

(d) The patient should be considered for liver transplantation.

(e) A third-generation cephalosporin is contraindicated.

Haematological Disease

6.1 The following statements are correct (page 353):
  (a) Plasma is the liquid component of blood which lacks soluble fibrinogen.
  (b) The liver and spleen are chief sites of haemopoiesis after the seventh month of gestation.
  (c) The bone marrow is the only source of blood cells in adult life.
  (d) In the adult haemopoiesis is confined to the central skeleton and proximal ends of long bones.
  (e) Stem cells have the capability for self-renewal, as well as differentiation.

6.2 An increased reticulocyte count occurs in (page 355):
  (a) Aplastic anaemia
  (b) Haemorrhage
  (c) Haemolysis
  (d) Response to treatment with haematinics
  (e) Pregnancy

6.3 The erythrocyte sedimentation rate (ESR) (page 355):
  (a) is increased in patients with polycythaemia vera
  (b) is a measure of the acute-phase response
  (c) when raised reflects an increase in the plasma concentration of large proteins
  (d) decreases with age
  (e) is higher in males

6.4 C-reactive protein (page 355):
  (a) is synthesized exclusively in the liver
  (b) is more useful than ESR in monitoring chronic inflammatory conditions
  (c) falls after trauma
  (d) is unaffected by the level of haemoglobin
  (e) follows the clinical state of the patient much more slowly than ESR

6.5 Correct statements about erythropoiesis include (page 356):
  (a) Reticulocytes are unable to synthesize haemoglobin.
  (b) Normoblasts are normally present in peripheral blood.
  (c) Ineffective erythropoiesis is substantially increased in megaloblastic anaemia.
  (d) Erythropoietin is produced mainly in the liver.
  (e) Inappropriate production of erythropoietin is seen in renal disease.

6.6 The following are required for normal erythropoiesis (page 356):
  (a) Iron
  (b) Folic acid
  (c) Vitamin D

(d) Androgens
(e) Vitamin B$_{12}$

6.7 The following statements about haemoglobin synthesis are correct (page 356, Fig 6.2):
(a) Protoporphyrins are byproducts of haemoglobin synthesis.
(b) Haemoglobin synthesis occurs in the mitochondria of a developing red cell.
(c) The major rate-limiting step in the synthesis of haemoglobin is the formation of δ aminolaevulinic acid.
(d) Each adult haemoglobin molecule, Hb A, consists of two β and two γ chains.
(e) Erythropoietin stimulates ALA synthetase.

6.8 Correct statements about haemoglobin function include (pages 356–357):
(a) An increase in the concentration of 2,3-diphosphoglycerate (2,3-DPG) shifts the haemoglobin oxygen dissociation curve to the left.
(b) The steepest part of the oxygen dissociation curve occurs at partial pressures of oxygen that occur in tissues.
(c) Sickle cell Hb shift the oxygen dissociation curve to the left.
(d) Hb F binds avidly to 2,3-DPG.
(e) During acclimatization to high altitude, 2,3-DPG levels decrease as a compensatory mechanism before erythropoietin produces an increase in the level of haemoglobin.

6.9 The following associations are correct (page 358):
(a) Koilonychia – haemolytic anaemia
(b) Jaundice – haemolytic anaemia
(c) Bone deformities – thalassaemia major
(d) Leg ulcers – sickle cell disease
(e) Clubbing – haemolytic anaemia

6.10 The following statements regarding the absorption of iron are correct (Table 6.2):
(a) Ferric iron is absorbed better than ferrous.
(b) It takes place in the duodenum and jejunum.
(c) Ascorbic acid reduces iron absorption.
(d) The formation of insoluble complexes with phytate increases iron absorption.
(e) There is decreased absorption in hereditary haemochromatosis.

6.11 Correct statements about iron metabolism include (page 361):
(a) Iron is transported in the plasma bound to ferritin.
(b) Iron is stored in the tissues as transferrin.
(c) Haemosiderin is more easily mobilized than ferritin for haemoglobin formation.

(d) When iron levels are high, the 'iron-responsive element-binding protein' increases ferritin synthesis and downregulates transferrin receptors.
(e) There is a diurnal rhythm for iron levels, with higher levels in the morning.

6.12 Causes of iron deficiency include (page 361):
(a) Hookworm infestation
(b) Menstrual loss
(c) *Giardia* infection
(d) Pregnancy
(e) Postgastrectomy

6.13 Features of iron deficiency include (page 361):
(a) Clubbing of nails
(b) Total iron-binding capacity falls compared with normal
(c) Macrocytic blood picture
(d) Plummer–Vinson syndrome
(e) The bone marrow shows erythroid hyperplasia with ragged normoblasts

6.14 Correct statements about the management of iron deficiency include (page 362):
(a) Intravenous iron is the treatment of choice.
(b) The addition of ascorbic acid to iron therapy is essential.
(c) If the patient has side effects from iron medication, reducing the dose is all that is required to reduce symptoms.
(d) The response to iron therapy can be monitored using the reticulocyte count.
(e) Oral iron therapy is necessary for 6 months to replenish iron stores.

6.15 Recognized causes of anaemia of chronic disease include (page 363):
(a) Infective endocarditis
(b) Tuberculosis
(c) Osteomyelitis
(d) Rheumatoid arthritis
(e) Inflammatory bowel disease

6.16 Recognized features of anaemia of chronic disease include (page 363):
(a) Increased release of iron from the bone marrow to developing erythroblasts
(b) Increased red cell survival
(c) Raised serum ferritin
(d) Stainable iron in the bone marrow
(e) Raised serum iron

6.17 Causes of sideroblastic anaemia include (Table 6.4):
(a) Isoniazid
(b) Secondary carcinoma

(c) Alcohol
(d) Iron-deficiency anaemia
(e) Myeloid leukaemia

6.18 Characteristic haematological features of lead poisoning include (page 364):
(a) Sideroblastic anaemia
(b) Haemolysis
(c) Punctate basophilia
(d) Howell–Jolly bodies
(e) Hypersegmented polymorphs

6.19 In thalassemia trait (Table 6.3):
(a) serum iron is reduced
(b) serum TIBC is reduced
(c) serum ferritin is reduced
(d) iron is absent in the bone marrow
(e) iron is absent in erythroblasts

6.20 Causes of microcytic anaemia include (Table 6.3):
(a) Thalassaemia
(b) Sideroblastic anaemia
(c) Anaemia of chronic disorder
(d) Sickle cell anaemia
(e) Sickle cell trait

6.21 Normocytic normochromic anaemia is seen in (page 364):
(a) Chronic renal failure
(b) Following acute blood loss
(c) Hypothyroidism
(d) Hypoadrenalism
(e) Rheumatoid arthritis

6.22 Vitamin B_{12} (page 365):
(a) is found in plants
(b) is usually destroyed by cooking
(c) deficiency may take 2 years or more after absorptive failure as the daily losses are small
(d) forms a complex with 'R' binder in the gut
(e) requires intrinsic factor for absorption

6.23 The following statements are correct (page 365):
(a) Methylcobalamin is a coenzyme for the methylation of homocysteine to methionine by methyltetrahydrofolate.
(b) Deoxyadenosylcobalamin is a coenzyme for the conversion of methylmalonyl CoA to succinyl CoA.
(c) Measurement of methylmalonic acid in the urine is used as a test for folic acid deficiency.

(d) Vitamin B_{12} in plasma is mainly bound to transcobalamin I.
(e) Vitamin B_{12} is transported from the enterocytes to the bone marrow and other tissues by transcobalamin II.

6.24 Causes of vitamin B_{12} deficiency include (Table 6.5):
(a) Gastrectomy
(b) Vegan diet
(c) Coeliac disease
(d) Zollinger–Ellison syndrome
(e) Fish tapeworm

6.25 Neurological features of vitamin B_{12} deficiency include (page 366):
(a) Motor neuron disease
(b) Ataxia
(c) Paraplegia
(d) Polyneuropathy
(e) Dementia

6.26 Causes of megaloblastic anaemia include (page 364):
(a) Azidothymidine (AZT)
(b) Iron-deficiency anaemia
(c) Folic acid deficiency
(d) Myelodysplasia
(e) Vitamin B_{12} deficiency

6.27 Correct statements about the biochemical basis of megaloblastic anaemia include (page 364):
(a) There is a block in DNA synthesis.
(b) In vitamin B_{12} and folate deficiency the common biochemical problem is an inability to methylate deoxyuridine monophosphate to deoxythymidine monophosphate.
(c) The methyl group is supplied by the folate coenzyme methylene tetrahydrofolate polyglutamate.
(d) Vitamin B_{12} deficiency hastens the demethylation of methyl tetrahydrofolate.
(e) Congenital forms of megaloblastic anaemia are due to interference with purine or pyrimidine synthesis.

6.28 The following statements are correct (page 367):
(a) Folates are present in food as monoglutamates.
(b) Methyl tetrahydrofolate is the main form of folate in serum.
(c) Vitamin B_{12} converts methyl tetrahydrofolate to tetrahydrofolate.
(d) Intracellular folates are active coenzymes in the transfer of single carbon units in amino acid metabolism and DNA synthesis.
(e) Cooking causes a substantial loss of folate.

6.29 Causes of folic acid deficiency include (Table 6.6):
- (a) Alcohol excess
- (b) Pregnancy
- (c) Haemolysis
- (d) Phenytoin
- (e) Trimethoprim

6.30 Investigations used to confirm folic acid deficiency include (page 368):
- (a) Schilling's test
- (b) Tests for achlorhydria
- (c) *Lactobacillus casei* methods of assaying serum folate, particularly in patients on antibiotics
- (d) Red cell folate
- (e) Serum transferrin levels

6.31 Causes of macrocytosis without megaloblastic changes include (page 368):
- (a) Pregnancy
- (b) Folic acid deficiency
- (c) Liver disease
- (d) Hypothyroidism
- (e) Vitamin B_{12} deficiency

6.32 Causes of aplastic anaemia include (Table 6.7):
- (a) Fanconi's anaemia
- (b) Hypersplenism
- (c) Benzene
- (d) Viral hepatitis
- (e) Pregnancy

6.33 Drugs associated with marrow aplasia include (page 369):
- (a) Chloramphenicol
- (b) Carbimazole
- (c) Chlorpromazine
- (d) Chlorpropamide
- (e) Phenytoin

6.34 Recognized features of aplastic anaemia include (page 369):
- (a) Activated cytotoxic T cells
- (b) Pancytopenia
- (c) Virtual absence of reticulocytes
- (d) Hypocellular bone marrow with increased fat spaces
- (e) Hypersplenism

6.35 Causes of pancytopenia include (Table 6.8):
- (a) Hodgkin's lymphoma
- (b) SLE
- (c) Myelofibrosis

    (d) Paroxysmal nocturnal haemoglobinuria
    (e) Overwhelming sepsis

6.36 In severe acquired aplastic anaemia (Fig 6.14):
    (a) Bone marrow transplantation is the treatment of choice for patients under 20 years of age who have an HLA-identical sibling donor.
    (b) Patients above the age of 45 are not eligible for bone marrow transplantation even when an HLA-identical donor is available.
    (c) Transplantation using unrelated donors is best restricted to children less than 6 years of age.
    (d) Immunosuppressive therapy should be avoided in patients over the age of 45.
    (e) Steroids are the drug of choice.

6.37 Causes of haemolytic anaemia include (Table 6.9):
    (a) Thalassaemia
    (b) Pyruvate kinase deficiency
    (c) Paroxysmal nocturnal deficiency
    (d) Valve prosthesis
    (e) Acquired spherocytosis

6.38 Features of hereditary spherocytosis include (page 373):
    (a) Leg ulcers
    (b) Positive Coombs' test
    (c) Aplastic anaemia
    (d) Pigment gall stones
    (e) Splenectomy reduces spherocytosis

6.39 The following suggest an intravascular site for haemolysis (page 372):
    (a) Elevated bilirubin
    (b) Haemosiderinuria
    (c) Excessive urinary urobilinogen
    (d) Low haptoglobin
    (e) Presence of methaemalbumin

6.40 Hereditary spherocytosis (page 373):
    (a) is inherited in an autosomal recessive manner
    (b) is associated with an increase in surface-to-volume ratio of erythrocytes
    (c) is associated with an excess of structural protein spectrin
    (d) patients can develop aplastic anaemia after parvovirus infection
    (e) patients develop megaloblastic anaemia as a result of folate depletion owing to the hyperactivity of the bone marrow.

6.41 The following statements about different types of haemoglobin are correct (Table 6.10):
    (a) Glycosylated haemoglobin is decreased in patients with uncontrolled diabetes.

(b) Hb A2 is decreased in patients with β-thalassaemia.
(c) Hb F is increased in β-thalassaemia.
(d) Hb H is found in α-thalassaemia.
(e) Hb Barts comprises 100% of haemoglobin in homozygous α-thalassaemia.

6.42 Recognized features of β-thalassaemia major include (Table 6.11):
(a) Excessive production of β-chains
(b) Rarely, requires blood transfusions
(c) Hepatosplenomegaly
(d) 'Hair on end' appearance on bone X-ray
(e) Gene deletions are commoner than point mutations

6.43 The following associations are correct (Table 375):
(a) Thalassaemia minor – symptomless heterozygous carrier state
(b) Haemoglobin Barts – is always fatal
(c) Homozygous α-thalassaemia – hydrops fetalis
(d) Haemoglobin H disease – incompatible with life
(e) Homozygous Haemoglobin Constant Spring – no clinical abnormality

6.44 Sickle cell crisis may be precipitated by (page 378):
(a) Infection
(b) Dehydration
(c) Cold
(d) Acidosis
(e) Hypoxia

6.45 Correct statements about sickle cell disease include (page 378):
(a) It is caused by a single-base mutation.
(b) Sickle cell trait protects against *Plasmodium falciparum.*
(c) Sickle cell syndrome usually presents in childhood.
(d) In older patients vaso-occlusive problems occur in sickle cell anaemia.
(e) Individuals with sickle cell trait have no symptoms unless they are subjected to anoxia.

6.46 Features of sickle cell crisis include (page 378):
(a) Pleuritic chest pain
(b) Bone pain
(c) Hemiparesis
(d) Priapism
(e) Haematuria

6.47 Long-term problems of sickle cell anaemia include (page 378):
(a) Salmonella osteomyelitis
(b) Leg ulcers
(c) Proliferative retinopathy

(d) Chronic renal disease
(e) Aseptic necrosis of the femoral heads

6.48 The following statements about sickle cell anaemia are correct (page 378):
  (a) Sickling of red cells on a blood film can be induced in the presence of sodium metabisulphite
  (b) A mixture of Hb S in a reducing solution such as sodium dithionite gives a turbid appearance owing to precipitation of Hb S, whereas normal haemoglobin gives a normal appearance.
  (c) Hb electrophoresis is usually not required to confirm the diagnosis.
  (d) The parents of the affected child will show features of sickle cell trait.
  (e) High reticulocyte count is rare.

6.49 The following statements are correct (page 379):
  (a) Individuals with sickle cell trait can develop symptoms when flying in non-pressurized aircraft.
  (b) Sickle cell trait protects against *Plasmodium falciparum* malaria.
  (c) The combination of β-thalassaemia trait and sickle cell trait resembles sickle cell anaemia.
  (d) Hydroxyurea should be avoided in sickle cell crisis.
  (e) Of the offspring of parents who both have either β-thalassemia or sickle cell trait, 25% will have β-thalassemia major or sickle cell anaemia.

6.50 Red cells (page 379):
  (a) have a nucleus
  (b) are able to synthesize proteins
  (c) have sodium and potassium pumps
  (d) have mitochondria
  (e) have ribosomes

6.51 In the red cell (Fig 6.22):
  (a) the Embden–Meyerhof pathway results in the production of ATP
  (b) the hexose monophosphate shunt maintains glutathione in a reduced state
  (c) 2,3-DPG is formed from the Rappaport–Luebering shunt of the glycolytic pathway
  (d) oxidation of the haemoglobin molecule, producing methaemoglobin and precipitation of globin chains, results in Heinz bodies
  (e) 2,3-DPG binds to the central part of the Hb tetramer, fixing it in the low-affinity state

6.52 The following statements are correct (page 381):
  (a) G6PD reduces glucose-6-phosphate to 5-phosphogluconate.
  (b) G6PD deficiency is rare in males.
  (c) Heterozygotes with G6PD deficiency have some protection against *Plasmodium falciparum.*

(d) In the Mediterranean type of G6PD deficiency the enzyme levels are low in both young and old red cells.

(e) Imbalanced lyonization can exaggerate the response to oxidant drugs if there is a large excess of G6PD-deficient cells in a heterozygote.

6.53 Drugs causing haemolysis in G6PD deficiency include (Table 6.13):
   (a) Acetylsalicylic acid
   (b) Chloroquine
   (c) Nitrofurantoin
   (d) Quinidine
   (e) Dapsone

6.54 Recognized features of G6PD deficiency include (page 381):
   (a) Favism
   (b) X-linked inheritance
   (c) Chronic haemolytic anaemia
   (d) Neonatal jaundice
   (e) Rapid extravascular jaundice

6.55 During an acute attack the blood film in G6PD deficiency may show (page 381):
   (a) Bite cells
   (b) Blister cells
   (c) Heinz bodies
   (d) Reticulocytosis
   (e) Howell–Jolly bodies

6.56 Immune destruction of red cells by autoantibodies occurs in (page 382):
   (a) Paroxysmal nocturnal haemoglobinuria
   (b) Prosthetic heart valves
   (c) Disseminated intravascular coagulation
   (d) Haemolytic disease of the newborn
   (e) Products of *Clostridium perfringens* infection

6.57 Features of warm autoimmune haemolytic anaemia include (Table 6.14):
   (a) Spherocytosis
   (b) IgM antibody
   (c) Thrombocytopenia
   (d) Corticosteroids should be avoided
   (e) Negative Coombs' test

6.58 Causes of warm autoimmune haemolytic anaemia include (Table 6.14):
   (a) Systemic lupus erythematosus
   (b) Lymphoid maligancy
   (c) Methyldopa
   (d) Rheumatoid arthritis
   (e) Carcinomas

6.59 Causes of cold autoimmune haemolytic anaemia include (Table 6.14):
(a) Infectious mononucleosis
(b) *Mycoplasma pneumoniae* infection
(c) Lymphomas
(d) Malaria
(e) Cytomegalovirus infection

6.60 Drugs causing haemolytic anaemia include (page 385):
(a) Quinine
(b) Penicillin
(c) Steroids
(d) Cyclophosphamide
(e) Methyldopa

6.61 Features of haemolytic disease of the newborn include (page 385):
(a) Hydrops fetalis
(b) Bile pigment stones
(c) Intrauterine death
(d) Kernicterus
(e) Cardiac failure

6.62 In haemolytic disease of the newborn a sample of cord blood shows (page 386):
(a) Polycythaemia
(b) Low reticulocyte count
(c) A negative direct antiglobulin test
(d) A raised bilirubin
(e) IgG antibodies

6.63 Management of haemolytic disease of the newborn includes (page 386):
(a) Intrauterine blood transfusion in severely affected fetuses before 33 weeks' gestation
(b) Phototherapy of the baby in mild cases
(c) Long-term anticoagulation
(d) In severe cases after 33 weeks' gestation labour should be induced
(e) Anti-D immunoglobulin to the fetus

6.64 Indications for exchange transfusion in haemolytic disease of the newborn include (page 386):
(a) A cord haemoglobin of >14 g dL^{-1}
(b) A cord bilirubin of >60 mmol L^{-1}
(c) A rapidly rising titre of IgG antibodies
(d) A rapidly rising bilirubin level
(e) A high reticulocyte count

6.65 Correct statements about the prevention of RhD immunization in the mother include (page 386):
(a) Anti-D is given just before delivery.

(b) Anti-D is given when the mother is RhD positive and the fetus is RhD negative.
(c) Anti-D is given only when mother's serum contains no detectable anti-D.
(d) Antenatal prophylaxis in susceptible women at 28 and 34 weeks' gestation has been shown to reduce the incidence of immunization.
(e) The Kleihauer test is used to assess the number of fetal cells in the maternal circulation.

6.66 Features of paroxysmal nocturnal haemoglobinuria include (page 386):
(a) Extravascular haemolysis
(b) Aplastic anaemia
(c) Defective production of glycosyl phosphatidylinositol
(d) Venous thrombotic episodes
(e) Red blood cells lyse more readily in acidified serum than do normal cells

6.67 Microangiopathic haemolytic anaemia occurs in (page 387):
(a) Eclampsia
(b) Malignant hypertension
(c) Thrombotic thrombocytopenic purpura
(d) Disseminated intravascular coagulation
(e) March haemoglobinuria

6.68 Correct statements about polycythaemia include (page 387):
(a) PCV is a more reliable indicator of polycythaemia than haemoglobin.
(b) In relative erythrocytosis there is an increase in plasma volume.
(c) Polycythaemia is defined as a decrease in haemoglobin, PCV and red cell count.
(d) Polycythaemia is a clonal stem cell disorder.
(e) Absolute erythrocytosis is due to primary polycythaemia or secondary polycythaemia.

6.69 Causes of polycythaemia include (Table 6.15):
(a) High altitude
(b) Left-to-right shunt in the heart
(c) Wilms' tumour
(d) Cerebellar haemangioblastoma
(e) Hepatocellular carcinoma

6.70 Clinical features of polycythaemia vera include (page 388):
(a) Hypertension
(b) Splenomegaly
(c) Severe itching after a bath
(d) Peptic ulceration
(e) Gout

6.71 Laboratory features of polycythaemia vera include (page 388):
(a) Decreased packed cell volume
(b) Elevated serum erythropoietin
(c) Aplasia of the bone marrow
(d) High leucocyte alkaline phosphatase score
(e) High vitamin B_{12}-binding proteins

6.72 Management of polycythaemia vera includes (page 388):
(a) Avoid venesection because it causes iron deficiency.
(b) Hydroxyurea is useful in treating associated thrombocytopenia.
(c) One dose of radioactive phosphorus may give control for up to 18 months.
(d) Cimetidine may be useful in relieving pruritus.
(e) Radioactive phosphorus therapy is confined to patients under the age of 70.

6.73 Myelodysplasia (page 390):
(a) is a group of acquired bone marrow disorders caused by a defect in stem cells
(b) mainly occurs in the young
(c) patients have hypercellular bone marrow despite pancytopenia
(d) transforms into acute myeloblastic anaemia in about 30% of cases
(e) is treated with bone marrow transplantation in patients over the age of 50 who have an HLA-identical sibling

6.74 Features of myelofibrosis include (page 389):
(a) Leucoerythroblastic anaemia
(b) Bone marrow shows markedly increased fibrosis
(c) The Philadelphia chromosome is present
(d) A low serum urate
(e) High white cell count

6.75 Common causes of death in myelofibrosis include (page 390):
(a) Leukaemic transformation
(b) Cardiovascular disease
(c) Infection
(d) Gastrointestinal bleeding
(e) Renal failure

6.76 Correct statements about the spleen include (page 390):
(a) The red pulp has a structure similar to lymphoid follicles.
(b) The leucocytes from the blood that enters the spleen preferentially pass to the red pulp.
(c) About one-quarter of the body's T lymphocytes are present in the spleen.
(d) The spleen shares the function of antibody production with other lymphoid tissues.
(e) Extramedullary haemopoiesis occurs in the spleen.

6.77 Features of hypersplenism include (page 391):
(a) Leucopenia
(b) Intravascular haemolysis
(c) Decreased plasma volume
(d) Aplasia of the bone marrow
(e) Thrombocytopenia

6.78 Common causes of massive splenomegaly include (page 391):
(a) Portal hypertension
(b) Kala-azar
(c) Myelofibrosis
(d) Acute malaria
(e) Gaucher's disease

6.79 Indications for splenectomy include (page 391):
(a) Sickle-cell disease
(b) Hodgkin's disease
(c) Autoimmune thrombocytopenic purpura
(d) Hypersplenism
(e) Coeliac disease

6.80 Haematological features of post-splenectomy include (page 391):
(a) Monocytosis
(b) Howell–Jolly bodies
(c) Pappenheimer bodies
(d) Target cells
(e) Thrombocytopenia

6.81 Correct statements about prophylaxis against infection after splenectomy include (page 391):
(a) Pneumococcal vaccination should be given 2–3 weeks before splenectomy.
(b) *Haemophilus influenzae* type B vaccine should be given, even in those who have previously been immunized.
(c) Meningococcal immunization is mandatory.
(d) Long-term prophylactic penicillin is recommended.
(e) Hepatitis A vaccination is recommended routinely.

6.82 Correct statements about blood transfusion include (page 393):
(a) A blood transfusion may immunize the recipient against donor antigens the recipient lacks.
(b) Repeated blood transfusions decrease the risk of the occurrence of alloimmunization.
(c) Transplacental passage of fetal blood cells during pregnancy may alloimmunize the mother against fetal antigens inherited from the father.

(d) The ABO blood group system involves naturally occurring IgG antibodies.

(e) The antibodies that develop in RhD-negative individuals after exposure to RhD-positive positive cells are IgM antibodies.

6.83 Immunological complications of blood transfusion include (Table 6.17):
(a) Haemolysis
(b) Iron overload
(c) Purpura
(d) Fever
(e) Urticaria

6.84 The following infections can be transmitted by blood transfusion (page 394):
(a) Hepatitis
(b) HIV
(c) CMV
(d) Malaria
(e) Toxoplasmosis

6.85 The following statements are correct (page 395):
(a) Whole blood has a shelf half-life of 5 weeks.
(b) Leucocyte-depleted red cell concentrates should be avoided in patients likely to receive repeated transfusions.
(c) Washed red cell concentrates should be avoided in patients with severe recurrent urticarial reactions.
(d) Fresh frozen plasma contains all the coagulation factors present in plasma.
(e) Albumin solutions should not be used to treat patients with malnutrition.

6.86 Causes of neutrophil leucocytosis include (Table 6.18 and Table 6.19):
(a) Corticosteroid therapy
(b) Myeloproliferative disorder
(c) Megaloblastic anaemia
(d) Felty's syndrome
(e) Typhoid

6.87 The following statements are correct (pages 396–398):
(a) A leukaemoid reaction is an overproduction of white cells with many immature cells.
(b) In leucoerythroblastic anaemia, nucleated red cells and white cell precursors are found in the peripheral blood.
(c) Eosinophils are smaller than neutrophils.
(d) Monocytes are smaller than neutrophils.
(e) The physiological role of the basophil is known.

6.88 Causes of eosinophilia include (Table 6.20):
  (a) *Ascaris* infestations
  (b) Hypoadrenalism
  (c) Bronchial asthma
  (d) Lymphoma
  (e) Sarcoidosis

6.89 Causes of lymphocytosis include (page 398):
  (a) Infectious mononucleosis
  (b) Tuberculosis
  (c) Syphilis
  (d) Lymphomas
  (e) HIV

6.90 Haemostasis depends on (page 398):
  (a) The vessel wall
  (b) Platelets
  (c) Coagulation factors
  (d) Neutrophils
  (e) Basophils

6.91 Correct statements about platelet adhesion include (page 398):
  (a) Platelets bind to collagen using glycoprotein Ib (GPIb).
  (b) Platelets bind to von Willebrand factor in plasma using glycoprotein Ia (GPIa).
  (c) Platelets bind to fibrinogen using the glycoprotein IIIb–IIIa (GPIIb–IIIa) receptor complex.
  (d) Following adhesion, platelets undergo a shape change from a disc to a sphere.
  (e) Following adhesion, platelets release the contents of their cytoplasmic granules.

6.92 Prostacyclin (PGI$_2$) (page 399):
  (a) is synthesized by the vascular endothelial cells
  (b) opposes the action of thromboxane A$_2$
  (c) lowers cyclic AMP levels
  (d) initiates platelet release reaction
  (e) prevents platelet aggregation

6.93 Correct statements about the formation of the haemostatic plug include (page 399):
  (a) Platelet adhesion is dependent on von Willebrand factor.
  (b) Tissue factor activates the extrinsic pathway.
  (c) Endothelial damage activates Factor XII.
  (d) The presence of thrombin encourages the fusion of platelets.
  (e) The release of ADP from platelets induces platelet aggregation.

6.94 Inhibitors of coagulation include (page 400):
  (a) Protein C
  (b) α_2-Macroglobulin
  (c) Antithrombin III
  (d) Protein S
  (e) α_1-Antitrypsin

6.95 The following statements about the fibrinolytic system are correct (page 401):
  (a) The fibrinolytic system is activated by the presence of fibrin.
  (b) The most important plasminogen activator is urokinase.
  (c) Plasmin breaks down fibrinogen and fibrin.
  (d) Degradation of fibrin yields D-dimer.
  (e) Fibrinolysis helps to restore vessel wall patency.

6.96 The following statements are correct (page 401):
  (a) The bleeding time is used to test the extrinsic pathway.
  (b) The prothrombin time is prolonged with abnormalities of the intrinsic pathway.
  (c) The partial thromboplastin time is prolonged with abnormalities of the extrinsic pathway.
  (d) The thrombin time is prolonged with fibrinogen deficiency.
  (e) Prolonged prothrombin time due to coagulation factor deficiency may be corrected by the addition of normal plasma to the patient's plasma.

6.97 The following statements about the extrinsic pathway are correct (page 401):
  (a) Activated Factor X inhibits the conversion of prothrombin to thrombin.
  (b) Thrombin hydrolyses the peptide bonds of fibrinogen, releasing fibrinopeptides A and B.
  (c) Factor XIII stabilizes the fibrin clot by cross-linking adjacent fibrin molecules.
  (d) The extrinsic pathway in vivo begins with the activation of Factor IX by Factor VIIa.
  (e) Factor XI only makes an important contribution after major trauma.

6.98 The following statements about bleeding disorders are correct (page 401):
  (a) The prothrombin time is measured by adding tissue thromboplastin in the form of animal brain extract and calcium to the patient's plasma.
  (b) In vascular/platelet disorders the bleeding is mainly from the skin.
  (c) Coagulation disorders are typically associated with haemarthroses.
  (d) Bleeding time measures platelet plug formation in vivo.
  (e) The partial thromboplastin time is prolonged with Factor VII deficiency.

6.99 Vascular disorders include (Table 6.21):
  (a) Osler–Weber–Rendu disease
  (b) Marfan's syndrome

(c) Henoch–Schönlein purpura
(d) Senile purpura
(e) Scurvy

6.100 Causes of thrombocytopenia include (Table 6.22):
(a) Leukaemia
(b) Co-trimoxazole
(c) Disseminated intravascular coagulation
(d) Haemolytic uraemic syndrome
(e) Myeloma

6.101 Chronic autoimmune thrombocytopenia is seen in (page 403):
(a) SLE
(b) Thyroid disease
(c) Evans' syndrome
(d) Chronic lymphatic leukaemia
(e) HIV

6.102 Features of chronic idiopathic thrombocytopenic purpura include (page 403):
(a) It is characteristically seen in adult women.
(b) Major haemorrhage is common.
(c) Splenomegaly is common.
(d) Spontaneous remissions are common.
(e) There are normal or increased numbers of megakaryocytes in the bone marrow.

6.103 Acquired forms of platelet dysfunction include (page 404):
(a) Myeloproliferative disorders
(b) Uraemia
(c) Liver disorders
(d) Paraproteinemia
(e) Drug-induced

6.104 The following associations are correct (page 404):
(a) Glanzmann's thrombasthenia – lack of platelet granules causing poor platelet aggregation.
(b) Storage pool disease – lack of platelet membrane glycoprotein IIb/IIIa complex.
(c) Glanzmann's thrombasthenia – defective fibrinogen binding.
(d) Bernard – Soulier syndrome – lack of platelet membrane glycoprotein IIb/IIIa.
(e) Bernard–Soulier syndrome – defective binding site for factor vWF.

6.105 The following statements about the inheritance of haemophilia A are correct (page 404):
  (a) If a female carrier has a son, he has a 50% chance of having haemophilia.
  (b) If a female carrier has a daughter, she has a 50% chance of being a carrier.
  (c) All daughters of haemophiliacs are carriers.
  (d) All sons of haemophiliacs are normal.
  (e) In approximately 50% of families with severe disease the defect is an inversion of the chromosome.

6.106 Features of haemophilia A include (page 404):
  (a) About one-third of cases are sporadic.
  (b) Haemarthroses are common.
  (c) The level of factor vWF is reduced.
  (d) Bleeding time is prolonged.
  (e) Bleeding is treated by administering factor oral Factor VIII concentrates.

6.107 The following statements about the management of haemophilia are correct (page 405):
  (a) The majority of severely affected patients are now given Factor VIII concentrate prophylaxis three times per week from early childhood in an attempt to prevent joint damage.
  (b) DDAVP causes a decrease in Factor VIII:c levels.
  (c) About 50% of haemophiliacs have antibodies to Factor VIII:C.
  (d) Factor VIII has a half-life of 36–48 hours.
  (e) Factor VIII concentrate is administered subcutaneously.

6.108 Features of von Willebrand disease include (page 406):
  (a) Haemarthroses are common.
  (b) There is defective platelet aggregation with ristocetin.
  (c) It is inherited as an autosomal dominant condition.
  (d) It is caused by a deficiency of Factor IX.
  (e) Bleeding time is normal.

6.109 The following associations between defective haemostasis and liver pathology are correct (page 407):
  (a) Vitamin K deficiency – cholestasis
  (b) Reduced synthesis of coagulation factors – hepatocellular damage
  (c) Thrombocytopenia – hypersplenism
  (d) Functional abnormalities of platelets – liver failure
  (e) Disseminated intravascular coagulation – acute liver failure

6.110 Causes of disseminated intravascular coagulation include (page 407):
  (a) Septicaemia
  (b) Disseminated malignant disease

    (c) Haemolytic transfusion reactions
    (d) Amniotic fluid embolism
    (e) *Falciparum* malaria

6.111 In severe disseminated intravascular coagulation (page 407):
    (a) prothrombin time is prolonged
    (b) thrombin time is prolonged
    (c) FDP level is depressed
    (d) plasma thromboplastin time with kaolin is prolonged
    (e) fibrinogen level is markedly raised

6.112 Lupus anticoagulants (page 408):
    (a) are associated with recurrent miscarriages
    (b) are directed against phospholipids
    (c) are seen in the majority of patients with systemic lupus erythematosus
    (d) lead to prolongation of partial thromboplastin time with kaolin
    (e) inhibit coagulation factor activity

6.113 The following statements are correct (page 409):
    (a) The risk of venous thrombosis is decreased in women with Factor V Leiden who are pregnant.
    (b) Antithrombin deficiency can be inherited as a X-linked recessive disorder.
    (c) Patients with antithrombin deficiency are markedly sensitive to heparin therapy.
    (d) Protein S deficiency results in venous thrombosis before the age of 40 years.
    (e) Low molecular weight heparin is equally effective and safe as unfractionated heparin in the immediate treatment of pulmonary embolism.

6.114 Risk factors for venous thrombosis include (Table 6.24):
    (a) Immobility
    (b) Malignancy
    (c) Oestrogen therapy
    (d) Antithrombin III deficiency
    (e) Protein C deficiency

6.115 The following associations are correct (page 410):
    (a) Abciximab – stimulates platelet IIb/IIIa receptors
    (b) Hirudin – inactivates thrombin bound to fibrin more efficiently than AT-III potentiated by heparin
    (c) Clopidogrel – inhibits platelet aggregation
    (d) Streptokinase – conformational change in circulating plasminogen
    (e) t-Pa – greater affinity for fibrin-bound plasminogen than circulating plasminogen

6.116 Prophylactic methods to prevent venous thrombosis include (page 411):
- (a) Elevation of legs
- (b) Compression stockings
- (c) Calf muscle stimulation
- (d) Passive calf muscle exercise during surgery
- (e) Low-dose heparin

6.117 Heparin (page 411):
- (a) is a mixture of polysaccharides
- (b) dosage is controlled by INR
- (c) potentiates the formation of complexes between antithrombin-III and serine proteases
- (d) induced bleeding may be neutralized with protamine
- (e) may cause osteoporosis

6.118 Low molecular weight heparins (page 411):
- (a) inhibit Factor Xa activity
- (b) can be given as a once-daily subcutaneous injection
- (c) produce little effect on tests over overall coagulation at standard doses for prophylaxis
- (d) are not fully neutralized by protamine
- (e) cause more inhibition of platelet function than unfractionated heparins

6.119 Oral anticoagulant (page 412):
- (a) dosage is controlled by partial thromboplastin time
- (b) acts by interfering with vitamin K metabolism
- (c) is a must before thrombolytic therapy
- (d) is contraindicated in venous thrombosis
- (e) induced bleeding is treated with fresh frozen plasma

6.120 Conditions requiring oral anticoagulants include (page 412):
- (a) Non-embolic strokes
- (b) Recurrent deep vein thrombosis
- (c) Pulmonary embolism
- (d) Cardiac prosthetic valves
- (e) Pregnancy

6.121 Relative contraindications to the use of oral anticoagulants include (page 412):
- (a) Severe hypertension
- (b) Arterial grafts
- (c) Peptic ulceration
- (d) Transient ischaemic attacks
- (e) Severe liver disease

6.122 Anticoagulant effects may be increased by (page 413):
  (a) Cimetidine
  (b) Rifampicin
  (c) Amiodarone
  (d) Barbiturates
  (e) Tricyclic antidepressants

6.123 A 28-year-old female patient has a platelet count of $60 \times 10^9/l$. The following statements are correct:
  (a) Intramuscular injections should be avoided.
  (b) Normal or increased megakaryocytes in the bone marrow aspirate suggest increased platelet destruction.
  (c) Dental foils can safely be used.
  (d) Prothrombin time is prolonged.
  (e) The blood picture occurs in about 10% of pregnancies.

6.124 A 35-year-old woman was diagnosed as having idiopathic thrombocytopenic purpura. The following statements are correct:
  (a) Major haemorrhage is rare.
  (b) The only blood count abnormality is thrombocytopenia.
  (c) Megakaryocytes are decreased in the bone marrow.
  (d) The detection of platelet autoantibodies is essential for confirmation of the diagnosis.
  (e) Transfused platelets survive twice as long as the patient's own platelets.

6.125 A 23-year-old male is diagnosed as having Factor VIII deficiency. The following statements are correct:
  (a) About one-third of cases are sporadic and have no family history of haemophilia.
  (b) The bleeding time is normal.
  (c) The prothrombin time is normal.
  (d) Recombinant Factor VIII concentrate is no longer used in the treatment.
  (e) Synthetic intranasal vasopressin produces a rise in Factor VIII:C proportional to the initial level of Factor VIII.

6.126 A young man with haemophilia A gives his family history. The following in his family could have the same inherited defect:
  (a) Son
  (b) Brother
  (c) Maternal uncle
  (d) Maternal grandfather
  (e) Maternal great grandfather

Medical Oncology

7.1 Environmental factors associated with the causation of cancer include (page 416):
(a) Tobacco
(b) Alcohol
(c) Diet
(d) Ultraviolet light
(e) Ionizing radiation

7.2 The following cancers have a low incidence in Asian countries compared to Europe and North America (page 417):
(a) Liver
(b) Lung
(c) Breast
(d) Colon
(e) Prostate

7.3 The frequency of the following cancers rises with increasing age (page 417):
(a) Hodgkin's disease
(b) Acute lymphoblastic leukaemia
(c) Lung
(d) Breast
(e) Colon

7.4 Smoking is associated with cancer of the (Table 7.2):
(a) Pharynx
(b) Oesophagus
(c) Bladder
(d) Pancreas
(e) Cervix

7.5 The risk of lung cancer is influenced by exposure to (page 416):
(a) Radon
(b) Mineral water
(c) Uranium
(d) Nickel
(e) Dietary fat intake

7.6 Dietary fat intake correlates with the incidence of cancer of the (page 416):
(a) Breast
(b) Colon
(c) Prostate
(d) Endometrium
(e) Pancreas

7.7 Ultraviolet light is known to increase the risk of (page 416):
(a) Liver cancer
(b) Basal cell carcinoma of the skin
(c) Squamous cell carcinoma of the skin
(d) Cutaneous melanomas
(e) Colonic cancer

7.8 Alcohol is known to increase the risk of cancer of the (Table 7.2):
(a) Mouth
(b) Pharynx
(c) Oesophagus
(d) Larynx
(e) Skin

7.9 The following associations are correct (Table 7.2):
(a) Asbestos – lung cancer
(b) Vinyl chloride – angiosarcoma of the liver
(c) Aromatic amines – bladder cancer
(d) Aflatoxin – liver cancer
(e) Oestrogens – endometrial carcinoma

7.10 The associations between the following cancers and infective agents are correct (page 416):
(a) T-cell leukaemia – retrovirus HTLV1
(b) Liver cancer – hepatitis B virus infection
(c) Stomach cancer – *Helicobacter pylori*
(d) Burkitt's lymphoma – Epstein–Barr virus
(e) Kaposi's sarcoma – HIV infection

7.11 Evidence for the genetic origin of cancer is based on the following (page 417):
(a) Most known carcinogens induce mutations.
(b) Many types of cancer are associated with chromosomal instability.
(c) Malignant tumours are clonal.
(d) Some tumours contain mutated oncogenes.
(e) Some cancers are inherited.

7.12 Autosomal recessive diseases that predispose to the development of cancer include (page 417):
(a) Marfan's syndrome
(b) Xeroderma pigmentosum
(c) Ataxia telangiectasia
(d) Bloom's syndrome
(e) Fanconi's anaemia

7.13 Inherited cancers that exhibit dominant inheritance include (page 418):
   (a) Retinoblastoma
   (b) Familial adenomatous polyposis
   (c) Wilms' tumour
   (d) Neuroblastoma
   (e) Neurofibromatosis

7.14 The following statements about the biology of the cancer are correct (page 418):
   (a) The activity of telomerase is essential to maintain the neoplastic state in cancer cells.
   (b) Angiostatin, an inhibitor of plasminogen, is used to inhibit cancer growth.
   (c) Loss of E-cadherin expression is associated with an increase in tumour invasion.
   (d) The attachment of tumour cells to the endothelial cells is partly through adhesion cells.
   (e) Certain tumours demonstrate upregulation of integrin receptors during tumour expression.

7.15 Recognized features of malignant lesions include (page 419):
   (a) Pleomorphism of cells
   (b) Increased numbers of mitoses
   (c) Nuclear aberration
   (d) Evidence of invasion into surrounding tissues
   (e) Increased production of angiostatin

7.16 Tumour markers include (page 420):
   (a) Creatinine kinase
   (b) Carcinoembryonic antigen
   (c) α-Fetoprotein
   (d) β-Human chorionic gonadotrophin
   (e) Prostate-specific antigen

7.17 Correct statements about the principles of chemotherapy include (page 421):
   (a) Drugs are not given intermittently because of their toxicity.
   (b) Tumours rapidly develop resistance to single agents given on their own.
   (c) With a chemosensitive tumour a relatively small increase in the dose may have a large effect on tumour cell kill.
   (d) Where cure is a realistic option the dose administered may be critical and may need to be maintained despite toxicity.
   (e) In situations where cure is not a realistic possibility and palliation is the aim, dose is less critical, particularly as quality of life becomes paramount.

7.18 Correct statements about the mechanism of action of cytotoxic drugs include (page 421):
(a) Alkylating agents cause the cross-linking of DNA strands.
(b) Antimetabolites interfere with normal synthesis of nucleic acids.
(c) Anti-tumour antibiotics acts by intercalating nucleotide pairs on the same strand of DNA.
(d) Vinca alkaloids promote microtubule formation.
(e) Epipodophyllotoxins produce DNA strand breaks.

7.19 The following associations regarding the side effects of cytotoxic drugs include (pages 423–424):
(a) Vomiting – cis-platinum
(b) Cardiac toxicity – doxorubicin
(c) Polyneuropathy – vinca alkaloids
(d) Cardiac toxicity – vinca alkaloids
(e) Hameorrhagic cystitis – cyclophosphamide

7.20 Recognized complications of chemotherapy include (page 423):
(a) Alopecia
(b) Bone marrow suppression
(c) Secondary malignancies
(d) Sterility
(e) Nephrotoxicity

7.21 Tumours with low levels of drug resistance include (page 423):
(a) Melanoma
(b) Testicular teratomas
(c) Hodgkin's disease
(d) Childhood acute leukaemia
(e) Squamous cell carcinomas

7.22 Correct statements about drug resistance with chemotherapy include (page 423):
(a) Drug resistance is one of the major obstacles of effecting cure with chemotherapy.
(b) One important mechanism for multidrug resistance concerns altered drugs binding to the enzyme topoisomerase II.
(c) Resistance to anthracycline drugs is mediated via decreased expression of P-glycoprotein, which mediates an efflux of cytotoxic drugs out of the cells.
(d) Anticancer drugs can themselves increase the rate of mutation.
(e) Resistance to anthracyclines is often associated with resistance to vinca alkaloids and epipodophyllotoxins.

7.23 Adjuvant chemotherapy has been shown to be of value in (page 424):
(a) Childhood renal sarcoma
(b) Wilms' tumour

(c) Breast cancer
(d) Colon cancer
(e) Mycetoma

7.24 Correct statements about endocrine therapy in cancer include (page 424):
(a) Oestrogens suppress the growth of breast cancer.
(b) Androgens suppress the growth of prostate cancer.
(c) Endometrial tumours frequently respond to progesterone.
(d) Hormonal therapy in general is curative.
(e) Aromatase inhibitors lack antitumour activity.

7.25 Recognized clinical features of acute leukaemias include (page 427):
(a) Hepatosplenomegaly
(b) Repeated sore throats
(c) Bruising
(d) Bleeding
(e) Lymph node enlargement

7.26 Correct statements about the 'tumour lysis' syndrome include (page 427):
(a) It tends to develop in leukaemias where the rate of cell division is very slow.
(b) It develops as a consequence of chemotherapy.
(c) It is characterized by hypercalcaemia.
(d) It is potentially life-threatening.
(e) It can usually be prevented by making sure that chemotherapy is given while the uric acid level is high.

7.27 Correct statements about acute leukaemias include (pages 427–430):
(a) Acute myelogenous leukaemia is an incurable disease.
(b) Acute promyelocytic leukaemia is associated with disseminated intravascular coagulation.
(c) All-trans-retinoic acid is useful in inducing remission in acute myelogenous leukaemia, except acute promyelocytic leukaemia.
(d) Acute lymphoblastic leukaemia is predominantly a disease of the elderly.
(e) Acute monoblastic leukaemia is characterized by gum infiltration.

7.28 Correct statements about chronic leukaemias include (pages 430–432):
(a) The majority of patients with chronic myeloid leukaemia live over a decade following diagnosis.
(b) Philadelphia chromosome is present in most patients with chronic myeloid leukaemia.
(c) Chronic lymphocytic leukaemia is a disease of older people.
(d) Infection is the predominant cause of death in chronic lymphocytic leukaemia.
(e) In hairy cell leukaemia the cells on a blood film have an irregular outline due to the presence of filament-like cytoplasmic projections.

7.29 The 'B' symptoms in the staging of Hodgkin's disease include (Table 7.13):
    (a) Pruritus
    (b) Alcohol-induced pain
    (c) Fever
    (d) Weight loss
    (e) Night sweats

7.30 Correct statements about the management of Hodgkin's disease include (page 432):
    (a) The long-term outcome is closely related to the stage.
    (b) Treatment is virtually always given with curative intent.
    (c) The majority of patients in stages IA and IIA are treated with chemotherapy.
    (d) Treatment is almost always given with curative intent.
    (e) Patients who develop recurrent Hodgkin's disease more than once will almost certainly die of Hodgkin's disease eventually.

7.31 Correct statements about non-Hodgkin's lymphoma include (pages 434–436):
    (a) The term non-Hodgkin's lymphoma encompasses many different histological subtypes.
    (b) High-grade lymphomas are incurable.
    (c) A high serum lactate dehydrogenase in high-grade lymphoma correlates with a good prognosis.
    (d) Recurrent high-grade lymphoma has a grave prognosis.
    (e) A lesion in the jaw is a recognized feature of Burkitt's lymphoma.

7.32 Indications for the use of myeloablative therapy with allogenic bone marrow transplantation include (pages 436–437):
    (a) Thalassaemia
    (b) Aplastic anaemia
    (c) Chronic myeloid leukaemia in the blast phase
    (d) Acute myeloid leukaemia in second chronic remission
    (e) Acute lymphoblastic leukaemia in second chronic remission

7.33 Indications for the use of myeloablative therapy with autologous bone marrow transplantation include (page 436, Table 7.17):
    (a) Acute myeloid leukaemia in first complete remission
    (b) Adult acute lymphoblastic leukaemia in first chronic remission
    (c) High-grade non-Hodgkin's lymphoma in second remission
    (d) Acute myeloid leukaemia in second chronic remission
    (e) High-grade non-Hodgkin's lymphoma in first remission in patients at high risk of recurrence

7.34 Recognized features of multiple myeloma include (page 437):
    (a) The presence of paraprotein in the serum
    (b) Bone marrow destruction

(c) Bone marrow infiltration
(d) Renal impairment
(e) Hypercalcaemia

7.35 Recognized features of Waldenstrom's macroglobulinaemia include
(page 439):
(a) Lymph node enlargement
(b) A bleeding tendency
(c) Visual disturbance
(d) Bone marrow infiltration
(e) Rouleau formation in the blood film

7.36 Correct statements about the management of solid tumours include
(page 439):
(a) It involves the combined use of surgery, radiotherapy and
chemotherapy.
(b) Metastatic testicular cancers can be cured by chemotherapy.
(c) In early laryngeal cancer radiotherapy can be used on its own with
curative intent.
(d) In the earlier stages surgery alone may be curative in many solid
tumours.
(e) Radiotherapy is a local treatment which can often be used after surgery
to reduce the chance of local recurrence.

7.37 Correct statements about breast cancer include (page 439):
(a) It is the commonest cancer in women.
(b) Despite surgical removal of the primary tumour most women will
eventually relapse with metastatic disease.
(c) Adjuvant chemotherapy reduces the death rate in postmenopausal
patients.
(d) Tamoxifen reduces the death rate in premenopausal node-positive
women.
(e) Patients with established metastatic disease are treated with hormonal
therapy or chemotherapy.

7.38 Breast cancers most likely to respond to hormonal treatment include
(page 440):
(a) Where there is an absence of oestrogen receptors
(b) Where there is a long interval from initial surgery to time of relapse
(c) Metastatic disease in bone and soft tissue
(d) Liver metastases
(e) Lymphangitis carcinomatosa

7.39 Hormonal manipulation for breast cancers in postmenopausal women
includes (pages 439–440):
(a) Oophorectomy
(b) Radiation-induced ablation

(c) LHRH analogue with downregulation of the pituitary
(d) Tamoxifen
(e) Progesterone

7.40 Correct statements about lung cancer include (page 440):
(a) It is the commonest cancer in females.
(b) Chemotherapy is the treatment of choice in non-small cell lung cancer.
(c) In non-small cell lung cancer surgery should be considered in all cases.
(d) Radiotherapy is curative in small cell lung cancer.
(e) In small cell lung cancer the disease is almost always disseminated by the time of diagnosis.

7.41 Correct statements about gastrointestinal cancer include (page 441):
(a) In early squamous cell carcinoma of the oesophagus radiotherapy is given as primary treatement.
(b) Adjuvant therapy is useful in gastric cancer.
(c) In Duke B and C colon cancer adjuvant chemotherapy following surgery is useful.
(d) Chemotherapy is based on 5-fluorouracil and cisplatinum in advanced gastric cancers.
(e) Chemotherapy is based on 5-fluorouracil and folinic acid in advanced colonic cancers.

7.42 Correct statements about ovarian cancers include (page 441):
(a) Surgery plays a major role in the treatment of ovarian cancer in all stages.
(b) Surgery can be curative when confined to the ovaries.
(c) In patients with advanced disease surgery has no role.
(d) The response to chemotherapy is enhanced if the tumour is debulked.
(e) Cisplatinum is used in treatment.

7.43 Correct statements about testicular cancers include (page 441):
(a) It is the commonest cancer in men over the age of 50.
(b) Seminomas are resistant to radiotherapy.
(c) Teratomas are slow-growing tumours.
(d) Teratomas often present with para-aortic and pulmonary metastases.
(e) The great majority of patients with teratomas can be cured with chemotherapy.

7.44 Correct statements about the management of cancers of an unknown primary site include (page 441):
(a) Breast cancers should be considered in women with axillary lymphadenopathy.
(b) In men prostatic cancers should always be considered.
(c) A subset of poorly differentiated carcinomas may be extremely responsive to chemotherapy.

(d) The most important primaries to exclude are those that respond well to treatment.

(e) Primary thyroid cancers have to be excluded in both men and women.

7.45 Correct statements about palliative medicine and symptom control include (page 442):

(a) Opioid drugs should be avoided in the management of cancer pain as they are addictive.

(b) Morphine will reduce the sensation of breathlessness in a proportion of patients.

(c) In constant burning dysaesthesias tricyclic antidepressants are helpful.

(d) Anticonvulsant drugs are useful in the management of lancinating neuropathic pain.

(e) Nausea and vomiting occur in up to two-thirds of cancer patients in the last 2 months of life.

7.46 A 38-year-old woman has breast cancer. The following statements are correct (page 440):

(a) Genetic factors account for about 5% or more of women with cancer breast.

(b) The gene *BRCA*-1 is inherited in an autosomal dominant fashion.

(c) The gene *BRCA*-2 is linked to breast cancer.

(d) The gene *BRCA*-1 is linked to ovarian cancer.

(e) The *BRCA*-2 gene is linked to male breast cancer.

7.47 A 62-year-old naval shipyard worker has a mass in the right middle lobe of the lung. Histology confirms adenocarcinoma. The following statements are correct (pages 440, 820):

(a) Smoking is not a risk factor.

(b) Adrenal metastases do not occur with adenocarcinoma.

(c) Bronchoalveolar carcinoma is a type of adenocarcinoma.

(d) Cisplatin is not used for chemotherapy because it is nephrotoxic.

(e) Surgical resection can be undertaken even when mediastinal lymph nodes are affected.

7.48 A 55-year-old man is diagnosed as having acute myelogenous leukaemia of the promyelocytic type. The following statements are correct (page 427):

(a) DIC often manifests after initiation of treatment.

(b) Chemotherapy is the only possible chance for a cure.

(c) Allopurinol is useful in reducing the severity of tumour lysis syndrome.

(d) Alkalization of urine with intravenous bicarbonate will decrease the precipitation of uric acid.

(e) He has the M3 subtype of the FAB (French–American–British) classification of acute leukaemia.

7.49 The pathology of a 62-year-old woman's surgical specimen shows a Duke stage C carcinoma of the transverse colon. The following statements are correct (page 441):
- (a) Patients treated with 5-fluorouracil and levamisole have a one-third reduction in death rate compared to those treated with no adjuvant chemotherapy.
- (b) Radiation therapy will improve survival benefit in these patients.
- (c) Radiation therapy may decrease local recurrence.
- (d) The mortality if untreated is 10%
- (e) Radiation therapy is contraindicated in those in whom systemic chemotherapy is contemplated.

7.50 A 52-year-old woman has ovarian cancer. The following statements are correct (page 441):
- (a) The risk of ovarian cancer is reduced in women who have had breast cancer.
- (b) The CA-125 test is elevated in only 50% of patients with detectable ovarian cancer.
- (c) The failure of CA-125 levels to return to normal by the fourth treatment is a bad prognostic sign.
- (d) Patients with residual disease after initial surgery have reduced survival.
- (e) It is reasonable to perform a second-look surgery in various clinical trials testing newer chemotherapeutic agents.

7.51 A 35-year-old man presents with rectal bleeding. Colonoscopy reveals several polyps throughout the colon and biopsy confirms a villous adenoma. The following statements are correct (page 441):
- (a) It can be inherited in an autosomal dominant manner.
- (b) It is recommended that all first-degree relatives have frequent proctosigmoidoscopy.
- (c) Associated gastric polyps tend to be more malignant than the colonic polyps.
- (d) The gene for this condition is the *APC* gene.
- (e) The presence of osteomas and desmoid tumours indicates that the patient has Gardner's syndrome.

7.52 The pathology of a 61-year-old man's nephrectomy shows renal cell carcinoma extending through Gerota's fascia. The following statements are correct:
- (a) The classic triad of pain, haematuria and abdominal mass occurs in over two-thirds of patients.
- (b) Metastases usually occur in the bone, lung and brain.
- (c) Adjuvant radiotherapy after surgery reduces mortality considerably.
- (d) Nephrectomy is useful even when the tumour has metasized because it reduces symptoms such as pain and haemorrhage.
- (e) Renal cell carcinoma is resistant to chemotherapy.

7.53 The histopathology of transrectal biopsy in a 65-year-old man with an elevated prostate-specific antigen (PSA) reveals an adenocarcinoma. The following statements are correct:
(a) PSA is more a sensitive test than serum acid phosphatase.
(b) PSA increases with age.
(c) In patients who undergo prostatectomy, the presence of detectable PSA 6–8 weeks after surgery indicates persistent disease.
(d) A PSA level that does not fall after radiation therapy predicts persistent disease.
(e) PSA is a more specific test than serum acid phosphatase.

7.54 A 29-year-old man has a single palpable lymph node in the right supraclavicular region. Histology of the biopsy sample shows a nodular sclerosing type of Hodgkin's disease. The following statements are correct (page 432):
(a) The Reed–Sternberg cell is pathgnomonic of Hodgkin's disease.
(b) The nodular sclerosing type has the best prognosis.
(c) The patient has stage I disease.
(d) The presence of night sweats, fever and weight loss indicates a worse prognosis.
(e) Patients with stage IB can be treated with radiation therapy alone.

Rheumatology and Bone Disease

8.1 The following statements about joint diseases are correct (pages 447–501):
- (a) Osteoarthritis commonly presents in the third decade.
- (b) Rheumatoid arthritis is commoner in men.
- (c) Reiter's syndrome is commoner in women.
- (d) Sickle cell arthropathy is common in Africans.
- (e) Occupation can be an important factor in soft-tissue rheumatism.

8.2 The following associations regarding joint pains are correct (page 448):
- (a) Long history – rheumatoid arthritis
- (b) Short history – gout
- (c) Sore throat – rheumatic fever
- (d) Diuretic therapy – gout
- (e) Sudden onset – gout

8.3 Correct statements about joint symptoms include (pages 448–450):
- (a) Morning stiffness is characteristic of inflammatory arthropathies.
- (b) Joint swelling always indicates local disease.
- (c) Recurrent attacks in the big toe are suggestive of gout.
- (d) Clicking and creaking of joints indicate an abnormal joint.
- (e) Spinal stiffness which is worse in the morning in a 20-year-old suggests ankylosing spondylitis.

8.4 Joint conditions that run in families include (page 449):
- (a) Osteoarthritis
- (b) Ankylosing spondylitis
- (c) Gout
- (d) Caisson disease
- (e) Septic arthritis

8.5 Correct statements about the investigation of joint diseases include (page 451):
- (a) ESR is characteristically raised in osteoarthritis.
- (b) Proteinase 3 (PR3-ANCA) is present in up to 90% of serum from patients with Wegener's granulomatosis.
- (c) Rheumatoid factors are IgA autoantibodies.
- (d) Antibodies against double-stranded DNA are seldom found in systemic lupus erythematosus.
- (e) Antibodies against soluble nuclear antigen are characteristic of mixed connective-tissue disease.

8.6 The following statements are correct (Information Box 8.2, pages 450–453):
- (a) A raised serum uric acid is diagnostic of gout.

(b) Polarized light microscopy reveals the presence of negatively birefringent crystals in gout.

(c) In pyrophosphate arthropathy, crystals of calcium pyrophosphate are weakly positively birefringent.

(d) HLA-B27 is found in most patients with ankylosing spondylitis.

(e) A high serum complement is characteristic of the active phase of SLE.

8.7 The following associations are correct (page 452):

(a) Anti-Ro (SS-A) – SLE + Sjögren's syndrome

(b) Anti-La (SS-B) – Sjögren's syndrome

(c) Anti-Sm – SLE

(d) Anti-U1-RNP – SLE

(e) Anti Jo-1 antibodies – polymyositis

8.8 Correct statements about the epidemiology of osteoarthritis include (page 466):

(a) It is the commonest type of arthritis.

(b) The pattern of development of joint disease is additive.

(c) Involvement of the hips and the knees is the commonest cause of disability in an elderly population.

(d) It is twice as common in men over the age of 55.

(e) Osteoarthritic hand involvement is commoner in black populations than in Caucasians.

8.9 Causes of secondary osteoarthritis include (Table 8.11):

(a) Perthes' disease

(b) Obesity

(c) Corticosteroid therapy

(d) Septic arthritis

(e) Haemochromatosis

8.10 Correct statements about the aetiology of osteoarthritis include (page 466):

(a) It is a result of active, sometimes inflammatory but potentially reparative, processes.

(b) It is the inevitable result of trauma and ageing.

(c) There is a breakdown of the collagen matrix in cartilage.

(d) Abnormal sclerotic bone is produced in an attempt to repair microfractures.

(e) It is associated with polymorphisms of the gene for human aggrecan.

8.11 Correct statements about the pathogenesis of osteoarthritis include (page 467):

(a) Matrix loss is caused by the action of metalloproteinases such as stromelysin, collagenase and gelatinase, which degrade collagen and proteoglycans.

(b) Synovial inflammation produce cytokines, which stimulate metalloproteinase production.

(c) Growth factors stimulate the repair of collagen.
(d) High intakes of vitamin C and antioxidants reduce the risk of osteoarthritis.
(e) In women, weight-bearing sports produce a two- to three-fold increase in the risk of osteoarthritis of the hip and knee.

8.12 Recognized clinical features of osteoarthritis include (page 468):
(a) Swan-neck deformity of the fingers
(b) Heberden's nodes
(c) Joint deformities
(d) Bouchard's nodes
(e) Rheumatoid nodules

8.13 Diagnostic markers for osteoarthritis include (page 469):
(a) Raised ESR
(b) Raised rheumatoid factor
(c) Antinuclear antibodies
(d) Crystals in synovial fluid
(e) Elevated C-reactive protein

8.14 Correct statements about the management of osteoarthritis include (page 469):
(a) Obese patients should be encouraged to lose weight.
(b) Penicillamine is effective.
(c) The application of heat to an affected joint may provide pain relief.
(d) A total hip replacement provides almost complete pain relief.
(e) The first metatarsophalangeal joint can also be replaced.

8.15 Correct statements about the epidemiology of rheumatoid arthritis include (page 470):
(a) It is uncommon in tropical countries compared to Britain.
(b) It is more common in men than in women.
(c) There is an increased incidence in those with a family history.
(d) It most often starts in the seventh decade.
(e) HLA-DR 4 is a common association.

8.16 Immunological disturbances seen in rheumatoid arthritis include (page 471):
(a) T-cell activation
(b) Immune complexes in synovial fluid
(c) Locally synthesized immunoglobulins in synovial fluid
(d) Impaired cell-mediated immunity
(e) Association with other organ-specific antibodies

8.17 Rheumatoid nodules occur in (page 471):
(a) Subcutaneous tissue
(b) Pleura

(c) Pericardium
(d) Lung
(e) Epidermis

8.18 Correct statements about rheumatoid arthritis include (page 472):
(a) The hip joint is usually affected at the onset of the disease.
(b) The distal interphalangeal joints are involved in most cases.
(c) The dorsal and lumbar spines are involved.
(d) Baker's cyst is a collection of fluid in the cubital fossa.
(e) Palindromic rheumatism describes widespread polyarticular involvement.

8.19 Non-articular features of rheumatoid arthritis include (page 475):
(a) Primary Sjögren's syndrome
(b) Amyloidosis
(c) Atlantoaxial subluxation
(d) Caplan's syndrome
(e) Felty's syndrome

8.20 Correct statements about the prognosis and management of rheumatoid arthritis include (page 476):
(a) It is not entirely consistent with a full, normal and busy life.
(b) Physical activity increases the rate of deterioration of the joints.
(c) Restriction of movement is particularly likely to occur in the shoulders.
(d) Flexion deformities are likely to occur in the knees.
(e) NSAIDs are more effective than simple analgesics in the relief of symptoms.

8.21 Indications for disease-modifying antirheumatic drug therapy in RA include (page 476):
(a) Progressive disease
(b) Troublesome extra-articular problems
(c) Failure of NSAIDs to control symptoms
(d) Excessive corticosteroid requirements
(e) In seropositive patients with a poor prognosis they should be used early, before the appearance of erosions on X-rays of the hands and feet.

8.22 Correct statements about disease-modifying antirheumatic drug therapy in RA include (page 476):
(a) These drugs act almost immediately.
(b) Improvement of joint symptoms is accompanied by a fall in ESR.
(c) Complete remission can be achieved.
(d) They mainly act through cytokine inhibition.
(e) Penicillamine is often the first choice for younger patients.

8.23 Spondyloarthropathies include (page 479):
(a) Rheumatoid arthritis

(b) Systemic lupus erythematosus
(c) Systemic sclerosis
(d) Reiter's disease
(e) Still's disease

8.24 Clinical features of ankylosing spondylitis include (page 479):
(a) The onset is typically in the sixth decade
(b) Low back pain
(c) Plantar fasciitis
(d) Loss of lumbar lordosis
(e) Increased chest expansion

8.25 Correct statements about the course and prognosis of ankylosing spondylitis include (page 479):
(a) The disease remits in pregnancy.
(b) Hip disease is more likely when the disease starts in teenagers.
(c) Women are more severely afflicted than men.
(d) Women are more likely to have peripheral joint disease.
(e) In severe cases the spine becomes completely fused.

8.26 Correct statements about the management of ankylosing spondylitis include (page 480):
(a) Slow-release indomethacin is often the best choice.
(b) An exercise programme is essential.
(c) Prophylactic radiotherapy is required in most patients.
(d) Hip replacement is common.
(e) Sulphasalazine is useful in spinal disease.

8.27 Clinical features of reactive arthritis (Reiter's syndrome) include (page 481):
(a) Urethritis
(b) Conjunctivitis
(c) Keratoderma blenorrhagica
(d) Plantar fasciitis
(e) Achilles tendinitis

8.28 Clinical features of psoriatic arthritis include (pages 480–481):
(a) Asymmetrical polyarthritis affecting the small joints of the hand
(b) Arthritis mutilans
(c) Skin lesions are minimal or absent
(d) Increased incidence of ankylosing spondylitis
(e) History of psoriasis in the family

8.29 Hyperuricaemia secondary to impaired excretion of uric acid is caused by (Table 8.17, page 483):
(a) Polycythaemia vera
(b) Leukaemia
(c) Thiazides

(d) High-dose aspirin
(e) Alcohol

8.30 Features of gout include (page 484):
(a) Tophi in the ears
(b) Vascular disease
(c) Hypertension
(d) Nephropathy
(e) Neuropathy

8.31 Drugs used in the management of acute attacks of gout include (page 484):
(a) Intramuscular corticotrophin
(b) Salicylates
(c) Colchicine
(d) Allopurinol
(e) Probenecid

8.32 Correct statements about septic arthritis include (page 485):
(a) *Neisseria* spp. are the commonest cause.
(b) The clinical features are similar for all different causative organisms.
(c) It is common in immunologically compromised individuals.
(d) Aspiration of the joint is the only important diagnostic manoeuvre.
(e) 'Blind' antibiotic therapy should be avoided even if identification of the organism is delayed.

8.33 Correct statements about specific types of bacterial arthritis include (page 486):
(a) In adults tuberculous arthritis is usually due to haematogenous spread from pulmonary or renal disease.
(b) Meningococcal arthritis usually occurs as a part of generalized meningococcaemia.
(c) Migratory polyarthritis is common in gonococcal arthritis.
(d) *Salmonella* arthritis is rarely polyarticular.
(e) Infective endocarditis may present with arthritis.

8.34 Correct statements about Lyme disease include (page 486):
(a) It was first described in Sweden.
(b) It is caused by a spirochaete.
(c) It is easily mistaken for Still's disease in children.
(d) The arthritis is characteristically episodic.
(e) Erythema chronicum migrans describes the characteristic headache seen in this condition.

8.35 Recognized causes of viral arthropathy include (page 486):
(a) Rubella vaccination
(b) Mumps
(c) Hepatitis B infection

(d) HIV infection
(e) Human parvovirus B_{19}

8.36 Fungal infestations which cause arthritis include (page 487):
(a) Candidiasis
(b) Actinomycosis
(c) Blastomycosis
(d) Coccidioidomycosis
(e) Histoplasmosis

8.37 Conditions in which arthritis is associated with an immunological reaction to infection include (page 487):
(a) Rheumatic fever.
(b) Henoch–Schönlein purpura
(c) Septic arthritis
(d) Systemic lupus erythematosus
(e) Systemic sclerosis

8.38 The term connective tissue disease includes (page 487):
(a) Marfan's syndrome
(b) Systemic lupus erythematosus
(c) Systemic sclerosis
(d) Polymyositis
(e) Ehlers–Danlos syndrome

8.39 Correct statements about the clinical features of SLE include (page 487):
(a) It is extremely variable in its manifestation.
(b) Most of the clinical features are due to the consequences of vasculitis.
(c) Mild cases may present only with arthralgia.
(d) Fever is rare in exacerbations.
(e) Joint involvement is rare.

8.40 Recognized features of SLE include (Fig 8.26, page 488):
(a) Glomerulonephritis
(b) Butterfly rash on the cheeks of the face
(c) Livedo reticularis
(d) Libman–Sacks endocarditis
(e) Raynaud's phenomenon

8.41 Neurological features of SLE include (Fig 8.26):
(a) Epilepsy
(b) Cerebellar ataxia
(c) Cerebrovascular accidents
(d) Peripheral neuropathy
(e) Cranial nerve lesions

8.42 Discoid lupus (page 489):
- (a) is malignant systemic lupus erythematosus
- (b) is another name for lupus vulgaris
- (c) causes lupus pernio
- (d) is characterized by the absence of skin involvement
- (e) is often cured by a course of antituberculous treatment

8.43 Drugs known to induce SLE include (page 489):
- (a) Paracetamol
- (b) Aspirin
- (c) Steroids
- (d) Hydralazine
- (e) Procainamide

8.44 Correct statements about investigations in SLE include (page 489):
- (a) ESR is raised in proportion to the disease activity.
- (b) C-reactive protein is elevated.
- (c) Double-stranded DNA binding is specific for SLE.
- (d) Serum complement levels are elevated during active disease.
- (e) Characteristic histological abnormalities are seen in renal biopsies.

8.45 Correct statements about the management of SLE include (page 489):
- (a) Systemic hydroxychloroquine therapy is the mainstay of treatment.
- (b) Active SLE should be treated with systemic steroids.
- (c) There is no evidence that treatment in remission alters the progression of disease.
- (d) Cyclophosphamide is reserved for patients with life-threatening disease.
- (e) Pregnancy is contraindicated in this condition.

8.46 Recognized features of antiphospholipid syndrome include (page 490):
- (a) Thrombocytopenia
- (b) Arterial and venous thromboses
- (c) Abortions
- (d) Migraine
- (e) Epilepsy

8.47 Cutaneous manifestations of systemic sclerosis include (page 491):
- (a) Raynaud's phenomenon
- (b) Calcinosis
- (c) Telangiectasia
- (d) Pigmentation
- (e) Depigmentation

8.48 Recognized features of diffuse systemic sclerosis include (page 491):
- (a) Antitopoisomerase-1 antibody
- (b) Dysphagia
- (c) Dilatation of small bowel

(d) Obliterative endarteritis of renal vessels
(e) Upper lobe fibrosis

8.49 Variants of systemic sclerosis include (pages 491–492):
(a) Lupus vulgaris
(b) Morphea
(c) CREST syndrome
(d) Mixed connective tissue disease
(e) Lupus pernio

8.50 Recognized features of dermatopolymyositis include (page 491):
(a) It presents with distal muscle weakness.
(b) It is associated with an increased incidence of carcinoma of the ovary.
(c) Dysphagia.
(d) EMG shows short polyphasic motor potentials with spontaneous fibrillation and high-frequency repetitive discharges.
(e) The muscle biopsy shows necrosis of muscle fibres.

8.51 Recognized features of primary Sjögren's syndrome include (page 492):
(a) Rheumatoid arthritis
(b) Dryness of mouth
(c) Parotid gland enlargement
(d) Renal tubular acidosis
(e) Anti-Ro (SSA) antibodies

8.52 Recognized features of the polyarteritis nodosa (PAN) group include (page 495):
(a) It usually presents in middle-aged men.
(b) It is associated with hepatitis B antigenaemia.
(c) Classic PAN characteristically involves the lung.
(d) The antineutropenic cytoplasmic antibody ANCA is present in the majority of patients.
(e) Microaneurysm formation.

8.53 Recognized features of the polyarteritis nodosa (PAN) group include (page 495)
(a) Mononeuritis multiplex
(b) Gastrointestinal haemorrhage
(c) Renal failure
(d) Myocardial infarction
(e) Livedo reticularis

8.54 ANCA-postive vasculitis includes (page 496):
(a) Wegener's granulomatosis
(b) Churg–Strauss granulomatosis
(c) Microscopic polyangiitis

(d) Henoch–Schönlein purpura
(e) Cryoglobulinaemic vasculitis

8.55 Characteristic features of Wegener's granuloma include (page 496):
(a) Upper respiratory tract involvement
(b) Fleeting pulmonary shadows
(c) Glomerulonephritis
(d) Cardiac failure
(e) Essential mixed cryoglobulinaemia

8.56 Features of polymyalgia rheumatica include (page 494):
(a) It is characterized by muscle stiffness, typically in the evenings.
(b) The onset is insidious.
(c) Tests for rheumatoid factor are positive.
(d) Elevated ESR despite appropriate treatment.
(e) Temporal artery biopsy shows giant cell arteritis in almost all the cases.

8.57 The differential diagnosis of arthritis in the elderly includes (page 497):
(a) Osteoarthritis
(b) Rheumatoid arthritis
(c) Pyrophosphate deposition
(d) Osgood–Schlatter's disease
(e) Still's disease

8.58 Features of Still's disease include (page 498):
(a) Positive tests for rheumatoid factor
(b) It usually begins in the fourth decade
(c) The disease is often episodic
(d) Characteristic rash
(e) Splenomegaly

8.59 Clinical features of Henoch-Schönlein purpura include (page 499):
(a) It is a childhood condition
(b) Rash localized to the buttocks
(c) Abdominal pain
(d) Symmetrical polyarthritis
(e) Glomerulonephritis

8.60 Pseudogout is associated with (page 485):
(a) Primary hyperparathyroidism
(b) Haemochromatosis
(c) Hypothyroidism
(d) Hypophosphatasia
(e) True gout

8.61 Gastrointestinal and liver diseases associated with arthritis include (page 499):
   (a) Autoimmune chronic active hepatitis
   (b) Primary biliary cirrhosis
   (c) Haemochromatosis
   (d) Whipple's disease
   (e) Ulcerative colitis

8.62 Correct statements about Charcot's joints include (page 500):
   (a) In tabes the knees and ankles are usually spared.
   (b) In diabetes mellitus the joints of the tarsus are involved.
   (c) In syringomyelia the shoulders are typically spared.
   (d) Leprosy is not associated with neuropathic joints, despite sensory impairment.
   (e) Neuropathic joints are not painful.

8.63 Haematological conditions associated with arthritis include (page 500):
   (a) Iron-deficiency anaemia
   (b) Haemophilia
   (c) Sickle cell crises
   (d) Acute leukaemia
   (e) Chronic leukaemia

8.64 The following statements are correct (page 500):
   (a) In Cushings's disease back pain is common.
   (b) Hypothyroid patients may complain of pain and stiffness in the proximal muscles.
   (c) In acromegaly about half the patients have arthritis.
   (d) In acromegaly the small joints of the hands and knees are typically spared.
   (e) Familial hypercholesterolaemia is associated with polyarthritis.

8.65 The following statements are correct (page 501):
   (a) In familial Mediterranean fever there is an increase in the production of pyrin.
   (b) In sarcoidosis the most common type of arthritis is associated with erythema nodosum.
   (c) In osteochondromatosis, foci of cartilage form within the synovial membrane.
   (d) Haemarthrosis is the main manifestation of pigmented villonodular synovitis.
   (e) In relapsing polyarthritis there is destruction of the cartilage in the ear.

8.66 Avascular necrosis occurs in the following systemic conditions (page 460):
   (a) Sickle cell disease
   (b) Alcohol abuse
   (c) Prolonged steroid therapy

(d) Systemic lupus erythematosus
(e) Caisson disease

8.67 Behçet's syndrome is characterized by (page 497):
    (a) Oral ulceration
    (b) Genital ulceration
    (c) Iritis
    (d) Polyarthritis
    (e) Cardiac failure

8.68 Features of familial Mediterranean fever include (page 501):
    (a) Pleurisy
    (b) Palindromic rheumatism
    (c) It can be prevented by colchicine
    (d) Pleurisy
    (e) Amyloidosis

8.69 Clinical features of palindromic rheumatism include (page 473):
    (a) Polyarticular arthritis
    (b) Between attacks the joints are normal
    (c) Almost always goes on to develop chronic rheumatoid arthritis
    (d) Rheumatoid factor is always positive
    (e) Recurrent attacks of arthritis

8.70 Causes of back pain include (pages 457–460):
    (a) Ankylosing spondylitis
    (b) Osteoporosis
    (c) Osteomalacia
    (d) Pregnancy
    (e) Myeloma

8.71 Correct statements about the investigation of back pain include (page 457):
    (a) Investigations are more important than the history and examination.
    (b) MRI scan is the investigation of choice in disc disease.
    (c) X-rays are of little use in excluding serious bone disease.
    (d) Normal X-rays invariably exclude metastases.
    (e) A very high ESR suggests myeloma.

8.72 Causes of referred back pain include (pages 457–459):
    (a) Dysmenorrhoea
    (b) Oesophagitis
    (c) Pancreatitis
    (d) Diverticulitis
    (e) Cholecystitis

8.73 Pyogenic organisms known to cause discitis include:
    (a) *Staphylococcus aureus*

(b) *Mycobacterium tuberculosis*
(c) Brucella
(d) Rotavirus
(e) *Staphylococcus alba*

8.74 Correct statements about acute disc disease include (page 458):
(a) It is predominantly a disease of the elderly.
(b) Lumbar lordosis is lost.
(c) Foot drop is a recognized feature
(d) Bladder dysfunction is a feature
(e) Most patients require surgery.

8.75 Spondylolisthesis (page 458):
(a) arises because of a defect in the pars interarticularis
(b) is characterized by the slipping forward of one vertebra on to another
(c) is almost always treated surgically
(d) must never be treated with a corset
(e) is characterized by pain which is present on waking in the morning

8.76 Causes of spinal stenosis include (page 459):
(a) Disc prolapse
(b) Bad posture
(c) Degenerative osteophyte formation
(d) Coccydynia
(e) Congenital

8.77 The following associations regarding soft-tissue rheumatism are correct (page 456):
(a) Olecranon bursitis – tennis elbow
(b) De Quervain's tenosynovitis – pain in the anatomical snuffbox
(c) Enthesitis – housemaid's knee
(d) Golfer's elbow – medial epicondyle
(e) Enthesitis – plantar fasciitis

8.78 Examples of nerve compression syndromes include (page 456):
(a) Carpal tunnel syndrome
(b) Morton's metatarsalgia
(c) Trochanteric syndrome
(d) Student's elbow
(e) Tinel's compression

8.79 Frozen shoulder (pages 454–455):
(a) usually occurs in adults
(b) is usually bilateral
(c) is characterized by pain, usually troublesome at night
(d) shows restriction of glenohumeral movement
(e) causes axillary nerve palsy

8.80 Conditions that arise from repetitive manual work include (page 455):
- (a) Tennis elbow
- (b) Tenosynovitis
- (c) Rheumatoid arthritis
- (d) Carpal tunnel syndrome
- (e) Repetitive strain syndrome

8.81 Bone metabolism and mineralization are dependent on (page 503):
- (a) Collagen synthesis
- (b) Calcium absorption
- (c) Vitamin A
- (d) Bone resorption
- (e) Vitamin E

8.82 Correct statements about vitamin D metabolism include (page 503):
- (a) Poor nutrition is of only small importance in producing vitamin D deficiency.
- (b) Measurement of blood 25-hydroxycholecalciferol is a good indicator of vitamin D bioavailability.
- (c) 1,25-Dihydroxycholecalciferol is produced in the liver.
- (d) 1,25-Dihydroxycholecalciferol production is independent of parathyroid hormone.
- (e) Cholecalciferol is produced in the skin.

8.83 Parathyroid hormone increases (page 504):
- (a) tubular reabsorption of calcium
- (b) excretion of phosphate
- (c) osteoclastic resorption of bone
- (d) intestinal absorption of calcium
- (e) synthesis of 1,25-dihydroxycholecalciferol

8.84 The following statements are correct (page 503):
- (a) Calcitonin levels rise with increasing plasma calcium.
- (b) Steroids inhibit bone resorption.
- (c) Androgens induce the puberty growth spurt.
- (d) Growth hormone stimulates the growth of cartilage.
- (e) Hypothyroidism leads to growth.

8.85 Markers of bone resorption include (page 505):
- (a) Serum alkaline phosphatase
- (b) Serum osteocalcin
- (c) Type I collagen propeptides
- (d) Urinary hydroxyproline
- (e) Urinary pyridinoline cross-links of collagen

8.86 Causes of osteomalacia include (Table 8.24):
- (a) Vitamin D deficiency

(b) Immobility in the elderly
(c) Coeliac disease
(d) Gastric surgery
(e) Barbiturate therapy

8.87 Causes of elevated serum calcium include (page 505):
(a) Osteoporosis
(b) Osteomalacia
(c) Paget's disease
(d) Hyperparathyroidism
(e) Multiple myeloma

8.88 Causes of elevated phosphate include (page 505):
(a) Multiple myeloma
(b) Osteoporosis
(c) Osteomalacia
(d) Paget's disease
(e) Hypoparathyroidism

8.89 Causes of elevated alkaline phosphatase include (Table 8.21):
(a) Osteoporosis
(b) Osteomalacia
(c) Paget's disease
(d) Hyperparathyroidism
(e) Multiple myeloma

8.90 Risk factors associated with osteoporosis include (Table 8.23):
(a) Excess of alcohol
(b) Cushing's disease
(c) Rheumatoid arthritis
(d) Chronic renal failure
(e) Hypogonadism

8.91 Factors thought to be important in the pathogenesis of type 2 osteoporosis include (page 507, Table 8.22):
(a) Excessive sunshine
(b) Low calcium intake
(c) Less vitamin D-containing foods
(d) Less vitamin D synthesis in the skin
(e) Oestrogen deficiency

8.92 Typical fracture sites in osteoporosis include (page 508):
(a) Vertebrae
(b) Distal radius
(c) Neck of femur
(d) Ribs
(e) Clavicle

8.93 Measures used for the prophylaxis of osteoporosis include (page 508):
(a) Oestrogen therapy
(b) Increased dietary calcium
(c) Bisphosphonates
(d) Exercises against gravity
(e) Fluoride

8.94 Recognized features of Paget's disease include (page 511):
(a) Bone pain
(b) Changes in the skull
(c) Bowed tibiae
(d) High cardiac output
(e) Osteogenic sarcoma

8.95 Drugs used to treat pain in Paget's disease include (page 511):
(a) Simple analgesics
(b) Bisphosphonates
(c) Calcitonin
(d) Mithramycin
(e) Fluoride

8.96 Causes of hypocalcaemia include (Table 8.26):
(a) Renal failure
(b) Postoperatively in parathyroidectomy
(c) Hyperparathyroidism
(d) DiGeorge syndrome
(e) Pseudohypoparathyroidism

8.97 Features of hypoparathyroidism include (page 515):
(a) Laryngeal stridor
(b) Tetany
(c) Positive Chvostek's sign
(d) Short QT interval
(e) Papilloedema

8.98 Causes of hypercalcaemia include (Table 8.25):
(a) Secondary hyperparathyroidism
(b) Milk alkali syndrome
(c) Thiazides
(d) Myeloma
(e) Hypertension

8.99 Features of hypercalcaemia include (page 513):
(a) Depression
(b) Bone pain
(c) Peptic ulceration

(d) Renal colic
(e) Prolonged QT interval

8.100 Malignant metastases causing hypercalcaemia commonly arise from tumours in (page 513):
  (a) Renal cell carcinoma
  (b) Bronchus
  (c) Breast
  (d) Thyroid
  (e) Prostate

8.101 Severe hypercalcaemia (3 mmol L^{-1}) is usually associated with (page 514):
  (a) Malignant disease
  (b) Hyperparathyroidism
  (c) Renal dialysis
  (d) Vitamin D therapy
  (e) Frusemide

8.102 Correct statements about the investigations in hypercalcaemia include (page 514):
  (a) Hyperphosphataemia is common in primary hyperparathyroidism.
  (b) Detectable levels of parathormone imply hyperparathyroidism.
  (c) In sarcoidosis plasma calcium is resistant to suppression by steroids.
  (d) Plasma chloride is elevated in primary hyperparathyroidism.
  (e) Hand X-rays may show subperiosteal erosions in the terminal phalanges.

8.103 Correct statements about osteomyelitis include (page 516):
  (a) *Salmonella* is the organism responsible for most cases of acute osteomyelitis.
  (b) *Salmonella* osteomyelitis may occur as a complication of sickle cell anaemia.
  (c) Brodie's abscess is a characteristic feature of acute osteomyelitis.
  (d) Tuberculous osteomyelitis is usually due to haematogenous spread from the lung.
  (e) Pott's disease is tuberculous osteomyelitis of the spine.

8.104 Primary bone tumours include (Table 8.27):
  (a) Multiple myeloma
  (b) Fibrosarcoma
  (c) Chondromas
  (d) Ewing's tumour
  (e) Wilms' tumour

8.105 The following statements about the investigations in bony tumours are correct (page 517):
  (a) Skeletal isotope scans are limited by the fact that they are unable to pick up bony metastases before radiological changes occur.
  (b) Osteosclerotic changes on X-ray are characteristic of prostatic metastases.
  (c) Serum alkaline phosphatase arising from bone is usually depressed.
  (d) Hypercalcaemia is seen in most patients.
  (e) Serum acid phosphatase is raised in prostatic metastases.

8.106 Mutations of fibrillar collagen result in (page 517):
  (a) Alport's disease
  (b) Osteogenesis imperfecta
  (c) Ehlers–Danlos syndrome
  (d) Epidermolysis bullosa
  (e) Marble bone disease

8.107 The following statements about connective tissue disorders are correct (page 518):
  (a) Achondroplasia is due to a defect in the fibroblast growth factor-3 (FGF-3) gene.
  (b) Blue sclera are a feature of osteogenesis imperfecta.
  (c) Leucoerythroblastic anaemia is a feature of marble bone disease.
  (d) Acid phosphatase is elevated in marble bone disease.
  (e) Infantile rickets is seen in hypophosphatasia.

8.108 A 39-year-old woman has a 4-year history of deteriorating rheumatoid arthritis despite treatment with NSAIDs and corticosteroids. The rheumatologist decides to initiate methotrexate. The following statements about methotrexate are correct:
  (a) The therapeutic effects are dramatic and the patient will experience clinical improvement within 36–40 hours.
  (b) The presence of a transient elevation of SGOT and alkaline phosphatase is an early indicator of the patient's likelihood of developing cirrhosis.
  (c) Women with childbearing potential should be recommended birth control because methotrexate is teratogenic.
  (d) Methotrexate therapy can result in cirrhosis.
  (e) Methotrexate can cause haemorrhagic cystitis.

8.109 A 77-year-old man gives a 2-year history of worsening pain in the right knee joint. Clinical examination reveals swelling of the joint without warmth, and crepitus with passive flexion and extension of the knee. A diagnostic arthrocentesis will show synovial fluid with the following characteristics:
  (a) Haemorrhagic effusion
  (b) Good viscosity

(c) A white blood cell count of 750 mm³
(d) A glucose level of 20 mg/dL
(e) Culture and sensitivity will reveal gonococci

8.110 A 38-year-old woman with a long history of seropositive rheumatoid arthritis complains of pain behind the left knee. Clinical examination reveals cystic swelling in the popliteal fossa. The differential diagnosis includes:
(a) Popliteal artery aneurysm
(b) Baker's cyst
(c) Deep venous thrombosis
(d) Gout
(e) Caplan's syndrome

8.111 A 38-year-old man with a 10-year history of chronic haemodialysis complains of tingling in the thumb and the lateral three fingers which is worse at night. Clinical examination reveals wasting of the muscle of the thenar eminence and decreased sensation in the affected fingers. The following statements are correct:
(a) He has ulnar nerve palsy.
(b) His symptoms are due to deposition of β_2-microglobulin in the carpal tunnel.
(c) In this condition the median nerve is typically spared.
(d) Tinel's sign may be positive.
(e) He has Felty's syndrome.

8.112 A 41-year-old woman on long-term oral corticosteroid therapy complains of pain in the right hip and difficulty in walking. X-ray of the hip shows no bony abnormality. The following statements are correct:
(a) The patient has rheumatoid arthritis.
(b) A normal X-ray of the hip excludes osteonecrosis.
(c) The patient is malingering.
(d) The patient has SLE.
(e) Magnetic resonance imaging is the next test be done to confirm the diagnosis.

8.113 A 90-year-old woman presents to the A and E department with pain in the right hip following a fall. Radiographs show a fracture of the neck of the femur and osteopenia. Recognized causes of her condition include:
(a) Smoking
(b) Low calcium intake
(c) Increased intake of ethanol
(d) Hormone replacement therapy
(e) Osgood–Schlatter syndrome

Renal Disease

9.1 The metabolic and endocrine functions of the kidney include (Table 9.1):
    (a) Excretion of waste products
    (b) Production of erythropoietin
    (c) Metabolism of vitamin D
    (d) Destruction of renin
    (e) Production of prostaglandins

9.2 Potassium (page 520):
    (a) is freely filtered at the glomerulus
    (b) is almost completely absorbed in the proximal tubule
    (c) is excreted in the distal tubule
    (d) is excreted in collecting ducts
    (e) elimination is less dependent on GFR than is the elimination of urea or creatinine

9.3 The following are excreted in the proximal tubule (page 520):
    (a) Water
    (b) Sodium
    (c) Potassium
    (d) Bicarbonate
    (e) Glucose

9.4 The following statements are correct (page 520):
    (a) A high filtration rate relates to the elimination of compounds present in low concentration.
    (b) Filtered hydrogen ion is largely reabsorbed.
    (c) The ability to excrete unwanted potassium is less dependent on glomerular filtration rate than is the elimination of urea.
    (d) The more tubular secretion of a compound occurs, the less dependent is elimination on the GFR.
    (e) Filtered bicarbonate is largely excreted.

9.5 Production of urea is increased by (Table 9.2):
    (a) Low-protein diet
    (b) Old age
    (c) Steroid therapy
    (d) Tetracyclines
    (e) Surgery

9.6 The elimination of urea is increased in (Table 9.2):
    (a) Pregnancy
    (b) Glomerular disease
    (c) Hypotension

(d) Dehydration

(e) Urinary obstruction

9.7 Drugs that reduce tubular secretion of creatinine include (page 522):

(a) Cimetidine

(b) Trimethoprim

(c) Spironolactone

(d) Amiloride

(e) Inulin

9.8 The following associations are correct (page 522):

(a) Incomplete absorption of a normal filtered load – renal glycosuria

(b) Defect in tubular reabsorption of amino acid – Fanconi's syndrome

(c) Tubular defects in reabsorption of water – nephrogenic diabetes insipidus

(d) Tubular defects in reabsorption of bicarbonate – proximal renal tubular acidosis

(e) Defective acidification of urine – distal renal tubular acidosis

9.9 Renin release is controlled by (page 523):

(a) Pressure changes in the efferent arteriole

(b) Parasympathetic tone

(c) Chloride concentration in the distal tubule

(d) Osmotic concentration in the distal tubule

(e) Local prostaglandin release

9.10 Erythropoietin secretion may be increased by (page 523):

(a) Loss of renal substance

(b) Polycystic renal disease

(c) Benign renal cysts

(d) Renal cell carcinoma

(e) Acute glomerulonephritis

9.11 Atrial natriuretric peptide (page 523):

(a) reduces glomerular filtration rate

(b) increases renin secretion

(c) increases aldosterone secretion

(d) opposes the action of angiotensin II

(e) opposes the sodium-retaining action of aldosterone on the renal tubule

9.12 The following statements are correct (page 525):

(a) Overt bleeding from the urethra is suggested when blood is seen at the start of voiding and then the urine becomes clear.

(b) Blood diffusely present throughout the urine comes from the bladder or above.

(c) Blood only at the end of micturition suggests bleeding from the prostate.

(d) The presence of red cell casts is diagnostic of bleeding from the kidney.
(e) Tamm–Horsfall glycoprotein indicates bleeding from the kidney.

9.13 The following statements about proteinuria are correct (page 526):
(a) Microalbuminuria is used as a predictor of the development of diabetic nephropathy.
(b) Increased urinary excretion of N-acetyl-β-glucosaminidase indicates glomerular damage.
(c) Increased excretion of β_2-microglobulin indicates proximal tubular damage.
(d) Increased excretion of retinol-binding protein indicates proximal tubular damage.
(e) Normal urine contains small quantities of albumin.

9.14 Causes of sterile pyuria include (page 527):
(a) Kidney stones
(b) Tubulointerstitial disease
(c) Papillary necrosis
(d) Tuberculosis
(e) Interstitial cystitis

9.15 The following statements about urinary casts are correct (page 527):
(a) Hyaline casts may be seen in normal urine.
(b) Coarsely granular casts occur with pathological proteinuria.
(c) Even one red cell cast indicates renal disease.
(d) White cell casts are seen in acute pyelonephritis.
(e) Tubular cell casts occur in acute tubular necrosis.

9.16 Correct statements about bacteria in urine include (page 527):
(a) The demonstration of bacteria on Gram staining of a random sample of urine suggests urinary tract infection.
(b) The presence of pyuria in the presence of bacteria may be accepted as evidence of urinary tract infection in a febrile patient.
(c) Urine for quantitative culture must be obtained prior to starting antibiotic treatment.
(d) Stix testing for blood is very useful in the diagnosis of urinary tract infection.
(e) Stix testing for protein is sensitive for the presence of bacturia.

9.17 Correct statements about imaging in renal disease include (page 528):
(a) A plain abdominal X-ray is always taken prior to urography.
(b) The main value of plain abdominal X-ray is to identify renal calcification.
(c) CT scan is useful in the diagnosis of retroperitoneal masses.
(d) Spiral CT scanning can be used to image the renal artery.
(e) Micturition cystourography is used to demonstrate vesicoureteric reflux.

9.18 Ultrasound is useful in defining (page 528):
  (a) Reflux nephropathy
  (b) Papillary necrosis
  (c) Renal cysts
  (d) Renal masses
  (e) Renal size

9.19 Dynamic scintigraphy (page 530):
  (a) is used to identify ectopic kidneys
  (b) is used to determine relative renal function
  (c) is used to assess renal blood flow in renal artery stenosis
  (d) can demonstrate the severity of obstruction
  (e) using gallium-67 is useful for localization of infection

9.20 Indications for renal biopsy include (Table 9.4):
  (a) Nephrotic syndrome
  (b) Failure to recover from assumed reversible acute renal failure
  (c) Single kidney
  (d) Small kidneys
  (e) Uncontrolled hypertension

9.21 Complications of transcutaenous renal biopsy include (Table 9.5):
  (a) Mortality of 1 in a 100
  (b) Microscopic haematuria
  (c) Perirenal haematoma
  (d) Arteriovenous malformation
  (e) Introduction of infection

9.22 Features of glomerulonephritis include (page 531):
  (a) It is usually unilateral.
  (b) It may be due to the deposition of immune complexes.
  (c) It may be due to the in situ formation of immune complexes.
  (d) It is usually due to the deposition of antiglomerular basement membrane antibody.
  (e) It is usually associated with pyelonephritis.

9.23 Secondary mechanisms of glomerular injury include (page 532):
  (a) Complement activation
  (b) Fibrin deposition
  (c) Platelet aggregation
  (d) Inflammation with neutrophil-dependent mechanisms
  (e) Activation of kinin systems

9.24 Causes of glomerulonephritis due to the deposition of antibasement membrane antibody include (Table 9.6):
  (a) Hepatitis B
  (b) Systemic lupus erythematosus

(c) Penicillamine
(d) Goodpasture's syndrome
(e) Cryoglobulins

9.25 The following correlations between the histological type of glomerulonephritis and the most common clinical presentation are correct (Table 9.7):
(a) Membranous glomerulonephritis – nephrotic syndrome in adults
(b) Minimal change nephropathy – absence of proteinuria
(c) Focal glomerulosclerosis – haematuria without proteinuria
(d) Crescent formation in proliferative glomerulonephritis – rapidly progressive renal failure
(e) IgA nephritis – asymptomatic haematuria

9.26 Focal segmental glomerulonephritis is a feature of (pages 533–534):
(a) Systemic lupus erythematosus
(b) Subacute infective endocarditis
(c) Shunt nephritis
(d) Henoch–Schönlein purpura
(e) IgA nephritis

9.27 Proliferative glomerulonephritis with crescent formation is a feature of (page 534):
(a) Microscopic polyarteritis
(b) Wegener's granulomatosis
(c) Goodpasture's syndrome
(d) Buerger's disease
(e) Hodgkin's disease

9.28 Features of type 2 mesangiocapillary glomerulonephritis include (page 534):
(a) Loss of subcutaneous fat.
(b) It may occur after measles.
(c) It does not affect young adults.
(d) It does not lead to chronic renal failure.
(e) The linear intramembranous deposits usually stain for C3 only.

9.29 Membranous glomerulonephritis is associated with (page 535):
(a) Systemic lupus erythematosus
(b) Hepatitis B infection
(c) Malignancy of the bronchus
(d) Penicillamine therapy
(e) *Plasmodium malariae*

9.30 Features of minimal-change glomerular lesions include (page 535):
(a) Glomeruli appear normal on light microscopy.
(b) It rarely occurs in children.
(c) It occurs in Hodgkin's disease.

(d) It usually leads to chronic renal failure.
(e) Patients have a higher incidence of asthma.

9.31 Features of IgA nephropathy include (page 535):
(a) Usually occurs in old age
(b) Recurrent haematuria
(c) Dismal prognosis
(d) It is sometimes related to the infection
(e) There is a similar pathological picture in Henoch–Schönlein purpura

9.32 Features of focal segmental glomerulosclerosis include (page 538):
(a) It may recur in the kidneys within hours of renal transplantation.
(b) It rarely presents as proteinuria.
(c) It is sensitive to steroid therapy.
(d) It does not lead to chronic renal failure.
(e) The deep glomeruli at the corticomedullary junction are affected first.

9.33 Steroid or immunosuppressive therapy is of benefit in glomerulonephritis complicating (page 539–540):
(a) Systemic lupus erythematosus
(b) Polyarteritis nodosa
(c) Wegener's granulomatosis
(d) Goodpasture's syndrome
(e) Cryoglobulinaemic renal disease

9.34 Life-threatening complications of glomerulonephritis include (page 537):
(a) Idiopathic epilepsy
(b) Myocardial infarction
(c) Hypertensive encephalopathy
(d) Pulmonary oedema
(e) Uraemia

9.35 Features of Goodpasture's syndrome include (page 536):
(a) Lung haemorrhage which responds to repeated plasma exchange and immunosuppressive therapy.
(b) Glomerulonephritis which responds dramatically to plasma exchange
(c) When oliguria occurs the renal failure is irreversible.
(d) Nephrotic syndrome is a common presenting feature.
(e) It is mediated by anti-glomerular basement membrane antibody.

9.36 Features of polyarteritis nodosa include (page 539):
(a) Aneurysmal dilatation of medium-sized arteries on renal arteriography.
(b) Focal proliferative glomerulonephritis.
(c) The condition is commoner in women.
(d) It is common in the elderly.
(e) Typically the patient is ANCA positive.

9.37 Features of haemolytic uraemic syndrome include (page 541):
  (a) Extravascular haemolysis
  (b) Red cell fragmentation
  (c) It follows a febrile illness
  (d) Recurrent episodes
  (e) Most children recover spontaneously

9.38 Renal impairment in multiple myeloma may be due to (page 541):
  (a) Acute tubular necrosis
  (b) Amyloidosis
  (c) Hypercalcaemia
  (d) Renal sepsis
  (e) Urinary tract obstruction

9.39 Causes of nephrotic syndrome include (Table 9.9, page 542):
  (a) Systemic lupus erythematosus
  (b) Diabetes mellitus
  (c) Amyloidosis
  (d) Renal tuberculosis
  (e) Polycystic kidneys

9.40 Causes of hypoalbuminaemia include (Table 9.10):
  (a) Protein – energy malnutrition
  (b) Liver disease
  (c) Nephrotic syndrome
  (d) Protein-losing enteropathy
  (e) Extensive burns

9.41 The following statements about investigations in nephrotic syndrome are correct (page 543):
  (a) Minimal-change lesions usually result in red cells in the urine.
  (b) Serum C3 complement concentrations increase in immune complex-mediated glomerulonephritis.
  (c) A selective protein leak is found in minimal-change nephropathy.
  (d) Measurement of selective protein leak is necessary before renal biopsy.
  (e) There is an approximate reciprocal relationship between serum albumin concentration and serum cholesterol concentration.

9.42 Renal biopsy is indicated in nephrotic syndrome in the following situations (page 544):
  (a) In male children who have a highly selective protein leak
  (b) In long-standing insulin-dependent diabetes with retinopathy
  (c) Patients on penicillamine therapy
  (d) In young children with no hypertension
  (e) In young children with no red cells or red cell casts in the urine

9.43 Complications of nephrotic syndrome include (page 545):
(a) Rapidly progressive hypertension
(b) Pneumococcal infections
(c) Renal vein thrombosis
(d) Hyperlipidaemia
(e) Oliguric renal failure

9.44 Correct statements about the management of nephrotic syndrome include (page 544):
(a) Children with minimal-change lesions rarely respond to steroid therapy.
(b) Infusion of albumin produces permanent relief.
(c) Spontaneous remission of membranous glomerulonephritis occurs in most patients.
(d) Amyloidosis usually responds to steroid therapy.
(e) Albumin infusion combined with mannitol may initiate diuresis in oliguric renal failure.

9.45 Organisms causing urinary tract infection in domiciliary practice include (Table 9.11):
(a) *Escherichia coli*
(b) *Klebsiella aerogenes*
(c) *Proteus mirabilis*
(d) *Streptococcus faecalis*
(e) *Staphylococcus epidermidis*

9.46 The following statements about the pathogenesis of urinary tract infection are correct (page 545):
(a) Infection is most often due to bacteria from the patient's bowel.
(b) Humoral immunity is known to maintain the sterility of the bladder.
(c) The first critical phase in the development of UTI is the entry and establishment of bacteria within the bladder.
(d) Transfer of bacteria along the urethra to the bladder is inhibited by sexual intercourse.
(e) Extension of infection up the ureters is prevented by vesicoureteric reflux.

9.47 Excretion urography in chronic pyelonephritis shows (page 547):
(a) Vesicoureteric reflux
(b) Irregular renal outlines
(c) Clubbed calyces
(d) A variable reduction in renal size
(e) Stenosis of the renal artery.

9.48 Relapse of a urinary tract infection occurs (page 547):
(a) as a result of reinvasion of a susceptible tract
(b) in renal stones
(c) in scarred kidneys

(d) in polycystic disease
(e) in bacterial prostatitis

9.49 Causes of abacteriuric frequency include (page 548):
(a) Post-coital bladder trauma
(b) Vaginitis
(c) Atrophic vaginitis
(d) Urethritis in the elderly
(e) Hunner's ulcer

9.50 The following statements about the investigation of urinary tract infection are correct (page 548):
(a) Excretion urography should be carried out in all females following a first proven episode of bacteriuria.
(b) Micturating cystography is indicated in children with an abnormal excretion urogram.
(c) Cystoscopy is invaluable in patients with known UTI.
(d) The diagnosis is based on quantitative culture of a clean-catch midstream specimen of urine.
(e) Absence of pyuria excludes the diagnosis of urinary tract infection.

9.51 Prophylactic measures to prevent reinfection of the urinary tract include (page 549):
(a) Avoidance of constipation
(b) Avoidance of bubble baths
(c) Voiding of urine before sexual intercourse
(d) Voiding at 2–3 hour intervals
(e) A 2-litre daily fluid intake

9.52 Features of xanthogranulomatous pyelonephritis include (page 550):
(a) It is most often due to *Proteus* spp.
(b) It is usually bilateral.
(c) It is associated with staghorn calculi.
(d) Antibacterial treatment usually eradicates infection.
(e) Nephrectomy is the treatment of choice.

9.53 Common causes of acute tubulointerstitial nephritis include (Table 9.13):
(a) Penicillins
(b) Sulphonamides
(c) Non-steroidal anti-inflammatory drugs
(d) Phenindione
(e) Allopurinol

9.54 Common causes of chronic tubulointerstitial nephritis include (Table 9.14):
(a) Chronic pyelonephritis
(b) Diabetes
(c) Alport's syndrome

(d) Sickle cell disease
(e) Hyperuricaemic nephropathy

9.55 Chronic analgesic abuse predisposes to (page 552):
(a) acute tubulo interstitial pyelonephritis
(b) chronic tubulo interstitial nephritis
(c) uroepithelial tumours
(d) glomerulonephritis
(e) Balkan nephropathy

9.56 Renal changes in benign essential hypertension include (page 553):
(a) Hyalinization of the vessel wall
(b) Onion-skin appearance of large vessels
(c) Fibrinoid necrosis of the afferent glomerular arterioles
(d) Reduction in the size of both kidneys
(e) Increased sclerotic glomeruli

9.57 The following statements regarding screening for unilateral renovascular disease are correct (page 544):
(a) Rapid sequence excretion urography is useful.
(b) Renal DTPA scan can demonstrate decreased renal perfusion on the affected side.
(c) Divided renal function studies that involve ureteric catheterization are frequently used.
(d) Renal arteriography is the gold standard for diagnosis.
(e) Micturating urography is a useful test.

9.58 Causes of urinary tract stone formation include (Table 9.16):
(a) Polycystic kidneys
(b) Hypocalcaemia
(c) Urinary tract infection
(d) Renal tubular acidosis
(e) Hyperuricaemia

9.59 Causes of hyperoxaluria include (page 556):
(a) Excessive dietary intake of calcium
(b) Excessive ingestion of spinach
(c) Crohn's disease
(d) Hyperuricaemia
(e) Uricosuria

9.60 Clinical features of urinary tract stones include (Table 9.17):
(a) Renal colic
(b) Haematuria
(c) Strangury
(d) Urinary tract infection
(e) Urinary tract obstruction

9.61 Causes of medullary calcification include (Table 9.18):
(a) Sarcoidosis
(b) Renal tubular acidosis
(c) Primary oxaluria
(d) Medullary sponge kidney
(e) Primary hyperparathyroidism

9.62 Causes of urinary tract obstruction include (Table 9.19):
(a) Bladder tumour
(b) Retroperitoneal fibrosis
(c) Phimosis
(d) Neuropathic bladder
(e) Prostatic obstruction

9.63 The following statements about the clinical features of urinary tract obstruction are correct (pages 561–562):
(a) Complete anuria may occur with complete obstruction of a single kidney.
(b) Polyuria may occur in partial obstruction.
(c) An enlarged hydronephrotic kidney may be palpable.
(d) In acute retention an enlarged bladder may be felt.
(e) Retention with overflow indicates obstruction of the ureters.

9.64 Correct statements about the investigation of urinary tract obstruction include (page 562):
(a) Ultrasound is an unreliable means of ruling out upper urinary tract dilatation.
(b) In obstructive uropathy the relative uptake may be normal on the side of obstruction.
(c) Excretion urography can usually exclude obstruction even in the presence of severe renal failure.
(d) Antegrade pyelography defines the site and cause of obstruction.
(e) Pressure–flow studies showing a high voiding pressure to maintain urinary flow indicates bladder flow obstruction.

9.65 Correct statements about the treatment of urinary tract obstruction include (page 564):
(a) Temporary external drainage of urine by nephrostomy must be avoided.
(b) Dialysis may be required in the ill patient before surgery.
(c) Permanent diversion may be achieved by ureteric anastomosis to an ileal conduit opening on to the abdominal wall.
(d) Diuresis rarely follows relief of obstruction at any site in the urinary tract.
(e) In obstruction due to untreatable malignant disease it is wise to consider carefully whether urinary diversion is justified, as this may exchange a pain-free death from renal failure for a painful one with malignant invasion of bones.

9.66 The following are associated with retroperitoneal fibrosis (page 565):
  (a) Retroperitoneal lymphoma
  (b) Carcinoma of the bladder
  (c) Abdominal aortic aneurysm
  (d) Prolonged exposure to methysergide
  (e) Carcinoma of the colon

9.67 Drugs causing acute tubular necrosis include (page 566):
  (a) Steroids
  (b) Aminoglycoside
  (c) Amphotericin B
  (d) Digitalis
  (e) Cephaloridine

9.68 Drugs known to increase serum concentration of urea include (Table 9.20):
  (a) Sodium valproate
  (b) Corticosteroids
  (c) Tetracycline
  (d) β-Blockers
  (e) Cimetidine

Water, Electrolytes and Acid-Base Homeostasis

10.1 The following statements are correct (page 597):
    (a) Water accounts for more than half the total body weight.
    (b) The percentage of water is more in women.
    (c) Two-thirds of the water is interstitial fluid.
    (d) The major intracellular solute is potassium.
    (e) The major extracellular solute is sodium.

10.2 Correct statements about osmotic pressure include (page 597):
    (a) Osmotic pressure is the primary determinant of distribution of water between the three major water compartments in the body.
    (b) Most of the intracellular magnesium is osmotically active.
    (c) A characteristic of an osmotically active solute is that it cannot freely leave its compartment.
    (d) The retention of urea in renal failure results in an alteration in the distribution of total body water.
    (e) Sodium ion is an important contributor to fluid distribution between the intersititium and plasma.

10.3 Correct statements about osmolality include (page 598):
    (a) It is determined by the concentration of osmotically active particles.
    (b) Fully ionized molecules have half the osmolality of undissociated particles.
    (c) The major determinant of plasma osmolality is sodium concentration.
    (d) Plasma osmolality can be approximated using plasma glucose and urea levels only.
    (e) Plasma alcohol concentration can be estimated by substracting calculated from measured osmolality.

10.4 The following statements are correct (page 598):
    (a) The distribution of extracellular water between the vascular and interstitial spaces is determined by the equilibrium between hydrostatic and oncotic pressures.
    (b) Water given intravenously as 5% dextrose is distributed equally in all compartments.
    (c) One litre of normal saline given intravenously remains in the extracellular compartment.
    (d) Colloid given intravenously remains in the vascular compartment.
    (e) The extracellular volume is controlled by the total body content of sodium.

10.5 Correct statements about the regulation of extracellular volume include (page 598):
(a) Effective arterial blood volume is the primary determinant of renal sodium and water excretion.
(b) Volume receptors in the cardiac atria control the release of atrial natriuretic hormone.
(c) Sodium concentration in the distal renal tubule alter renin release from juxtaglomerular cells.
(d) Prostaglandin I_2 modulates the sodium-retaining effect of angiotensin II.
(e) A salt load increases the secretion of renin.

10.6 Correct statements about the regulation of body sodium content include (page 598):
(a) Most of the body's sodium is in the intracellular compartment.
(b) Bone is devoid of sodium.
(c) Changes in renal sodium excretion are achieved by changes in sodium concentration.
(d) Changes in afferent arteriolar pressure in the juxtaglomerular apparatus affect sodium excretion.
(e) Activation of barorecepetors in the vascular tree affects body sodium content.

10.7 Renal sodium excretion is increased by (page 599):
(a) Atrial distension
(b) Aldosterone
(c) Oestrogens
(d) Raised arterial pressure
(e) Exogenous cardiac glycosides

10.8 Correct statements regarding the regulation of body water content include (page 600):
(a) Changes in water balance respond to changes in sodium concentration rather than primarily changes in volume.
(b) Water intake normally exceeds the amount that is required for physiological functioning.
(c) Thirst is suppressed by angiotensin-II.
(d) Water excretion is governed largely by serum osmolality.
(e) Water excretion is increased by antidiuretic hormone.

10.9 Stimuli which may decrease ADH release even if serum osmolality is normal include (page 601):
(a) Hypovolaemia
(b) Surgery
(c) Nausea
(d) Psychiatric illness
(e) Potassium depletion

10.10 Vasopressin (page 601):
   (a) increases the permeability of the renal collecting ducts to water
   (b) causes the formation of concentrated urine
   (c) effects on the kidney are counterbalanced by locally generated prostaglandin E_2
   (d) increases water intake by causing thirst
   (e) decreases sodium excretion

10.11 Pathological decreases in water excretion are a result of (page 601):
   (a) Decreased renal sensitivity to ADH
   (b) Syndrome of inappropriate ADH secretion
   (c) Oxytocin
   (d) Alcohol
   (e) Heart failure

10.12 Correct statements about the mechanism of action of ADH include (Fig 10.4):
   (a) It acts on V2 (vasopressin) receptors located on the basolateral surface of principal cells of the cortical collecting tubule.
   (b) It initiates a sequence of events which leads to preformed cytoplasmic vesicles that contain aquaporin.
   (c) When the ADH effect is worn off, water channels aggregate in clathrin-coated pits.
   (d) A defect in the function of the water channel results in central diabetes insipidus.
   (e) It also influences potassium reabsorption.

10.13 The following are caused by disturbances of extracellular volume control (page 602):
   (a) Ankle oedema due to venous thrombosis
   (b) Leg oedema due to immobility
   (c) Arm oedema due to subclavian thrombosis
   (d) Facial oedema due to superior vena caval obstruction
   (e) Lymphoedema

10.14 Extracellular volume expansion may cause (page 603):
   (a) Pulmonary oedema
   (b) Pleural effusion
   (c) Ascites
   (d) Pericardial effusion
   (e) Raised jugular venous pressure

10.15 The following mechanisms of oedema are correct (page 603):
   (a) Heart failure – increase in effective circulatory volume
   (b) Hypoalbuminaemia – increase in plasma oncotic pressure
   (c) Hepatic cirrhosis – peripheral vasodilatation due to increase nitric oxide generation

(d) Renal impairment – excess sodium loss

(e) Nifedipine – increased capillary pressure owing to relaxation of precapillary arterioles

10.16 Drugs that may cause renal sodium excretion include (page 603):

(a) Mineralocorticoids

(b) Liquorice

(c) Non-steroidal anti-inflammatory drugs

(d) Frusemide

(e) Thiazides

10.17 Increased capillary permeability to proteins causes oedema in (page 603):

(a) Septicaemia

(b) Association with therapeutic doses of interleukin-II

(c) Ovarian hyperstimulation syndrome

(d) Association with nifedipine

(e) Complement-deficiency syndrome

10.18 Loop diuretics (page 604):

(a) stimulate excretion of sodium chloride

(b) stimulate excretion of water

(c) increase venous capacitance

(d) prevent gout

(e) cause allergic tubulointerstitial nephritis

10.19 Thiazides (page 604):

(a) are stronger diuretics than loop diuretics

(b) are useful in diabetes insipidus

(c) are useful in patients with idiopathic hypercalciuria

(d) cause urate excretion

(e) cause hyperkalaemia

10.20 The following uses of diuretics are correct (page 604–605):

(a) Acetazolamide – metabolic acidosis

(b) Acetazolamide – glaucoma

(c) Thiazides – hypercalciuria

(d) Potassium-sparing diuretics – Bartter's syndrome

(e) Loop diuretics – SIADH

10.21 Features of loss of circulating volume include (page 606):

(a) Loss of skin turgor

(b) Postural hypotension

(c) Low jugular venous pressure

(d) Tachycardia

(e) Peripheral venoconstriction

10.22 Causes of postural hypotension include (Table 10.4):
(a) Shy–Drager syndrome
(b) Tricyclic antidepressants
(c) Nitrates
(d) Calcium channel blockers
(e) α-Adrenergic receptor blockers

10.23 Causes of extracellular volume depletion include (Table 10.5):
(a) Burns
(b) Leaking aortic aneurysm
(c) Ileostomy losses
(d) Diuretics
(e) Diarrhoea

10.24 Correct statements regarding sodium concentration include (page 608):
(a) Disturbances of sodium concentration are caused by disturbances of water balance.
(b) The serum sodium concentration reflects body's total sodium content.
(c) Hyponatraemia indicates that sodium must be replaced.
(d) In spurious hyponatraemia the serum osmolality is normal.
(e) Severe hyponatraemia is treated initially with intravenous normal saline.

10.25 Causes of hyponatraemia with normal extracellular volume include (Tables 10.7, 10.8, 10.10):
(a) Hypothyroidism
(b) Chlorpropamide
(c) Superior vena caval obstruction
(d) Heart failure
(e) Addison's disease

10.26 Low serum sodium concentrations are seen (pages 607–610):
(a) when a sample is taken upstream from an intravenous infusion of 5% dextrose
(b) in hypertriglyceridaemia
(c) in hyperproteinemia
(d) in water retention
(e) in hyperosmolar diabetic coma

10.27 The following statements about the treatment of hyponatraemia are correct (page 610):
(a) Hyponatraemia is almost always actively treated.
(b) It should be corrected rapidly if there is good evidence it developed rapidly.
(c) Rapid treatment of hyponatraemia can result in central pontine myelinolysis.

(d) Restriction of water intake is useful.
(e) Hypertonic saline may be used.

10.28 Causes of hypernatraemia include (Table 10.11):
(a) Lithium
(b) Tetracyclines
(c) Acute tubular necrosis
(d) Diabetes insipidus
(e) Total parenteral nutrition

10.29 Uptake of potassium into cells is stimulated by (page 611):
(a) Insulin
(b) Cell damage
(c) Theophyllines
(d) α-Adrenergic stimulation
(e) Acidosis

10.30 Causes of hypokalaemia include (Table 10.12):
(a) Liquorice
(b) Bartter's syndrome
(c) Salbutamol
(d) Villous adenoma of the colon
(e) Insulin treatment in diabetic ketoacidosis

10.31 Features of Bartter's syndrome include (pages 611–612):
(a) Elevated blood pressure
(b) High urinary potassium
(c) Low plasma renin
(d) Hyperplasia of the juxtaglomerular apparatus
(e) Impairment of sodium and chlorine reabsorption in the thick ascending limb of Henle

10.32 Features of Liddle's syndrome include (page 612):
(a) Hyperkalaemia
(b) Alkalosis
(c) High aldosterone production
(d) Low blood pressure
(e) Potassium wasting

10.33 Correct statements about the management of hypokalaemia include (pages 611–612):
(a) Acute hypokalaemia may correct spontaneously.
(b) Cardiac arrhythmias may require treatment with intravenous potassium.
(c) Intravenous potassium is usually given rapidly.

(d) Failure to correct hypokalaemia may be due to concurrent hypomagnesaemia.

(e) Oral potassium supplements cause gastrointestinal irritation.

10.34 Drugs causing hyperkalaemia include (Table 10.14):
(a) Amiloride
(b) Angiotensin-converting enzyme inhibitors
(c) Cyclosporin
(d) Heparin
(e) Non-steroidal anti-inflammatory drugs

10.35 The following mechanisms of hyperkalaemia are correct (page 613):
(a) Hyporeninaemic hypoaldosteronism – decreased excretion of potassium
(b) Digoxin poisoning – decreased sodium–potassium – ATPase activity
(c) Vigorous exercise – increased release of potassium from cells
(d) Transfusion of stored blood – decreased renal excretion
(e) Tumour lysis – decreased sodium–potassium ATPase activity

10.36 Causes of hyperkalaemia include (Table 10.14):
(a) Addison's disease
(b) Diabetic ketoacidosis
(c) Rhabdomyolysis
(d) Renal failure
(e) Alkalosis

10.37 Causes of spurious hyperkalaemia include (Table 10.14):
(a) Vigorous fist clenching during phlebotomy
(b) Hyporeninaemic hypoaldosteronism
(c) Leukaemia
(d) Thrombocytosis
(e) Digoxin poisoning

10.38 Management of hyperkalaemia includes (Practical box 10.1):
(a) Intravenous calcium gluconate
(b) Dextrose without insulin
(c) Salbutamol
(d) Calcium resonium
(e) Haemodialysis

10.39 Causes of hypomagnesaemia include (Table 10.15):
(a) Diuretics
(b) Alcohol excess
(c) Haemodialysis with high-magnesium dialysate
(d) Digoxin
(e) Prolonged nasogastric suction

10.40 Causes of hypophosphataemia include (Tables 10.17 and 10.18):
   (a) After parathyroidectomy
   (b) Hyperparathyroidism
   (c) Tumour lysis
   (d) Aluminium hydroxide
   (e) Chronic renal failure

10.41 The following statements are correct (pages 616–617):
   (a) In the presence of carbonic anhydrase, carbonic acid dissociates to carbon dioxide and water.
   (b) Maintenance of normal plasma bicarbonate does not depend on the reabsorption of bicarbonate filtered across the glomerular capillaries.
   (c) Proximal tubular bicarbonate reabsorption is catalysed by the sodium–potassium–ATPase pump.
   (d) More acid is secreted into the proximal tubule than into any other nephron segment.
   (e) Most dietary hydrogen ions come from sulphur-containing amino acids.

10.42 The following statements are correct (page 618):
   (a) Secretion of hydrogen ions from the cortical collecting tubule is indirectly linked to sodium reabsorption.
   (b) Aldosterone has several facilitating effects on hydrogen ion secretion.
   (c) Phosphoric acid is the usual titratable urinary buffer.
   (d) In pathophysiological conditions the ammonia buffer system is far more important than titratable acids.
   (e) Glutamine is the primary source of ammonia.

10.43 Correct statements about the anion gap include (page 620):
   (a) It allows identification of whether the acidosis is due to retention of hydrochloric acid or another acid.
   (b) There are more cations than unmeasured anions.
   (c) Albumin makes up the largest portion of unmeasured anions.
   (d) If the anion gap is normal in the presence of acidosis, this suggests that hydrochloric acid is being lost or that sodium bicarbonate is being retained.
   (e) A fall in albumin concentration may increase the anion gap.

10.44 The following associations about the various causes of metabolic acidosis are correct (Table 10.21):
   (a) Acetazolamide – increased gastrointestinal bicarbonate loss
   (b) Hyperparathyroidism – increased gastrointestinal bicarbonate loss
   (c) Increased catabolism of arginine – increased hydrochloric acid production
   (d) Distal tubular renal acidosis – increased renal bicarbonate loss
   (e) Type 4 renal tubular acidosis – increased renal bicarbonate loss

10.45 Causes of proximal renal tubular acidosis include (Table 10.23):
(a) Wilson's disease
(b) Multiple myeloma
(c) Vitamin D deficiency
(d) Lead poisoning
(e) Hyperparathyroidism

10.46 Causes of distal tubular acidosis include (Table 10.24):
(a) Sjögren's syndrome
(b) Medullary sponge kidney
(c) Lithium carbonate
(d) Sickle cell anaemia
(e) Renal transplant rejection

10.47 Causes of metabolic acidosis with a normal anion gap include (Table 10.21):
(a) Uraemia
(b) Diabetic ketoacidosis
(c) Lactic acidosis
(d) Salicylate overdose
(e) Starvation

10.48 Factors that stimulate bicarbonate reabsorption and hydrogen ion excretion despite the presence of alkalosis include (page 623):
(a) Extracellular volume depletion
(b) Potassium excess
(c) Excess mineralocorticoids
(d) Thiazide diuretics
(e) Loop diuretics

10.49 Correct statements about the management of metabolic acidosis include (page 623):
(a) Rapid correction may result in tetany.
(b) The administration of sodium bicarbonate may lead to extracellular volume depletion.
(c) Bicarbonate therapy decreases carbon dioxide production.
(d) Bicarbonate therapy may worsen intracellular acidosis.
(e) Intravenous sodium bicarbonate is routinely given during cardiac arrest.

Cardiovascular Disease

11.1 Correct statements about the cellular basis of myocardial contraction include (page 625):
(a) Each myofibril is made up of a series of sarcomeres.
(b) During cardiac contraction the length of the actin and myosin molecules decreases.
(c) Troponin promotes actin–myosin interaction.
(d) Calcium ions activate troponin C.
(e) Calcium is made available during the plateau phase (phase 2) of the action potential.

11.2 The following statements about Starling's law of the heart are correct (page 626):
(a) It states that the pressure within a sphere is inversely proportional to its radius.
(b) It states that the pressure within a sphere is proportional to the wall stress.
(c) It explains the increase in stroke volume as ventricular end-diastolic volume is raised.
(d) It states that the heart rate is inversely proportion to the blood pressure.
(e) It describes the rate of depolarization in the sinoatrial node.

11.3 Correct statements regarding the conducting system of the heart include (page 626):
(a) The natural heart beat begins in the atrioventricular node.
(b) The His bundle connects the sinoatrial node to the atrioventricular node.
(c) The right bundle has two divisions.
(d) Conduction in the atria is slower than that in the atrioventricular node.
(e) The sinoatrial node is located at the junction of the inferior vena cava and right atrium.

11.4 Correct statements about the nerve supply to the cardiovascular system include (page 627):
(a) The vagus supplies mainly the sinoatrial and atrioventricular nodes.
(b) Adrenergic nerves supply the fibres of the atria, ventricle and conducting system.
(c) β_1 receptors predominate in the vascular smooth muscle.
(d) Cholinergic nerves from the vagus supply mainly the ventricular myocardium via M2 muscarinic receptors.
(e) Under basal conditions vagal inhibitory effects predominate over the sympathetic excitatory effects.

11.5 The following statements about coronary circulation are correct (page 627):
(a) The right coronary artery supplies the posterior left ventricular wall.

(b) The interventricular septum is supplied by both the posterior descending coronary artery and the left anterior descending artery.
(c) The atrioventricular node is usually supplied by the left coronary artery.
(d) The right coronary artery usually supplies the majority of the left ventricle.
(e) The left circumflex artery gives branches to the left atrium.

11.6 In the fetus (page 629):
(a) Pulmonary circulation is important for the oxygenation of blood.
(b) Systemic venous return is a mixture of oxygenated and deoxygenated blood.
(c) Venous blood to the right atrium is deflected through the foramen ovale to the left atrium.
(d) Blood from the pulmonary arteries is diverted to the aorta through the ductus arteriosus.
(e) At birth, inspiration constricts pulmonary arterioles, resulting in a dramatic increase in pulmonary vascular resistance.

11.7 The following statements regarding the normal cardiac cycle are correct (page 629, Fig 11.6):
(a) Atrial contraction precedes atrial depolarization.
(b) PR interval precedes ventricular activation.
(c) Right ventricular contraction starts before left ventricular contraction.
(d) The atrioventricular valves close when the ventricular pressures exceed the atrial pressures.
(e) The tricuspid and mitral valves open after the ventricular pressures have fallen below right and left atrial pressures.

11.8 Dyspnoea (page 630):
(a) is an awareness of breathing
(b) does not occur in healthy people
(c) can be due to respiratory causes
(d) occurring in left ventricular failure is due to a fall in left atrial pressure
(e) is an increase in respiratory rate

11.9 Orthopnoea (page 630):
(a) is breathlessness that occurs with chest pain
(b) occurs because flat posture results in an increased central and pulmonary blood volume
(c) is made worse by abdominal contents pushing up against the diaphragm
(d) improves on lying flat
(e) is a form of paroxysmal nocturnal dyspnoea

11.10 Correct statements about PND include (page 630):
(a) It occurs as a result of the accumulation of fluid in the lungs.
(b) PND is NYHA grade 4.

(c) PND can be excluded if the patient is aroused from sleep.
(d) It can result in blood-tinged sputum.
(e) It is easily discriminated from bronchial asthma by history.

11.11 Cheyne–Stokes respiration is (page 630):
(a) seen in severe heart failure
(b) seen in the elderly without obvious heart failure
(c) seen after morphine administration
(d) related to stimulation of the respiratory centre
(e) alternate hyperventilation and apnoea

11.12 The following statements regarding angina pectoris are correct (pages 630–631):
(a) It literally means a strangling sensation in the chest.
(b) A similar pain that occurs at rest is felt in myocardial infarction.
(c) Sharp pains over the heart are not usually angina.
(d) It may radiate to the teeth, back or abdomen.
(e) It may be associated with heaviness of one or both arms.

11.13 The following statements about chest pain are correct (page 631):
(a) The pain of pericarditis is aggravated by posture.
(b) In da Costa's syndrome anxiety is associated with a left submammary stabbing pain.
(c) Mitral valve prolapse can cause a 'precordial catch'.
(d) Central chest pain similar to angina can occur with pulmonary hypertension.
(e) Chest pain due to oesophageal disease is easily differentiated from that due to heart disease.

11.14 Causes of chest pain include (page 631):
(a) Pulmonary hypertension
(b) Pneumothorax
(c) Pulmonary embolism
(d) Mediastinitis
(e) Costochondritis

11.15 Causes of palpitations include (page 631):
(a) Tachycardia
(b) Bradycardia
(c) Irregular heart rhythm
(d) Lying on the left side
(e) Anxiety

11.16 The following statements regarding premature beats are correct (page 631):
(a) They are usually felt as 'missed beats'.
(b) They are followed by a pause before the next normal beat.

(c) The normal beat following a premature beat is forceful.
(d) They often occur in clusters.
(e) The normal beat following a premature beat has a shorter diastolic filling period.

11.17 Symptoms associated with paroxysmal tachycardias include (page 631):
(a) Presyncope
(b) Syncope
(c) Chest pain
(d) Dyspnoea
(e) Polyuria

11.18 Causes of syncope include (page 631, Table 11.4):
(a) Vasovagal attack
(b) Complete heart block
(c) Aortic stenosis
(d) Rapid supraventricular tachycardia
(e) Mitral regurgitation

11.19 Recognized features of vasovagal syncope include (page 631):
(a) Cough
(b) Bradycardia
(c) Seizures
(d) Recovery within a few seconds
(e) Peripheral vasoconstriction

11.20 Causes of fatigue in cardiovascular practice include (page 631):
(a) β-Blockers
(b) Persistent cardiac arrhythmias
(c) Cyanotic heart disease
(d) Infective endocarditis
(e) Heart failure

11.21 Oedema of heart failure (page 631):
(a) is due to water retention
(b) is due to salt retention
(c) is worse at night
(d) is seen over the sacrum in ambulant patients
(e) in severe cases may be associated with pleural effusion or ascites

11.22 Causes of clubbing include (page 632):
(a) Acute infective endocarditis
(b) Fallot's tetralogy in neonates
(c) Bronchiectasis
(d) Fibrosing alveolitis
(e) Essential hypertension

11.23 The following statements about cyanosis are correct (page 632):
  (a) It is a dusky blue discoloration of the skin and mucous membranes.
  (b) It is due to the presence of unoxygenated haemoglobin.
  (c) It is more readily provoked in the presence of polycythaemia.
  (d) It is more readily provoked when anaemia is present.
  (e) It is a feature of methaemoglobinaemia.

11.24 Causes of central cyanosis include (page 632):
  (a) The presence of sulphaemoglobin
  (b) Essential hypertension
  (c) Secondary hypertension
  (d) Chronic bronchitis
  (e) Left to right cardiac shunts

11.25 The pulse is irregular in (page 633):
  (a) Ventricular tachycardia
  (b) Atrial fibrillation
  (c) Premature beats
  (d) Intermittent heart block
  (e) Sinus arrhythmia

11.26 A small-volume pulse may be felt in (page 633):
  (a) Cardiac failure
  (b) Tachycardia
  (c) Aortic regurgitation
  (d) Shock
  (e) Obstructive vascular disease

11.27 Causes of collapsing pulse include (page 633):
  (a) Aortic stenosis
  (b) Persistent ductus arteriosus
  (c) Thyrotoxicosis
  (d) Anaemia
  (e) Fever

11.28 Recognized causes of pulsus paradoxus include (page 633):
  (a) Cardiac tamponade
  (b) Severe asthma
  (c) Constrictive pericarditis
  (d) Severe heart failure
  (e) Combined aortic stenosis and regurgitation

11.29 The following statements regarding pulsus alternans are correct (page 633):
  (a) The rhythm is irregular.
  (b) Alternate beats are weak and strong.
  (c) When it is due to cardiac failure it indicates a poor prognosis.

(d) When associated with abnormal tachycardia it does not indicate a poor prognosis.
(e) It is a synonym for pulsus bigeminus.

11.30 Correct statements about pulsus bisferiens include (page 634):
(a) It is a palpable double pulse.
(b) It may be seen in hypertrophic obstructive cardiomyopathy.
(c) It may be seen in aortic regurgitation with aortic stenosis.
(d) The first wave is due to transmission of the left ventricular pressure.
(e) The second peak is caused by recoil of the vascular bed.

11.31 The following statements regarding 'normal blood pressure' are correct (page 634):
(a) There is no single blood pressure that is normal in all subjects.
(b) In the resting adult systolic blood pressure does not usually exceed 150 mmHg.
(c) In children pressures are usually higher than adults.
(d) In the elderly rigidity of the arteries produces an increase in diastolic pressure.
(e) Exertion reduces blood pressure.

11.32 The following statements about blood pressure cuffs are correct (page 634):
(a) A small cuff leads to an underestimation of the pressure.
(b) A standard arm cuff is 12 cm wide.
(c) The usual thigh cuff is 15 cm wide.
(d) If an arm cuff is used on the thigh the femoral pressure will be less than the brachial pressure.
(e) A standard arm cuff used in an obese patient will underestimate the pressure.

11.33 The following statements about variations in blood pressure are correct (page 634):
(a) Systolic blood pressure varies by up to 10 mmHg between the right and the left arm.
(b) Standing causes an increase in diastolic pressure.
(c) Standing causes a reduction in systolic pressure.
(d) Blood pressure is variable in atrial fibrillation.
(e) In orthostatic hypotension there is a fall in both systolic and diastolic pressure.

11.34 Pulsatile jugular venous pulse is produced by (page 635):
(a) Superior vena caval obstruction
(b) Constrictive pericarditis
(c) Hypovolaemia
(d) Cardiac tamponade
(e) Heart failure

11.35 The following statements about the jugular venous pressure wave are correct (page 636):
  (a) The *v* wave is produced by ventricular systole.
  (b) The *a* wave occurs immediately after the carotid pulsation.
  (c) The *a* wave is prominent in atrial fibrillation.
  (d) Giant *v* waves are seen in tricuspid regurgitation.
  (e) Steep *y* descent is seen in constrictive pericarditis.

11.36 The following associations are correct (page 636):
  (a) Tapping apex beat – mitral regurgitation
  (b) Thrusting apex beat – aortic regurgitation
  (c) Heaving apex beat – hypertension
  (d) Heaving apex beat – aortic stenosis
  (e) Double apex beat – hypertrophic obstructive cardiomyopathy

11.37 Impalpable apex beat is a feature of (page 636):
  (a) Aortic regurgitation
  (b) Obesity
  (c) Emphysema
  (d) Pleural effusion
  (e) Pericardial effusion

11.38 The following statements about the use of the stethoscope are correct (Table 11.5):
  (a) The bell is useful for high-frequency sounds.
  (b) Early diastolic murmurs are best heard with a diaphragm.
  (c) The fourth heart sound is best heard with a bell.
  (d) The third heart sound is best heard with a diaphragm.
  (e) The opening snap is best heard with a bell.

11.39 The following statements are correct (page 636):
  (a) The first heart sound is best heard at the point which the apex beat is felt.
  (b) The pulmonary component of the second heart sound is best heard in the second interspace just to the right of the sternum.
  (c) The tricuspid area is in the fourth interspace, just to the left of the sternum.
  (d) The murmur of aortic stenosis is best transmitted to the second intercostal space immediately to the right of the sternum.
  (e) The third and fourth right ventricular sounds are heard well in the tricuspid area.

11.40 Causes of a loud first heart sound include (page 634):
  (a) Long PR interval
  (b) Pericardial effusion
  (c) Hyperdynamic circulation

    (d) Mitral stenosis
    (e) Emphysema

11.41 Causes of reverse splitting of the second heart sound include (page 637):
    (a) Left bundle branch block
    (b) Atrial septal defect
    (c) Left ventricular failure
    (d) Aortic stenosis
    (e) In young healthy adults

11.42 The following mechanisms of production of heart sounds are correct (pages 637–638):
    (a) Third heart sound – rapid ventricular filling as soon as the atrioventricular valves open
    (b) Fourth heart sound – ventricular filling that accompanies atrial systole
    (c) Ejection click – sudden opening of a deformed but mobile aortic or pulmonary valve
    (d) Midsystolic click – sudden prolapse of the mitral valve into the left atrium during ventricular systole
    (e) Pericardial knock – early, sudden and marked halting of ventricular filling due to constriction

11.43 Causes of continuous murmurs include (page 639, Table 11.8):
    (a) Venous hum in the neck
    (b) High mammary blood flow in lactating women
    (c) Collateral circulation of coarctation of aorta
    (d) Patent ductus arteriosus
    (e) Atrial septal defect

11.44 The following statements about cardiac murmurs are correct (page 639):
    (a) Austin Flint murmur is due to pulmonary regurgitation.
    (b) Diastolic murmurs are always associated with disease.
    (c) Systolic murmurs occur synchronously with carotid pulsation.
    (d) The intensity of an ejection systolic murmur is greatest in midsystole.
    (e) Early diastolic murmurs are high-pitched in quality.

11.45 The cardiothoracic ratio in a PA chest film may be >50% in (page 640):
    (a) Neonates
    (b) Infants
    (c) Athletes
    (d) Scoliosis
    (e) Funnel chest

11.46 The following associations regarding patterns of specific chamber enlargement seen on chest X-ray are correct (page 641):
    (a) Left atrial dilatation – double atrial shadow to the right of the sternum
    (b) Large left atrium – splaying of the carina of the trachea

(c) Right ventricular enlargement – anterior enlargement on lateral chest X-ray

(d) Left ventricular enlargement – posterior enlargement on lateral chest X-ray

(e) Ascending aortic dilatation – prominence of the aortic shadow to the left of the mediastinum

11.47 Correct statements about calcification in the cardiovascular system include (page 641):

(a) Pericardial calcification results from tuberculous pericarditis.

(b) Left ventricular aneurysms are characteristically devoid of calcification.

(c) Calcification in the descending aorta signifies syphilis.

(d) The pulmonary and tricuspid valves are the most commonly affected.

(e) Coronary arterial calcification is associated with coronary atheroma.

11.48 Causes of pulmonary oligaemia on the chest X-ray include (page 642):

(a) Left to right cardiac shunt

(b) Fallot's tetralogy

(c) Pulmonary stenosis

(d) Pulmonary embolism

(e) Aortic stenosis

11.49 Recognized features of pulmonary venous hypertension on the chest X-ray include (page 642):

(a) Pruning of the pulmonary arteries

(b) Dilatation of the lower lobe pulmonary veins

(c) Kerley B lines

(d) Mottling of the lung fields

(e) Pleural effusion

11.50 The following statements about the ECG are correct (page 644):

(a) The P wave is caused by atrial repolarization.

(b) The PR interval is the length of time from the end of the P wave to the start of the QRS complex.

(c) The QT interval extends from the end of the QRS complex to the end of the T wave.

(d) The ST segment is the period between the end of the QRS complex and the start of the T wave.

(e) The T wave results from ventricular repolarization.

11.51 Indications for exercise electrocardiography include (Table 11.10):

(a) Evaluation of treatment of angina

(b) Unstable angina

(c) Recent myocardial infarction

(d) Severe aortic stenosis

(e) Provocation of cardiac arrhythmias

11.52 The following statements about echocardiography are correct (page 649):
   (a) Congenitally abnormal bicuspid aortic valves show a 'dome' shape in systole.
   (b) In mitral stenosis, the M mode shows restriction and reversal of direction of the posterior leaflet motion.
   (c) In infective endocarditis vegetations less than 2 mm can be detected.
   (d) In hypertrophic obstructive cardiomyopathy there is a displacement of the mitral valve apparatus towards the septum in systole.
   (e) Pericardial effusions cannot be detected.

11.53 In ischaemic heart disease echocardiography is used to diagnose (page 650):
   (a) Abnormalities in coronary artery anatomy
   (b) Left ventricular thrombus
   (c) Mitral papillary muscle rupture
   (d) Abnormalities in ventricular wall motion
   (e) Left ventricular aneurysm

11.54 The following statements are correct (page 651):
   (a) Thallium behaves like potassium.
   (b) A persistent cold spot on thallium redistribution image implies infarction.
   (c) Thallium is taken up by damaged myocardium.
   (d) ^{99m}Tc-labelled sestamibi is a sensitive method of measuring viability.
   (e) Exercise is best avoided during the scan.

11.55 Causes of 'hot spots' in a technetium pyrophosphate scan include (page 652):
   (a) Calcified costal cartilage
   (b) Breast tissue
   (c) Unstable angina
   (d) Complete occlusion of the coronary vessels supplying the infarcted myocardium
   (e) Bone

11.56 The following statements about radionuclide ventriculography are correct (page 652):
   (a) A multigated acquisition scan is obtained by tagging the patient's red blood cell with technetium-99 m.
   (b) A first pass study images the heart as a bolus of isotope makes a single pass through the circulation.
   (c) It allows a crude estimation of the ejection fraction.
   (d) It allows visualization of wall motion.
   (e) A deterioration on exercise suggests ischaemic heart disease or myocardial abnormality.

11.57 The following echocardiographic associations are correct (pages 647–650):
   (a) Congenital aortic stenosis – 'dome'-shaped aortic valves in systole
   (b) Hypertrophic cardiomyopathy – asymmetric septal hypertrophy
   (c) Hypertrophic cardiomyopathy – systolic anterior motion
   (d) Pericardial effusion – echo-free region between myocardium and pericardium
   (e) Aortic aneurysm – dilatation of the aortic root

11.58 Recognized causes of sudden cardiac death include (Information box 11.1, page 645):
   (a) Pulmonary hypertension
   (b) Ventricular fibrillation
   (c) Atrial fibrillation
   (d) Aortic dissection
   (e) Severe bradyarrhythmias

11.59 The following statements about cardiac resuscitation are correct (page 654):
   (a) Single rescuer – cardiac compression at 80 beats/min with two respirations after 15 compressions.
   (b) Two rescuers – continuous compressions at 60 beats/min and one respiration given every five compressions.
   (c) If an intravenous line cannot be established adrenaline may be administered via the endotracheal tube.
   (d) When due to ventricular fibrillation adrenaline is contraindicated.
   (e) Calcium chloride is useful in the management of ventricular fibrillation.

11.60 The main mechanisms of sudden unexpected cardiac arrest include (Information box 11.1):
   (a) Atrial fibrillation
   (b) First-degree heart block
   (c) Asystole
   (d) Ventricular fibrillation
   (e) Electromechanical dissociation

11.61 Correct statements about defibrillation in ventricular fibrillation include (page 655):
   (a) Electrical energy is used for converting to sinus rhythm.
   (b) Initially 200 J are used.
   (c) The patient should be held down by staff during the procedure.
   (d) Two paddles are placed on the chest wall.
   (e) It can convert asystole into sinus rhythm.

11.62 Indications for DC cardioversion include (page 656):
   (a) First-degree AV block
   (b) Bradyarrhythmias
   (c) Atrial flutter

(d) Atrial fibrillation
(e) Ventricular tachycardia

11.63 Right heart bedside catheterization is performed to (page 657):
(a) Improve cardiac output
(b) Treat unstable angina pectoris
(c) Measure cardiac output
(d) Remove fluid from the pericardial space
(e) Measure pulmonary artery wedge pressure

11.64 Tachyarrhythmias (page 658):
(a) of ventricular origin are less symptomatic than supraventricular tachycardias
(b) may occur in apparently normal hearts
(c) with underlying poor cardiac function tend to be more life-threatening
(d) are those in which the heart rate is >72 beats/min
(e) result in hypertension

11.65 The following associations are correct (page 658):
(a) Accelerated automaticity – sinus tachycardia
(b) Triggered activity – ventricular arrhythmia in long QT syndrome
(c) Accelerated automaticity – escape rhythms
(d) Triggered activity – digoxin-induced atrial tachycardias
(e) Re-entry or circus movement – paroxysmal tachycardias

11.66 Sinus arrhythmia (page 659):
(a) is a quickening in the heart rate on inspiration and a decrease in the rate on expiration
(b) results from a fall in parasympathetic tone on inspiration
(c) is due to phasic changes of the sinus discharge rate resulting from fluctuations in autonomic tone
(d) is treated with β-blockers
(e) may be seen in children and young adults

11.67 Recognized features of sick sinus syndrome include (page 660):
(a) Long intervals between consecutive P waves on the ECG
(b) Block at sinoatrial level
(c) Sinus arrest
(d) A combination of fast and slow supraventricular rhythms
(e) Thromboembolism

11.68 The following statements about atrioventricular block are correct (page 660):
(a) First-degree block means that the PR interval is prolonged.
(b) All forms of second-degree block have a similar prognosis.
(c) Wenckebach block is characterized by a progressive increase in the PR interval until a P wave fails to conduct.

(d) Mobitz type II block occurs when some P waves do not conduct, and is not preceded by a progressive increase in the PR interval.
(e) Patients with second-degree atrioventricular block are usually symptomatic.

11.69 The following statements regarding complete heart block are correct (page 661):
(a) Disease in the proximal bundle of His is associated with a narrow QRS complex.
(b) Treatment is essential in narrow complex complete heart block.
(c) Broad complex complete heart block is due to a lesion in the Purkinje network.
(d) Cannon waves are seen in the jugular venous pulse.
(e) A permanent pacemaker should always be inserted in broad complex heart block even if the patient is asymptomatic.

11.70 Recognized features of left bundle branch block include (page 662):
(a) Tall late R waves in leads I and V6
(b) Abnormal Q waves
(c) Deep S wave in lead V1
(d) Widely split second heart sound
(e) Chest pain

11.71 Causes of left bundle branch block include (Table 11.12):
(a) Hyperkalaemia
(b) Aortic regurgitation
(c) Right ventriculotomy
(d) Cardiomyopathy
(e) Ostium secundum atrial septal defect

11.72 Causes of right bundle branch block include (Table 11.12):
(a) Aortic stenosis
(b) Hypertension
(c) Ventricular septal defect
(d) Recurrent pulmonary embolism
(e) Cardiomyopathy

11.73 The following statements about atrial fibrillation are correct (page 664):
(a) It occurs in at least one-third of patients over 65 years of age.
(b) It tends to be paroxysmal in those under the age of 65.
(c) The irregularly irregular pulse is not maintained during exercise.
(d) Thyroid function tests are mandatory in unaccounted atrial fibrillation.
(e) Anticoagulation is advised in patients with underlying mitral valve disease.

11.74 Causes of atrial fibrillation include (page 665):
(a) Hypothyroidism

(b) alcohol toxicity
(c) rheumatic mitral stenosis
(d) pneumonia
(e) no cause

11.75 Carotid sinus massage (Practical box 11.4, page 666):
(a) stimulates vagal efferent discharge
(b) is performed simultaneously on both sides in resistant tachycardias
(c) results in a severe rise in blood pressure in carotid sinus hypersensitivity
(d) is useful in supraventricular tachycardias
(e) is useful in revealing the P-wave pattern of an atrial tachyrhythmia

11.76 In Wolff–Parkinson–White syndrome (pages 667–668):
(a) There is abnormal myocardial bundle connecting the atrium and the ventricle.
(b) The PR interval is prolonged.
(c) Digoxin is the drug of choice to treat associated atrial fibrillation.
(d) Intravenous verapamil will terminate most of the tachycardias.
(e) Amiodarone is ineffective in treating atrial fibrillation.

11.77 Ventricular tachycardia is more likely than a supraventricular tachycardia with a bundle branch block when there is (Table 11.16):
(a) A narrow QRS complex
(b) Atrioventricular dissociation
(c) An upright, bifid QRS complex having a taller second peak in V1
(d) A deep S wave in V6
(e) QRS polarity which is the same in all chest leads

11.78 Features of torsades de pointes include (page 670):
(a) Short duration
(b) Spontaneous conversion of sinus rhythm
(c) Rapid irregular ventricular complexes which change shape and position from upright to an inverted position
(d) Shortened QT interval on ECG between spells of tachycardia
(e) Syncope

11.79 The following statements about anti-arrhythmics are correct (pages 671–673):
(a) Lignocaine increases the rate of sodium entry into the cell.
(b) The mortality in patients treated with flecainide was twice that of controls in post-infarction patients.
(c) Class II drugs enhance the action of catecholamines on the cardiac action potential.
(d) Amiodarone widens action potential duration.
(e) Calcium channel blockers reduce the plateau phase of the action potential.

11.80 The following statements concerning ventricular arrhythmias are correct (page 670):
   (a) If the attack of ventricular fibrillation occurs during the first day or two of an acute myocardial infarction, it is probable that prophylactic therapy will be unnecessary.
   (b) The Lown classification of ventricular premature beats is designed in the setting of an acute myocardial infarction.
   (c) Ventricular ectopics may be ignored in the absence of heart disease.
   (d) An implantable cardioverter–defibrillator device has cut sudden death rate in serious ventricular arrhythmias.
   (e) Verapamil is the drug of choice in ventricular tachycardias.

11.81 The following statements regarding cardiac failure are correct (pages 674–676):
   (a) It is estimated that about 10% of those over the age of 65 have heart failure.
   (b) About half the patients with severe heart failure die within 5 years.
   (c) Myocardial hypertrophy is one of the major adaptations to haemodynamic overload of the left ventricle.
   (d) Apoptosis or programmed cell death occurs in the heart of idiopathic dilated cardiomyopathy.
   (e) Plasma endothelin is depressed in patients with heart failure.

11.82 Causes of high-output cardiac failure include (page 674):
   (a) Aortic stenosis
   (b) Beri beri
   (c) Anaemia
   (d) Thyrotoxicosis
   (e) Paget's disease

11.83 Atrial natriuretic peptides (page 675):
   (a) are potent vasoconstrictors
   (b) are short-chain peptides
   (c) are secreted by the atria in response to distension
   (d) enhance sodium and water retention
   (e) levels falls in heart failure

11.84 Causes of right heart failure include (page 677):
   (a) Chronic lung disease
   (b) Mitral stenosis
   (c) Pulmonary embolism
   (d) Right to left cardiac shunts
   (e) Tricuspid valve disease

11.85 Recognized features of right heart failure include (page 677):
   (a) Raised jugular venous pressure
   (b) Hard nodular hepatomegaly

(c) Dependent pitting oedema
(d) Ascites
(e) Pleural exudate

11.86 Causes of left ventricular failure include (page 677):
(a) Mitral stenosis
(b) Mitral regurgitation
(c) Left ventricular aneurysm
(d) Atrial septal defect
(e) Pulmonary hypertension

11.87 Factors aggravating heart failure include (page 674):
(a) Anaemia
(b) Thyrotoxicosis
(c) Adjustment of heart failure therapy
(d) Pregnancy
(e) Infective endocarditis

11.88 The following statements are correct (page 677):
(a) The most common cause of systolic ventricular dysfunction is hypertension.
(b) Diastolic dysfunction is rarely associated with hypertension.
(c) Diastolic dysfunction and systolic dysfunction rarely coexist.
(d) Cardiac cachexia is associated with an increase in the cytokine tumour necrosis factor-α.
(e) In acute heart failure, severe cardiac failure can occur with relatively normal heart size.

11.89 The following statements regarding the treatment of heart failure are correct (pages 678–680):
(a) Prolonged bed rest is useful.
(b) A low-sodium diet is of questionable value.
(c) Diuretics improve survival in heart failure.
(d) Intravenous administration of frusemide relieves pulmonary oedema by arteriolar vasodilatation reducing afterload, an effect that is independent of its diuretic effect.
(e) Enalapril markedly improve survival in heart failure.

11.90 The following statements regarding the treatment of heart failure are correct (pages 678–680):
(a) Metolazone, a thiazide diuretic, is used in combination with loop diuretics to treat severe and resistant heart failure.
(b) Spironolactone is used in combination with ACE inhibitors when patients have hyperkalaemia.
(c) Combined therapy with hydralazine and oral nitrates is useful when ACE inhibitors are contraindicated.

(d) Amlodipine, a calcium channel blocker, is used in the treatment of cardiac failure of non-ischaemic aetiology.

(e) Reduction of filling pressure using nitrates does not significantly enhance cardiac output.

11.91 The following statements regarding the treatment of heart failure are correct (pages 681–682):

(a) ACE inhibitors are contraindicated in patients with bilateral renal artery stenosis.

(b) Cough due to ACE inhibitors is a result of inhibition of bradykinin metabolism.

(c) Losartan is contraindicated in the elderly.

(d) Carvedilol, a β-blocker, is contraindicated in heart failure.

(e) Intermittent dobutamine therapy may produce long-lasting improvements in symptoms and exercise tolerance at the cost of increased mortality.

11.92 The following statements about digoxin are correct (page 681):

(a) It is a negative inotrope.

(b) It acts by competitive inducement of sodium–potassium–ATPase.

(c) Trough serum levels are monitored to avoid toxicity.

(d) It is particularly beneficial in atrial fibrillation to control atrial rate.

(e) Digoxin toxicity is more prone to occur in liver failure.

11.93 Recognized features of digitalis toxicity include (page 681):

(a) Nausea

(b) Visual disturbances

(c) Ventricular bigeminy

(d) Ventricular tachycardia

(e) Atrioventricular block

11.94 Phosphodiesterase inhibitors (page 682):

(a) promote the breakdown of cyclic AMP

(b) produce an increase in myocardial contractility

(c) cause peripheral vasodilatation

(d) include xamoterol

(e) are deleterious to the myocardial cells when administered long term

11.95 The following statements are correct (page 683):

(a) Heart failure is associated with a fourfold increase in the risk of a stroke.

(b) Patients with asymptomatic left ventricular dysfunction are at risk of progressive deterioration and should be treated with prophylactic ACE inhibitor therapy.

(c) Myocardial hibernation is persistent ventricular dysfunction due to reduced myocardial perfusion, which is sufficient to maintain viability of the heart muscle, i.e. blood flow matches function.

(d) Myocardial stunning is reversible ventricular dysfunction that persists following an episode of ischaemia when blood flow has returned to normal.

(e) It is recommended that all patients with clinical heart failure should receive treatment with diuretics.

11.96 The following statements regarding cardiac transplantation are correct (page 683):

(a) It is the treatment of choice for patients with intractable heart failure whose life expectancy is more than 6 months.

(b) It is a treatment reserved for the elderly.

(c) Less than half the patients survive by the end of 1 year.

(d) Five-year survival following transplantation is less than one-third.

(e) Allograft coronary atherosclerosis is a major cause of long-term graft failure.

11.97 The following statements about the treatment of pulmonary oedema are correct (page 684):

(a) The patient is placed in the supine position.

(b) High-concentration oxygen should not be administered as it causes carbon dioxide retention.

(c) Aminophylline should be avoided in patients with bronchospasm.

(d) Glyceryl trinitrate produces prompt relief by reducing afterload.

(e) Morphine should not be given when the blood pressure is less than 90 mmHg.

11.98 In cardiogenic shock (page 684):

(a) The mortality is high.

(b) The pulmonary capillary wedge pressure is low.

(c) Fluid is administered if the wedge pressure is below 18 mmHg.

(d) Dopamine improves coronary perfusion.

(e) Intra-aortic balloon pump improves long-term mortality.

11.99 Myocardial ischaemia occurs despite normal coronary arteries in (page 685):

(a) Syndrome X

(b) Anaemia

(c) Hypotension

(d) Aortic stenosis

(e) Thyrotoxicosis

11.100 The following statements about atheroma are correct (pages 686–687):

(a) Males are less likely to have atheroma than are premenopausal women.

(b) It affects medium-sized arteries.

(c) Low values of high-density lipoproteins are strongly associated with atheroma.

(d) Angiographic studies suggest that lowering the serum cholesterol can not only slow the progression of coronary atherosclerosis, but can also cause regression of the disease.

(e) The risk from smoking declines to almost normal 2 years after cessation.

11.101 Features of Prinzmetal's angina include (page 687):
(a) It occurs more frequently in men.
(b) It occurs at rest.
(c) Coronary vasodilatation.
(d) ST elevation occurs during pain.
(e) Heart blocks and ventricular tachycardia.

11.102 Features of unstable angina include (Table 11.28):
(a) Worsening angina
(b) Angina at rest
(c) Elevated troponin I
(d) Transient ECG changes
(e) Untreated, a large proportion of such patients develop a myocardial infarction within weeks

11.103 Decubitus angina (page 687):
(a) occurs when the patient sits up
(b) occurs in association with impaired left ventricular function
(c) is associated with severe coronary artery disease
(d) is relieved by standing up
(e) is not relieved by glyceryl trinitrate

11.104 The following statements about resting ECG in angina are correct (page 688):
(a) It is abnormal between attacks.
(b) Transient ST segment depression occurs during an attack.
(c) T-wave inversion occurs during an attack.
(d) A normal ECG between attacks or even during an attack excludes angina pectoris.
(e) Tall, pointed upright T waves occur during an attack.

11.105 Correct statements about exercise ECG include (page 688):
(a) ST segment depression greater than or equal to 1 mm suggests myocardial ischaemia.
(b) The severity of the ECG changes indicate the extent of coronary artery disease.
(c) In the majority of patients with severe coronary artery disease the test is negative.
(d) Stress testing is more reliable in women.
(e) A normal stress test excludes coronary disease.

11.106 The following statements about thallium-201 scanning are correct (page 688):
  (a) It is of little use when the exercise test is equivocal.
  (b) It is useful in deciding whether stenotic vessels on angiography are giving rise to ischaemic areas on exercise.
  (c) A normal perfusion scan after exercise makes significant coronary artery disease unlikely.
  (d) Thallium is taken up by damaged myocardium.
  (e) A persistent cold spot indicates infarction.

11.107 Indications for coronary angiography include (Table 11.26):
  (a) Angina refractory to medical therapy
  (b) Severely abnormal exercise ECG
  (c) Unstable angina
  (d) Angina occurring after myocardial infarction
  (e) Myocardial infarction in patients under 50 years of age

11.108 The following statements about coronary angioplasty are correct (page 690):
  (a) It is a technique for dilating atheromatous obstructions of the coronary artery using a balloon.
  (b) It is useful for isolated, proximal, non-calcified atheromatous obstruction.
  (c) Multiple lesions cannot be treated by this procedure.
  (d) One-third of patients develop restenosis within 6 months after the procedure.
  (e) Intracoronary stents are used for the primary treatment of coronary stenoses.

11.109 Correct statements about coronary artery bypass surgery include (page 691):
  (a) It is performed by mobilizing the left internal mammary artery and implanting it into the left anterior descending artery distal to the obstruction.
  (b) Surgery provides dramatic relief from angina in only a small number of those operated on.
  (c) Surgery is not indicated when the left main stem is the only vessel affected.
  (d) When the ventricular function is normal surgical mortality is low.
  (e) There is evidence that diabetic patients have a better 5-year survival after treatment with bypass surgery than with PTCA.

11.110 The following statements regarding the treatment of variant angina are correct (page 689):
  (a) β-Blockers are useful.
  (b) Calcium antagonists should be avoided.
  (c) Surgery is the treatment of choice in such patients.

(d) Arrhythmias provoked by spasm are best ignored.
(e) Nitrates are useful.

11.111 Correct statements regarding the treatment of unstable angina include (page 692):
    (a) It should not be treated vigorously as it has a benign prognosis.
    (b) Aspirin decreases the incidence of both death and myocardial infarction.
    (c) Early coronary artery angiography is desirable.
    (d) Heparin is best avoided in such patients.
    (e) Infusion of glycoprotein IIb/IIIb inhibitors is contraindicated.

11.112 Myocardial infarction (pages 692–693):
    (a) is the most common cause of death in the UK
    (b) is painless in about a fifth of patients
    (c) occurs because of sudden coronary thrombosis
    (d) is associated with polymorphonuclear leucocytosis
    (e) is associated with a raised ESR

11.113 Silent myocardial infarction is seen in (page 693):
    (a) healthy, young individuals
    (b) the elderly
    (c) hypertensives
    (d) diabetics
    (e) smokers

11.114 Creatine kinase (page 694):
    (a) peaks within 24 hours after an infarct
    (b) returns to normal before 48 hours
    (c) has an MM fraction which is specific for heart muscle damage
    (d) intramuscular injections causes a rise in CK–MB levels
    (e) cardioversion can increase both the total CK and the MB isoenzyme fraction

11.115 Correct statements about cardiac troponins include (page 695):
    (a) They have a very high specificity for cardiac injury.
    (b) They are released within 2–4 hours after cardiac injury.
    (c) They can persist up to 7 days after injury.
    (d) They are not raised in unstable angina.
    (e) They are increased in hypertension.

11.116 Abnormal Q wave is a recognized feature of (page 693):
    (a) Wolff–Parkinson–White syndrome
    (b) A normal ECG in lead a VL
    (c) Subendocardial infarction
    (d) Left bundle branch block
    (e) Ventricular tachycardia

11.117 Correct statements about streptokinase in myocardial infarction include (page 695, Table 11.30):
(a) It achieves an early reperfusion rate in 50–70% of patients.
(b) Proliferative diabetic retinopathy is a contraindication.
(c) It achieves a 25% reduction in mortality if administered within 4 hours following the onset of symptoms.
(d) A good history of myocardial infarction is sufficient to administer this drug.
(e) Aspirin should be avoided with this drug as it increases the risk of fatal bleeding.

11.118 The following statements about left ventricular aneurysm are correct (page 698):
(a) It should be suspected if there is persistent ST segment elevation in the ECG.
(b) Diagnosis is confirmed by M-mode echocardiography.
(c) It is an early complication of myocardial infarction.
(d) Aneurysectomy may be necessary if embolic complications occur.
(e) It may be a source of arrhythmias.

11.119 Correct statements about the eligibility to drive vehicles after myocardial infarction include (page 696):
(a) All patients should have an exercise test before resuming driving.
(b) Car driving is not permitted for 6 weeks following myocardial infarction.
(c) Heavy goods vehicle driving licences are withdrawn pending evaluation of the patient's status.
(d) It is the physician's duty to notify the DVLC that the patient has had an MI.
(e) There are no restrictions on driving after myocardial infarction in those under the age of 55.

11.120 The non-cardiac features of rheumatic fever include (page 611):
(a) Fleeting polyarthritis
(b) Arthralgia
(c) Chorea
(d) Erythema marginatum
(e) Subcutaneous nodules

11.121 Treatment of acute rheumatic fever includes (page 700):
(a) Bed rest
(b) Parenteral penicillin, even if nasal or pharyngeal swabs do not culture streptococci
(c) Low-dose aspirin
(d) Systemic steroids if carditis is present
(e) Oral phenoxymethyl penicillin

11.122 Mitral stenosis (page 700):
   (a) is almost always due to rheumatic heart disease
   (b) is more common in women
   (c) is usually symptomatic when the valve orifice area is reduced to 2 cm^2
   (d) is the most common valve lesion due to rheumatic fever
   (e) is associated with malar flush

11.123 Complications of mitral stenosis include (page 701):
   (a) Atrial fibrillation
   (b) Systemic embolization
   (c) Left ventricular failure
   (d) Chest infection
   (e) Pulmonary hypertension

11.124 Auscultatory features of mitral stenosis include (page 702):
   (a) Midsystolic murmur
   (b) Soft first heart sound
   (c) Presystolic murmur
   (d) Opening snap
   (e) Loud second heart sound

11.125 The following statements regarding the treatment of mitral stenosis are correct (page 703):
   (a) Closed valvotomy is preferred to open valvotomy.
   (b) Mild mitral stenosis may not need treatment other than therapy for acute attacks of bronchitis.
   (c) Atrial fibrillation should not be anticoagulated unless there is evidence of thromboembolism.
   (d) Closed valvotomy is advised when the valves are mobile, non-calcified, and there is no associated regurgitation.
   (e) Cardiopulmonary bypass is required for closed valvotomy.

11.126 Indications for valve replacement in mitral stenosis include (page 703):
   (a) Associated mitral regurgitation
   (b) Severely calcified valve
   (c) Associated systemic hypertension
   (d) Pulmonary hypertension
   (e) Tricuspid stenosis

11.127 Causes of mitral regurgitation include (pages 703–704):
   (a) Myocardial infarction
   (b) Rheumatic heart disease
   (c) Infective endocarditis
   (d) Hypertrophic cardiomyopathy
   (e) Collagen disorders

11.128 Physical signs of mitral regurgitation include (page 704):
  (a) Loud first heart sound
  (b) Pansystolic murmur
  (c) Tapping apex beat
  (d) Prominent third heart sound
  (e) Mid-diastolic murmur

11.129 The following statements about mitral valve prolapse are correct (page 705):
  (a) Mild forms should be regarded as a normal variant.
  (b) It is more common in young men.
  (c) It is also known as Barlow's syndrome.
  (d) It is seen in hypertrophic cardiomyopathy.
  (e) It is seen in rheumatic heart disease.

11.130 Recognized clinical features of mitral valve prolapse include (page 705):
  (a) Atypical chest pain
  (b) Palpitations
  (c) Mid-diastolic click
  (d) Ejection systolic murmur
  (e) Pansystolic murmur

11.131 Causes of valvular aortic stenosis include (page 706):
  (a) Bicuspid aortic valve
  (b) Rheumatic fever
  (c) Infective endocarditis
  (d) Calcification of the aortic valve
  (e) Hypertrophic cardiomyopathy

11.132 Clinical features of aortic stenosis include (page 706):
  (a) Pansystolic murmur
  (b) Systolic ejection click
  (c) Syncope
  (d) Reversed splitting of second heart sound
  (e) Prominent fourth heart sound

11.133 The following statements about the treatment of aortic stenosis are correct (page 708):
  (a) Patients should be encouraged to participate in a strenuous fitness programme.
  (b) Angina is treated with β-blockade.
  (c) Nitrates are the cornerstone of treatment for associated angina.
  (d) Antibiotic prophylaxis against infective endocarditis is not essential.
  (e) Valve replacement in severe aortic stenosis is recommended even if the patient is asymptomatic.

11.134 Causes of chronic aortic regurgitation include (Table 11.36):
- (a) Ankylosing spondylitis
- (b) Rheumatic heart disease
- (c) Syphilis
- (d) Rheumatoid arthritis
- (e) Marfan's syndrome

11.135 Causes of acute aortic regurgitation include (Table 11.36):
- (a) Osteogenesis imperfecta
- (b) Ruptured sinus of Valsalva aneurysm
- (c) Aortic dissection
- (d) Acute rheumatic fever
- (e) Reiter's syndrome

11.136 The following associations are correct (page 708):
- (a) Quincke's sign – capillary pulsation in the nailbeds
- (b) De Musset's sign – head nodding with each heartbeat
- (c) Duroziez's sign – systolic bruit over the femoral arteries when the stethoscope is applied lightly
- (d) Pistol-shot femorals – a sharp bang over the femoral arteries in time with each heartbeat
- (e) Austin Flint murmur – mid-diastolic murmur

11.137 Causes of tricuspid regurgitation include (pages 709–710):
- (a) Systemic hypertension
- (b) Infective endocarditis
- (c) Carcinoid syndrome
- (d) Blunt trauma to the chest
- (e) Ebstein's anomaly

11.138 Extracardiac manifestations of infective endocarditis include (page 712):
- (a) Arthralgia
- (b) Focal glomerulonephritis
- (c) Roth's spots
- (d) Splenic infarcts
- (e) Osler's nodes

11.139 Organisms known to cause infective endocarditis include (page 711):
- (a) *Staphylococcus aureus*
- (b) *Staphylococcus epidermidis*
- (c) *Coxiella burnetii*
- (d) *Streptococcus viridans*
- (e) *Enterococcus faecalis*

11.140 Indications for surgery in infective endocarditis include (page 714):
- (a) Extensive damage to a valve
- (b) Worsening heart failure

(c) Worsening renal failure
(d) Failure to culture an organism and the infection persists
(e) Large vegetations

11.141 The following associations regarding aetiological factors of congenital cardiac disease are correct (page 714):
(a) Paternal rubella – persistent ductus arteriosus
(b) Maternal rubella – pulmonary stenosis
(c) Maternal alcohol abuse – septal defects
(d) Turner's syndrome – coarctation of the aorta.
(e) Down's syndrome – mitral valve defect

11.142 Clinical features of Eisenmenger's reaction include (pages 714–715):
(a) Clubbing of fingernails
(b) Paradoxical embolism
(c) Growth retardation
(d) Syncope
(e) Squatting

11.143 Ventricular septal defect (page 715):
(a) is the commonest congenital cardiac malformation
(b) is known as *maladie de Roger* when the defect is large
(c) when small can close spontaneously
(d) is usually due to a defect in the muscular part of the interventricular septum
(e) causes a long loud diastolic murmur

11.144 The following statements about atrial septal defect are correct (page 716):
(a) It is more common in men.
(b) It causes a wide and fixed split second heart sound.
(c) It is characterized by left bundle branch block.
(d) It is treated surgically once secondary pulmonary hypertension develops.
(e) It is complicated by atrial arrhythmias.

11.145 Persistent ductus arteriosus (page 716):
(a) is associated with paternal rubella
(b) is more common in males
(c) is more common in premature babies
(d) is treated with indomethacin in premature infants
(e) is treated surgically only if it fails to close by the age of 5

11.146 Recognized features of coarctation of the aorta include (page 717):
(a) More common in women
(b) Association with Turner's syndrome
(c) Bicuspid aortic valve

(d) Claudication
(e) Hypertension

11.147 The following are the features of Fallot's tetralogy (page 718):
(a) Hypertension
(b) Right ventricular hypertrophy
(c) Right ventricular outflow obstruction
(d) Overriding aorta
(e) Central cyanosis

11.148 Causes of pulmonary hypertension include (page 642):
(a) Chronic lung disease
(b) Increased pulmonary blood flow because of a right to left shunt
(c) Left ventricular failure
(d) Pulmonary thromboembolic disease
(e) Mitral valve disease

11.149 Clinical features of pulmonary hypertension include (page 722):
(a) Exertional chest pain
(b) Heaving apex beat
(c) Loud second heart sound
(d) Prominent *v* waves in the jugular venous pulse
(e) Graham–Steell murmur

11.150 Conditions predisposing to pulmonary emboli include (page 719):
(a) Pelvic and lower limb fractures
(b) Malignant disease
(c) Factor V Leiden deficiency
(d) Oral contraceptives
(e) Atrial fibrillation

11.151 Clinical features of pulmonary emboli include (page 720):
(a) Central chest pain
(b) Systemic hypertension
(c) Tachypnoea
(d) Syncope
(e) Bradycardia

11.152 Causes of cor pulmonale include (Table 11.39):
(a) Morbid obesity
(b) Poliomyelitis
(c) Pulmonary stenosis
(d) Recurrent pulmonary emboli
(e) Sleep apnoea syndrome

11.153 Clinical features of atrial myxoma are (page 723):
(a) Fever

(b) Syncope
(c) Third heart sound
(d) Soft first heart sound
(e) Elevated ESR

11.154 Factors causing myocarditis include (page 723):
  (a) Coxsackie virus
  (b) *Toxoplasma gondii*
  (c) Lead
  (d) *Cornybacterium diphtheriae*
  (e) *Trypanosoma cruzi*

11.155 Dilated cardiomyopathy is associated with the following (page 724):
  (a) Friedreich's ataxia
  (b) Haemochromatosis
  (c) Doxorubicin therapy
  (d) Pompe's disease
  (e) Systemic sclerosis

11.156 Hypertrophic cardiomyopathy is associated with (Table 11.40, page 726):
  (a) Mutations of β-myosin
  (b) Noonan's syndrome
  (c) Friedreich's ataxia
  (d) Mitrochondrial myopathies
  (e) Glycogen storage disease

11.157 Causes of pericarditis include (page 727):
  (a) Coxsackie B virus
  (b) Tuberculosis
  (c) Malignancy
  (d) Uraemia
  (e) *Haemophilus influenzae*

11.158 Recognized clinical features of constrictive pericarditis include (page 727):
  (a) Ascites
  (b) Hepatomegaly
  (c) Dependent oedema
  (d) Kussmaul's sign
  (e) Friedreich's sign

11.159 Causes of hypertension include (pages 730–731):
  (a) Addison's disease
  (b) Hypopituitarism
  (c) Conn's syndrome
  (d) Phaeochromocytoma
  (e) Obesity

11.160 ACE inhibitors (page 735):
  (a) are best avoided in the presence of bilateral renal artery stenosis
  (b) act by blocking the conversion of angiotensin I to angiotensinogen
  (c) are potent vasoconstrictors
  (d) are used in the treatment of heart failure
  (e) are used in the treatment of hypotension

11.161 Side effects of ACE inhibitors include (page 735):
  (a) Cough
  (b) Metallic taste
  (c) Glycosuria
  (d) First-dose hypotension
  (e) Leucocytosis

11.162 Relative contraindications to β-blockers include (page 735):
  (a) Diabetes
  (b) Asthma
  (c) Bradycardia
  (d) Heart block
  (e) Peripheral vascular disease

11.163 Side effects of methyldopa include (page 736):
  (a) Dry mouth
  (b) Impotence
  (c) Positive Coombs' test
  (d) Chronic active hepatitis
  (e) Fluid retention

11.164 The risk from hypertension is worse in (pages 730–736):
  (a) Those with a high HDL
  (b) Younger patients rather than the old
  (c) Women rather than men
  (d) Those with renal impairment
  (e) The presence of retinal changes

11.165 The following may be regarded as normal in the elderly (page 737):
  (a) A fourth heart sound
  (b) A systolic ejection murmur
  (c) Left axis deviation
  (d) Short PR interval
  (e) Loud first heart sound

11.166 The following conditions are largely confined to the elderly (pages 737–738):
  (a) Atrial fibrillation
  (b) Aortic sclerosis
  (c) Mitral annulus calcification

(d) Fibrosis and calcification of the His–Purkinje conduction system
(e) Non-infective endocarditis

11.167 In pregnancy (page 738):
(a) The cardiac output increases from the second month.
(b) The blood volume decreases from 8 weeks up to the 30th week.
(c) The pulse pressure falls.
(d) A third heart sound may be heard.
(e) The diastolic pressure may be lower owing to vasodilatation.

11.168 Pregnancy (page 738):
(a) should be terminated before the 16th week in severe mitral stenosis
(b) is poorly tolerated in patients with small septal defects
(c) in patients with pulmonary hypertension has a high mortality
(d) in those with prosthetic valves will require a change from oral anticoagulants to heparin
(e) can cause hypertension

11.169 Management of chronic ischaemia of the legs includes (page 739):
(a) Anticoagulants
(b) Aspirin.
(c) Local heat to the limbs
(d) Surgery within 3 months of the onset of symptoms to prevent the rapid progression of disease to gangrene
(e) Vasodilators

11.170 Abdominal aortic aneurysms (page 740):
(a) are usually due to atheroma
(b) should be ignored if they are asymptomatic
(c) may cause epigastric pain
(d) have a low mortality even when they rupture
(e) can present with back pain

11.171 Dissection of the aorta (page 740):
(a) in the majority of cases starts in the ascending aorta
(b) presents with chest pain which is easily distinguishable from that of myocardial infarction
(c) is less likely in pregnancy
(d) may cause widening of the mediastinum on the chest X-ray
(e) results in elevation of cardiac enzymes

11.172 Raynaud's phenomenon (page 741):
(a) consists of spasm of the arteries of the digits
(b) can result in gangrene in severe cases
(c) is seen in systemic sclerosis
(d) can occur in cryoglobulinaemia
(e) is treated using β-blockers

11.173 Anticoagulants in deep vein thrombosis (page 742):
- (a) are controversial for below-knee thrombi
- (b) do not affect the thrombus that is already present
- (c) are beneficial in patients with thrombi above the knee
- (d) are administered to promote clot lysis
- (e) are administered for about 3 months.

Respiratory Disease

12.1 The diaphragm (page 748):
   (a) lacks the slow-twitch type of muscle fibre
   (b) is supplied by both the phrenic nerves
   (c) has muscle fibres that arise from the lower ribs
   (d) is relatively resistant to fatigue
   (e) consists predominantly of smooth muscle fibres

12.2 The nose (page 749):
   (a) moistens and heats the inhaled air
   (b) removes particulate matter greater than 10 μm
   (c) secretes many protective proteins in the form of antibodies, lysozomes and interferon
   (d) removes most noxious gases almost completely during nasal breathing
   (e) has cilia which are vestigial

12.3 Neural stimuli influencing respiration arise from (Fig. 12.7):
   (a) Limb receptors
   (b) Pulmonary stretch receptors
   (c) Capillary juxtapulmonary receptors
   (d) Receptors in muscles and joints of the chest wall
   (e) the brain stem

12.4 The following chemicals stimulate respiration (Fig. 12.7):
   (a) Nitrogen
   (b) Carbon dioxide
   (c) Oxygen
   (d) Hydrogen ions in the venous blood
   (e) Sulphur dioxide

12.5 The airway tone (page 750):
   (a) is maintained by vagal efferent nerves
   (b) is highest in the mid-afternoon
   (c) is influenced by catecholamines, although the sympathetic fibres do not directly innervate the airways
   (d) is not reduced by atropine or β-adrenoreceptor agonists in a normal subject
   (e) shows an exaggeration of normal responsiveness in asthma with no change in circadian rhythm

12.6 The airways (pages 750–751):
   (a) affected in chronic bronchitis are the small airways
   (b) distend slightly during quiet breathing
   (c) at the periphery close completely along with central airways during a cough

(d) at the periphery are prevented from collapsing by pursed lip respiration in emphysema
(e) are hyperreactive in asthma

12.7 Causes of finger clubbing include (Table 12.3):
(a) Cyanotic heart disease
(b) Cirrhosis
(c) Pulmonary fibrosis
(d) Bronchiectasis
(e) Chronic bronchitis

12.8 Causes of collapse of the lung include (Table 12.4):
(a) Postoperative retention of secretions
(b) Emphysema
(c) Tumours
(d) Chronic bronchitis
(e) Inhaled foreign bodies

12.9 Causes of round shadows in the lung on chest X-ray include (Table 12.5):
(a) Lung abscess
(b) Aspergilloma
(c) Carcinoma of the bronchus
(d) Arteriovenous malformation
(e) Lipoma

12.10 Causes of miliary mottling include (page 760):
(a) Pneumoconiosis
(b) Tuberculosis
(c) Sarcoidosis
(d) Fibrosing alveolitis
(e) Pulmonary microlithiasis

12.11 CT scan of the chest is useful in (page 760):
(a) Assessing intrathoracic spread of bronchial carcinoma
(b) Diagnosis of lymphangitis carcinomatosa
(c) Diagnosis of bronchiectasis
(d) Assessing whether the patient with carcinoma of the bronchus is suitable for surgery
(e) Determining the aetiology of mediastinal lymph node enlargement

12.12 Radioisotope lung scanning (page 761):
(a) using macroaggregated human albumin is useful in determining lung ventilation
(b) using Xenon-133 at the same time as a perfusion scan allows comparison of ventilation and perfusion
(c) with a ventilation perfusion scan is useful in detecting pulmonary emboli

(d) is the gold standard in the diagnosis of pulmonary emboli
(e) is of particular value in detecting pulmonary emboli when the chest X-ray is normal in suspected pulmonary embolism

12.13 Peak expiratory flow rate (page 762):
(a) records maximum expiratory flow rate within the first 2 ms of expiration
(b) is an accurate measure of airflow limitation
(c) detects restrictive lung defects
(d) is measured using a mini-Wright peak-flow meter
(e) is an expensive test and is measured only in cases where the diagnosis is difficult

12.14 Forced expiratory volume in 1 second (page 762):
(a) is a good measure of the residual volume
(b) is expressed as a percentage of the forced vital capacity
(c) in normal subjects is around 75%
(d) is reduced in the same proportion as the forced vital capacity in restrictive lung disease
(e) is measured using a mini-Wright peak-flow meter

12.15 Transfer factor (page 764):
(a) reflects the uptake of oxygen from the alveolus into the red blood cell
(b) is measured using carbon monoxide
(c) is unaffected by lung volume in health
(d) is increased in emphysema and lung fibrosis
(e) is useful in the early detection of sarcoidosis

12.16 The indications for fibreoptic bronchoscopy include (page 766):
(a) Sarcoidosis
(b) Recurrent laryngeal nerve palsy
(c) Mediastinal tumours
(d) Haemoptysis
(e) Collection of bronchial secretions for cytology and bacteriology

12.17 The dangers of cigarette smoking include (Table 12.7):
(a) Increased birthweight in infants
(b) Bladder cancer
(c) Memory problems
(d) An increase in abnormal spermatozoa
(e) Carcinoma of the oesophagus

12.18 Foreign bodies (page 773):
(a) usually impact in the left main bronchus
(b) cause lung abscess
(c) are commonly inhaled after excess alcohol consumption

(d) produces a polyphonic wheeze

(e) in the trachea may be removed in an emergency using the Heimlich manoeuvre

12.19 Influenza (page 773):

(a) virus belongs to the orthomyxovirus group

(b) virus B is the cause of worldwide pandemics

(c) can cause prolonged debility and depression

(d) rarely causes post infectious encephalomyelitis

(e) vaccine produces lasting protection

12.20 Chronic bronchitis (page 775):

(a) is defined as a productive cough for at least 3 months in a year for 2 successive years

(b) patients tend to be 'pink puffers'

(c) predominantly affects the small airways

(d) rarely causes cor pulmonale, unlike emphysema

(e) when severe leads to carbon dioxide retention

12.21 Emphysema (page 776):

(a) is abnormal dilatation and destruction of lung tissue distal to the terminal bronchioles

(b) does not cause airflow limitation as it is associated with the dilatation of the airways

(c) results in α_1-antitrypsin deficiency

(d) results in increased total lung capacity

(e) results in increased gas transfer

12.22 Cor pulmonale (pages 719–723):

(a) is characterized by left ventricular failure secondary to lung disease

(b) results in central cyanosis due to right to left shunt

(c) is rarely associated with pulmonary hypertension

(d) is seen in long-standing mitral stenosis

(e) is complicated by acute left ventricular failure

12.23 The recognized physical findings of hypercapnia include (page 777):

(a) Peripheral vasoconstriction

(b) Papilloedema

(c) Asterixis

(d) Coma

(e) Collapsing pulse

12.24 The sensation of breathlessness can be reduced by (page 780):

(a) Paracetamol

(b) Promethazine

(c) Dihydrocodeine

(d) A combination of dihydrocodeine and oxygen
(e) Morphine in terminal cases

12.25 The mechanisms of nocturnal hypoxia in COPD are (page 780):
(a) Inhibition of intercostal and accessory muscles in REM sleep
(b) Shallow breathing in REM sleep
(c) Increased upper airway resistance
(d) Bronchodilatation
(e) Stimulation of the respiratory centre

12.26 Recognized clinical features of obstructive sleep apnoea include (Table 12.11):
(a) Hypersomnolence
(b) Restless sleep
(c) Morning headache
(d) Impotence
(e) Apposition of the tongue and palate to the posterior pharyngeal wall

12.27 Bronchiectasis is a complication of (Table 12.12):
(a) Chronic bronchial sepsis
(b) 'Immotile cilia' syndrome
(c) Cystic fibrosis
(d) Measles
(e) Whooping cough

12.28 Antibiotics found to be useful in *Pseudomonas aeruginosa* infections include (page 782):
(a) Ampicillin
(b) Oral gentamicin
(c) Carbenicillin
(d) Tobramycin
(e) Inhaled ceftazidime

12.29 Complications of bronchiectasis include (page 782):
(a) Cerebral abscess
(b) Pneumonia
(c) Empyema
(d) Pneumothorax
(e) Massive haemoptysis

12.30 Cystic fibrosis (page 783):
(a) is a dominantly inherited disorder
(b) has a carrier frequency of 1 in 2000 in Caucasians
(c) results from a gene mutation on the short arm of chromosome 7
(d) results from a deletion of the codon for phenylalanine
(e) patients have a defective transmembrane regulator protein

12.31 Recognized clinical features of cystic fibrosis include (page 784):
  (a) Structurally abnormal lungs at birth
  (b) Nasal polyps
  (c) Cirrhosis
  (d) Accelerated puberty in males
  (e) Cholesterol gall stones

12.32 The diagnosis of cystic fibrosis in adults depends on the clinical history, together with (page 784):
  (a) A sweat sodium concentration below 60 mmol/L
  (b) Intact epididymis and vas deferens
  (c) A family history of α_1-antitrypsin deficiency
  (d) Blood DNA analysis of the gene defect
  (e) Increased sodium levels in bronchial secretions

12.33 Recognized features of asthma include (pages 785–786):
  (a) Reversible obstruction to airflow in the intrathoracic airways
  (b) More frequent as individuals become more 'westernized'
  (c) Left ventricular failure
  (d) Hypercholesterolaemia
  (e) Systemic hypertension

12.34 Recognized precipitating factors of asthma include (Fig 12.31):
  (a) Isocyanates
  (b) Aspirin
  (c) Cold air
  (d) Rhinovirus infections
  (e) Emotion

12.35 Atopy includes a group of disorders (page 786):
  (a) that run in families
  (b) that have common wealing skin reactions to common allergens in the environment
  (c) that have circulating antibody in their serum which could be transferred to the skin of the non-sensitized individual
  (d) readily develop antibodies of the IgG class against common materials present in the environment
  (e) such as hay fever

12.36 Allergens precipitating asthma (page 787):
  (a) are similar to those in rhinitis
  (b) include the faeces of the house dust mite
  (c) include spores from *Aspergillus fumigatus*
  (d) are derived from the use of 'biological' washing powders
  (e) include those from flour and grain

12.37 Recognized causes of airway hyperreactivity to methacholine include (page 787):
(a) Exercise-induced asthma
(b) Wheeze following viral infection
(c) Allergic rhinitis
(d) Asthma provoked by pollen
(e) Sarcoidosis

12.38 Extrinsic asthma (page 786):
(a) implies no causative agent
(b) occurs in atopic individuals
(c) is often seen with eczema in childhood
(d) positive skin tests to inhaled allergens tend to be more common in adults than in children
(e) usually starts in middle age

12.39 Recognized clinical features of asthma include (page 790):
(a) Symptoms that are virtually identical to those suffering from airflow limitation caused by COPD
(b) Nocturnal cough
(c) Polyuria
(d) Wheeze
(e) Cough as the predominating symptom

12.40 The following statements about investigations in asthma are correct (page 790):
(a) Peak expiratory flow charts are useful to study the effect of work exposure.
(b) Exercise tests have been used in the diagnosis of asthma in children.
(c) Methacholine bronchial provocation tests should be limited to those with a FEV_1 <1.5 l.
(d) A substantial improvement in severe airway limitation on treatment with steroids excludes the presence of an asthmatic component.
(e) There are no diagnostic features of asthma on the chest X-ray.

12.41 Management of asthma includes (page 791):
(a) Children should be prevented from taking part in games because of their asthma.
(b) Rehousing of those with severe uncontrollable asthma to high altitudes where mites cannot survive.
(c) Rapid identification of extrinsic causes of asthma and their removal wherever possible (e.g. the family pet).
(d) Avoidance of aspirin in all asthmatics.
(e) Hyposensitization, which is a very effective form of treatment, as for allergic rhinitis.

12.42 Drug treatment in asthma (pages 793–795):
  (a) by the effective use of inhalers ensures that most of the aerosolized material enters the respiratory tract
  (b) is best delivered as aerosols, avoiding first-pass metabolism in the liver and resulting in lower doses and fewer side effects
  (c) with aerosols in the 1960s resulted in an increase in sudden deaths, as this is an ineffective method of administering bronchodilators
  (d) includes the use of β-adrenoceptor blockers
  (e) with ketotifen should be reserved for severe asthma

12.43 Correct statements about the management of asthma include (page 793):
  (a) Leukotriene receptor antagonists are contraindicated.
  (b) Methotrexate improves lung function in some steroid-dependent asthmatics.
  (c) Antibiotics are helpful in the management of patients who suffer from properly diagnosed asthma.
  (d) Inhaled corticosteroids can result in subcapsular cataract formation.
  (e) Yellow or green sputum containing eosinophils and bronchial epithelial cells in acute asthma indicates infection and antibiotic therapy must be instituted.

12.44 Inhaled steroids in asthma (page 793):
  (a) should be reserved for those not responding to oral steroid therapy
  (b) may result in hoarseness of voice due to the effect of corticosteroids on laryngeal muscle
  (c) cause no significant long-term unwanted effects
  (d) are indicated in those who continue to have symptoms in spite of treatment with a β_2-adrenoceptor agonist and sodium cromoglycate
  (e) can cause oral candidiasis

12.45 Patients with severe asthma may have (page 793):
  (a) bradycardia
  (b) pulsus alternans
  (c) silent chest
  (d) peak expiratory flow rate < 50% of predicted normal or best
  (e) wheeze

12.46 Pneumonia (page 794):
  (a) is defined as an inflammation of the lungs
  (b) is usually caused by bacteria
  (c) presents as a chronic illness with cough, purulent sputum and fever
  (d) associated mortality has dramatically decreased with the advent of antibiotics
  (e) is described as atypical when caused by agents such as *Mycoplasma*, influenza A virus, *Chlamydiae* and *Coxiella burnetii*.

12.47 Recognized precipitating factors of pneumonia include (page 795):
    (a) Cigarette smoking
    (b) Alcohol
    (c) Parainfluenza viral infection
    (d) Cystic fibrosis
    (e) Oesophageal obstruction

12.48 Recognized clinical features of pneumonia caused by *Streptococcus pneumoniae* include (page 795):
    (a) A preceding history of viral pneumonia
    (b) Herpes labialis
    (c) Dry cough
    (d) Rust-coloured sputum
    (e) Pleural rub

12.49 The following are true of chest X-rays in pneumonia (page 795):
    (a) X-ray changes may be minimal at the start of the illness.
    (b) Consolidation may remain on the chest X-ray for several weeks after the patient is clinically cured.
    (c) The chest X-ray always returns to normal within 6 weeks, except in patients with severe airflow limitation.
    (d) Persistent changes on chest X-ray after 6 weeks suggest a bronchial abnormality such as carcinoma.
    (e) Chest X-rays should be repeated at least two or three times a week during the acute illness.

12.50 *Mycoplasma* pneumonia patients (page 796):
    (a) are uncommon in the teens and 20
    (b) may have headache and malaise precede the chest symptoms
    (c) show a strong correlation between the X-ray appearances and their clinical state
    (d) have an elevated white blood cell count
    (e) may have cold agglutinins

12.51 Extrapulmonary manifestations of *Mycoplasma* pneumonia include (page 796):
    (a) Myocardial infarction
    (b) Erythema multiforme
    (c) Vomiting and diarrhoea
    (d) Haemolytic anaemia
    (e) Meningoencephalitis

12.52 *Haemophilus influenzae* pneumonia (page 796):
    (a) tends to occur in those with chronic bronchitis and emphysema
    (b) can be diffuse or confined to one lobe
    (c) has special features that separate it from other bacterial causes of pneumonia

(d) responds well to treatment with cefaclor
(e) causes haemoptysis during exacerbation of chronic bronchitis

12.53 *Chlamydia psittaci* pneumonia (page 797):
(a) typically occurs in those working with infected parrots
(b) has a very low-grade course over several months
(c) may cause rose spots on the abdomen
(d) is confirmed by the demonstration of a rising titre of complement-fixing antibody
(e) is treated with tetracycline as the antibiotic of choice

12.54 Recognized clinical features of staphylococcal pneumonia include (page 797):
(a) Patchy areas of consolidation
(b) Pneumothorax
(c) Empyema
(d) Metastatic abscesses in other organs
(e) Pleural effusion

12.55 Q-fever (page 797):
(a) is caused by *Branhamella catarrhalis*
(b) rarely has systemic symptoms
(c) can be complicated by endocarditis
(d) is associated with multiple lesions on the chest X-ray
(e) diagnosis is made by an increase in the titre of complement-fixing antibody

12.56 *Legionella* pneumonia tends to occur (page 797):
(a) In immunocompromised individuals
(b) In fit individuals living in accommodation where shower facilities have been contaminated with the organism
(c) Sporadically
(d) In elderly male smokers
(e) In hospitals

12.57 Recognized features of *Legionella pneumophilia* infection include (page 798):
(a) Dry cough
(b) Confusion
(c) Diarrhoea
(d) Hypernatraemia
(e) Lymphopenia with marked leucocytosis

12.58 *Klebsiella* pneumonia usually occurs in the elderly with a history of (page 798):
(a) Heart disease
(b) Lung disease

    (c) Diabetes
    (d) Alcohol excess
    (e) Malignancy

12.59 Recognized features of *Klebsiella* pneumonia include (page 798):
    (a) The lower lobes are more commonly affected
    (b) Sudden onset
    (c) Bloodstained sputum
    (d) Bulging of the fissures on the lateral chest X-ray
    (e) Low mortality

12.60 *Pseudomonas aeruginosa* (page 798):
    (a) infection correlates with a worsening clinical condition in those with cystic fibrosis
    (b) infection may be seen after cytotoxic chemotherapy
    (c) may simply represent contamination from the upper airways
    (d) is treated with a combination of tobramycin and piperacillin
    (e) can also be treated with ciprofloxacin

12.61 Recognized features of *Pneumocystis carinii* pneumonia include (pages 798–799):
    (a) Diarrhoea
    (b) Weight loss
    (c) Shortness of breath
    (d) Marked hypercapnia
    (e) Diffuse alveolar and interstitial shadowing beginning in the perihilar region

12.62 Shadows on the chest X-ray in patients with AIDS can result from (page 799):
    (a) Kaposi's sarcoma
    (b) *Mycobacteria avium intracellulare*
    (c) Cytomegalovirus
    (d) Non-specific interstitial pneumonitis
    (e) Lymphoid interstitial pneumonia

12.63 Mendelson syndrome (page 799):
    (a) is the acute regurgitation of gastric contents into the oesophagus
    (b) can be fatal
    (c) can complicate anaesthesia
    (d) occurs more often in pregnancy
    (e) can be severe owing to the destructiveness of gastric acid

12.64 Predisposing factors for aspiration pneumonia include (page 800):
    (a) Reflux oesophagitis
    (b) Oesophageal stricture
    (c) Bulbar palsy

(d) Sleep
(e) Tracheo-oesophageal fistula

12.65 Pathological features of tuberculous granulomas include (page 802):
(a) Peripheral caseation
(b) Epithelioid cells
(c) Langhans' giant cells
(d) Predominantly neutrophil infiltration
(e) Lymphocytes

12.66 Recognized clinical features of primary tuberculosis include (page 802):
(a) Collapse
(b) Bronchiectasis
(c) Meningitis
(d) Cavitation
(e) Miliary tuberculosis

12.67 The Mantoux test (page 802):
(a) is of value in the diagnosis of TB
(b) is used for contact tracing
(c) is positive in sarcoidosis
(d) is based on cell-mediated immunity
(e) uses old tuberculin for testing

12.68 Tuberculous acid-fast bacilli (page 804):
(a) are cultured on Dover's medium
(b) are cultured on Lowenstein–Jensen medium
(c) require at least 4–8 weeks to be cultured
(d) cultures to determine antibiotic sensitivity require about 7–12 weeks
(e) are stained with Ziehl–Nielsen stain

12.69 BCG (page 805):
(a) is a non-virulent bovine strain of *Mycobacterium tuberculosis*
(b) decreases the risk of developing tuberculosis by about 70%
(c) is only given to individuals who are tuberculin positive
(d) vaccination is not recommended until the age of 13 years
(e) vaccination is an important reason why the Mantoux test is of little value in clinical practice for the subsequent diagnosis of active disease

12.70 When the tuberculin test (page 806):
(a) is positive in an adult and the chest X-ray is negative, nothing more need be done
(b) is positive in a child antituberculous treatment is instituted
(c) is negative in a child it is repeated at 6 weeks; if it remains negative then BCG is administered

(d) is positive in a patient with HIV infection who has not had BCG, chemoprophylaxis with isoniazid is given
(e) is positive in a child it is repeated at 6 weeks

12.71 Greater emphasis is placed on contact tracing in TB (page 806):
(a) Of all close family members who share the same kitchen and bathroom facilities
(b) In those over the age of 35
(c) In Irish
(d) In Asians
(e) In Scots

12.72 Correct statements about the management of tuberculosis include (page 804):
(a) Bed rest improves the outcome of the disease.
(b) Pyrazinamide is valuable in preventing subsequent relapse.
(c) In pulmonary TB a combination of isoniazid and rifampicin is given for 6 months.
(d) Primary drug resistance is seen in immigrants to the UK.
(e) In HIV-infected patients treatment is with conventional therapy, but using four rather than three adverse drugs.

12.73 The following associations between these drugs and unwanted effects are correct (page 805):
(a) Isoniazid – stains body secretions pink
(b) Rifampicin – induces liver enzymes
(c) Pyrazinamide – hepatic toxicity
(d) Ethambutol – dose-related retrobulbar neuritis
(e) Isoniazid – damage to the vestibular nerve

12.74 Causes of pulmonary granulomas include (page 806):
(a) Sarcoidosis
(b) Talc
(c) Tuberculosis
(d) Helminthic infections
(e) Fungal infections

12.75 Aetiological factors suggested for sarcoidosis include (page 807):
(a) Atypical mycobacteria
(b) *Mycobacterium tuberculosis*
(c) Epstein–Barr virus
(d) Pine pollen
(e) Fungus

12.76 Immunopathological features of sarcoidosis include (page 807):
(a) Decreased CD4 helper cells in bronchoalveolar lavage
(b) Low circulating T lymphocytes

(c) Depressed cell-mediated reactivity to *Candida* spp.
(d) Overall lymphocytosis
(e) Increased alveolar macrophages but they represent a reduced percentage of the total number of cells.

12.77 Recognized features of sarcoidosis include (page 807):
(a) Bilateral hilar lymphadenopathy on chest X-ray
(b) Erythema marginatum
(c) Lupus vulgaris
(d) Parotid enlargement
(e) Anterior uveitis

12.78 The following statements about sarcoidosis are correct (page 808):
(a) Chest X-ray is normal with abnormal lung function tests.
(b) Lung infiltration may be present on chest X-ray, with lung function tests in the normal range.
(c) Sarcoidosis is the most common cause of erythema nodosum.
(d) The association of bilateral hilar lymphadenopathy with erythema nodosum occurs only in sarcoidosis.
(e) The Kveim test is more sensitive and more specific than transbronchial biopsy.

12.79 Lung function tests in pulmonary sarcoidosis show (page 808):
(a) An increase in total lung capacity
(b) A decrease in FEV_1
(c) An increase in FVC
(d) An increase in residual capacity
(e) A decrease in gas transfer

12.80 Death from sarcoidosis can result from (page 809):
(a) Renal damage
(b) Myocardial damage
(c) Cor pulmonale
(d) Respiratory failure
(e) Lupus pernio

12.81 Clinical manifestations of neurosarcoidosis include (pages 808, 1077):
(a) Myopathy
(b) Peripheral neuropathy
(c) Chronic meningo encephalitis
(d) Bilateral seventh-nerve palsies
(e) Myelopathy

12.82 The following statements about the management of sarcoidosis are correct (page 808):
  (a) Hilar lymphadenopathy on its own with no evidence of chest X-ray involvement of the lungs or decrease in lung function tests does not require treatment.
  (b) Persisting infiltration on the chest X-ray or abnormal lung function tests are unlikely to improve without corticosteroid treatment.
  (c) Steroids are contraindicated in neurosarcoidosis.
  (d) Severe erythema nodosum of sarcoidosis will respond to prednisolone therapy.
  (e) Controlled trials have clearly demonstrated that steroids are beneficial in sarcoidosis that is not improving spontaneously.

12.83 Recognized features of eosinophilic granuloma include:
  (a) It is a fatal disease of infancy
  (b) Dyspnoea and cough
  (c) Decreased gas transfer
  (d) Recurrent pneumothorax
  (e) Granulomas in the bone

12.84 Recognized features of Hand–Schüller–Christian disease include:
  (a) It begins over the age of 5 years
  (b) Bony defects
  (c) Exophthalmos
  (d) Diabetes insipidus
  (e) Diffuse nodular shadows and hilar adenopathy on the chest X-ray

12.85 Recognized features of Wegener's granulomatosis include (page 810):
  (a) Nasal mucosal ulceration
  (b) Migratory pulmonary infiltrates on chest X-ray
  (c) Cavitation on chest X-ray
  (d) Necrotizing glomerulonephritis
  (e) Benign prognosis and most cases do not require treatment

12.86 Pulmonary manifestations of rheumatoid arthritis include (Fig 12.40):
  (a) Obliterative bronchiolitis
  (b) Small airways disease
  (c) Diffuse fibrosing alveolitis
  (d) Cavitation on the chest X-ray
  (e) Pleural thickening

12.87 Correct statements about ANCA include (page 810):
  (a) They are characteristically absent in vasculitides associated with neutrophil infiltration of the vessel wall.
  (b) Proteinase-3 ANCA produce a perinuclear stain.

(c) When MPO ANCA are positive in patients with anti glomerular membrane progressive glomerulonephritis they are more likely to suffer from pulmonary haemorrhage.

(d) ANCA are more likely to be negative in Wegner's granulomatosis limited to the respiratory tract.

(e) ANCA are usually positive in Churg–Strauss syndrome.

12.88 Pulmonary manifestations of systemic sclerosis include (page 810):

(a) Diffuse fibrosis of alveolar walls on autopsy

(b) Honeycomb lung on chest X-ray

(c) Poor gas transfer

(d) Granulomas

(e) Aspiration pneumonia

12.89 Allergens implicated in pulmonary eosinophilia include (page 811):

(a) *Ascaris lumbricoides*

(b) *Strongyloides*

(c) Aspirin

(d) Penicillin

(e) Nitrofurantoin

12.90 Diseases caused by *Aspergillus fumigatus* include (Fig 12.41):

(a) Proximal bronchiectasis

(b) Fungus ball in an old cavity

(c) Recurrent segmental collapse

(d) Upper lobe fibrosis

(e) Chronic bronchitis

12.91 Recognized features of Churg–Strauss syndrome include (page 810):

(a) Usually occurs in females

(b) Asthma

(c) Vasculitis of the small arteries and veins

(d) ANCA are usually negative

(e) Eosinopenia

12.92 Recognized features of Goodpasture's syndrome include (page 813):

(a) Acute glomerulonephritis

(b) Haemoptysis

(c) Renal failure

(d) Antiglomerular basement membrane antibodies are found in the serum

(e) Liver failure

12.93 Pulmonary fibrosis may (page 813):

(a) follow unresolved pneumonia

(b) be seen in tuberculosis

(c) be due to busulphan

(d) be due to propranolol

(e) be idiopathic

12.94 Clinical features of fibrosing alveolitis include (pages 813–815):

(a) Systemic hypertension

(b) Cor pulmonale

(c) Clubbing

(d) Fine end-inspiratory crackles

(e) Wheeze

12.95 Diseases associated with fibrosing alveolitis include (page 813):

(a) Chronic active hepatitis

(b) Coeliac disease

(c) Renal tubular acidosis

(d) Systemic sclerosis

(e) Primary pulmonary hypertension

12.96 Histological features of cryptogenic fibrosing alveolitis include (page 813):

(a) Cellular infiltration of the alveolar walls

(b) Thining of the alveolar walls

(c) Fibrosis of the alveolar walls

(d) Increased type I pneumocytes within the alveolar space

(e) Increased macrophages within the alveolar space

12.97 Growth factors implicated in the pathogenesis of cryptogenic fibrosing alveolitis include (page 813):

(a) Fibronectin

(b) Platelet-derived growth factor

(c) Transforming growth factor-β

(d) Insulin-like growth factor I

(e) Glucagon

12.98 Recognized features of cystic fibrosis include:

(a) Respiratory function tests show an obstructive defect.

(b) Gas transfer is increased.

(c) Blood gases show normal $P_a\text{co}_2$.

(d) Blood gases show decreased $P_a\text{co}_2$.

(e) ESR is elevated.

12.99 Causes of honeycomb lung include (Table 12.16):

(a) Tuberous sclerosis

(b) Neurofibromatosis

(c) Histiocytosis X

(d) Berylliosis

(e) Asbestosis

12.100 Recognized features of extrinsic allergic alveolitis include (page 815):
   (a) Raised polymorphonuclear leucocyte count in acute cases
   (b) Precipitating antibodies in the serum
   (c) Decreased gas transfer
   (d) Increased lymphocytes and granulocytes on bronchoalveolar lavage
   (e) Honeycomb lung

12.101 Drugs known to precipitate asthma include (Table 12.18):
   (a) Amiodarone
   (b) Busulphan
   (c) Tartrazine
   (d) Iodine-containing contrast media
   (e) Aspirin

12.102 Drugs known to induce pulmonary eosinophilia include (Table 12.18):
   (a) Phenytoin
   (b) Carbamazepine
   (c) Chlorpropamide
   (d) Tetracycline
   (e) Sulphonamides

12.103 Drugs known to induce an SLE-like syndrome include (Table 12.18):
   (a) Propranolol
   (b) Hydralazine
   (c) Procainamide
   (d) Isoniazid
   (e) Para-aminosalicylic acid

12.104 Progressive massive fibrosis (page 817):
   (a) can develop even after exposure to coal dust has ceased
   (b) shows a mixed restrictive and obstructive ventilatory defect
   (c) is due to *Mycobacterium tuberculosis*
   (d) may have positive rheumatoid factor
   (e) may have antinuclear factor

12.105 Asbestos (page 819):
   (a) is a mixture of silicates of iron, magnesium, nickel, cadmium and aluminium
   (b) particularly blue asbestos, has been implicated in the development of mesotheliomas
   (c) and cigarette smoking together increase the risk of bronchial carcinoma fivefold
   (d) can cause mesothelioma 40 years after exposure
   (e) induced mesothelioma patients are eligible for compensation

12.106 The following statements about byssinosis are correct (page 819):
   (a) It is caused by exposure to pure cotton.

(b) It starts on the first day back at work after a break.
(c) It worsens as the duration of exposure increases.
(d) There is progressive dilatation of the airways.
(e) It is due to endotoxins from bacteria present on raw cotton.

12.107 Metastatic complications of bronchogenic carcinoma include (page 821):
(a) Bone pain
(b) Pathological fractures
(c) Gynaecomastia
(d) A change in personality
(e) Epilepsy

12.108 Non-metastatic endocrine manifestations of bronchogenic carcinoma include (Table 12.22):
(a) Ectopic prednisolone secretion
(b) Syndrome of inappropriate secretion of antidiuretic hormone
(c) Hypocalcaemia
(d) Hypoglycaemia
(e) Thyrotoxicosis

12.109 Non-metastatic neurological manifestations of bronchogenic carcinoma include (Table 12.22):
(a) Cerebellar degeneration
(b) Peripheral neuropathy
(c) Myasthenic syndrome
(d) Polymyopathy
(e) Myelopathy

12.110 The following statements about the treatment of bronchogenic carcinoma are correct (page 822):
(a) Surgery is the only treatment of value for localized non-small cell carcinoma.
(b) Radiotherapy should be avoided as it causes devastating radiation pneumonitis.
(c) Chemotherapy increases survival in small cell carcinoma.
(d) Prednisolone is given in terminally ill patients to improve appetite.
(e) Morphine should not be dispensed regularly as it leads to drug addiction.

12.111 Primary sites for metastatic lung tumours include (page 824):
(a) Kidney
(b) Cervix
(c) Ovary
(d) Bone
(e) Prostate

12.112 Causes of a solitary round shadow on chest X-ray include (page 824):
  (a) Secondary from renal carcinoma
  (b) Primary bronchial carcinoma
  (c) Tuberculoma
  (d) Hydatid cyst
  (e) Cardiac failure

12.113 Bornholm's disease (page 825):
  (a) is also known as epidemic myalgia
  (b) is caused by Coxsackie B virus
  (c) is common in young adults
  (d) causes pleuritic chest pain
  (e) the chest X-ray is normal

12.114 Causes of transudate include (page 825):
  (a) Hypothyroidism
  (b) Bacterial pneumonia
  (c) Constrictive pericarditis
  (d) Nephrotic syndrome
  (e) Heart failure

12.115 Causes of exudate include (page 825):
  (a) Meig's syndrome
  (b) Carcinoma of the bronchus
  (c) Pulmonary infarction
  (d) Yellow nail syndrome
  (e) Tuberculosis

12.116 Spontaneous pneumothorax (page 826):
  (a) usually occurs in young females
  (b) occurs in short and fat individuals
  (c) occurs in those with underlying emphysema
  (d) occurs as a complication of bronchial asthma
  (e) occurs as a complication of bronchogenic carcinoma

12.117 Causes of unilateral diaphragmatic paralysis include (page 826):
  (a) Poliomyelitis
  (b) Carcinoma of the bronchus
  (c) Herpes zoster
  (d) Syphilis
  (e) Subclavian vein puncture

12.118 Causes of bilateral diaphragmatic paralysis include (page 826):
  (a) Multiple sclerosis
  (b) Motor neurone disease
  (c) Guillain–Barré syndrome

(d) Traumatic quadriplegia
(e) Subclavian vein puncture

12.119 A 38-year-old man is seen in the respiratory clinic with shortness of breath and a dry cough. Pulmonary function tests are as follows: FVC 1.8 L, 40% predicted; FEV_1 1.6 L, 49% predicted; FEV_1/FVC 85%, TLC 2.6, 40% predicted; residual volume 0.78, 41% predicted; and D_LCO 4.5, 15% predicted. The following investigations are appropriate (pages 745–828):
(a) Methacholine test for bronchial hyperreactivity
(b) Gallium scan of the lungs
(c) Antinuclear antibody
(d) Open lung biopsy
(e) Arterial blood gas

12.120 A 61-year-old smoker and alcoholic presents to A and E and his PA and lateral chest X-rays reveal an infiltrate in the right posterior lower lobe. His job involves excavation at an old building site. The history excludes the following as the cause of his infiltrate (pages 745–828):
(a) *Staphylococcus aureus*
(b) Anaerobic organisms
(c) *Legionella* spp.
(d) Bronchogenic carcinoma
(e) Tuberculosis

12.121 A 71-year-old man presents with a chronic recurrent cough. Recognized causes of this condition are (pages 745–828):
(a) Congestive cardiac failure
(b) Bronchial asthma
(c) Gastro-oesophageal reflux
(d) Postnasal drip
(e) Duodenal ulcer

12.122 In a 70-year-old man with wheeze the arterial blood gas analysis showed PO_2 60 mmHg, PCO_2 76 mmHg, bicarbonate 25 mEq/L, and pH 7.2. His blood pressure was 260/110 mmHg. The following statements are correct (pages 745–828):
(a) This patient has respiratory acidosis.
(b) He should be treated with 90–100% oxygen.
(c) This patient has an acute exacerbation of chronic bronchitis.
(d) His blood pressure should be treated with atenolol.
(e) A V/Q scan will confirm pulmonary emboli.

12.123 The follow statements regarding the prognosis of sarcoidosis are correct (pages 806–809):
(a) It is worse in American blacks.
(b) The disease remits by 2 years in over two-thirds of patients with hilar adenopathy alone.

(c) The disease remits by 2 years in approximately half the patients with X-ray evidence of pulmonary infiltration without any demonstrable lymphadenopathy.

(d) The disease remits by 2 years in only one-third of patients with hilar adenopathy plus chest X-ray appearance of pulmonary infiltration.

(e) It is worse in those with increased gas transfer.

12.124 Long-term oxygen therapy will benefit patients who (pages 779–780):

(a) have a P_aCO_2 of more than 8 kPa

(b) have COAD with an FEV$_1$ of less than 1.2 L

(c) have carboxyhaemoglobin of less than 3%

(d) have a P_aO_2 of less than 9 kPa

(e) are administered oxygen therapy for 19 hours a day

12.125 The following statements about the respiratory tree are correct (page 746):

(a) The trachea is 10–12 cm in length.

(b) There are about 25 divisions in all between the trachea and alveoli.

(c) Cartilage is present in the first seven divisions of the bronchioles.

(d) The term small airways refers to bronchioles of less than 2 mm.

(e) There are 30 000 small airways in an average lung.

12.126 The following statements about the respiratory alveoli are correct (pages 746–747):

(a) There are approximately 300 million alveoli in each lung.

(b) The total surface area of the alveoli is 40–80 m^2.

(c) Type II pneumocytes are thought to be the source of surfactant.

(d) The alveoli of adjoining lobules communicate by the pores of Kohn.

(e) Each respiratory bronchiol supplies 200 alveoli.

12.127 The following statements about a typical normal adult at rest are correct (page 750):

(a) The pulmonary blood flow of 5 L/min carries 11 mmol/min of oxygen from the lungs to the tissues.

(b) The normal pressure of oxygen in arterial blood is between 11 and 13 kPa (83 and 98 mmHg).

(c) The normal pressure of carbon dioxide in arterial blood is between 4.8 and 6 kPa (36–45 mmHg).

(d) Ventilation at about 6 L/min carries 9 mmol/min of carbon dioxide out of the body.

(e) Respiratory rate is less than 22 per minute.

12.128 Transtracheal aspiration (page 759):

(a) involves pushing a needle through the cricothyroid membrane, through which a catheter is threaded to a position just above the carina

(b) rarely, induces coughing

(c) is useful for assessing lower respiratory tract infection

(d) is a technique used to induce anaesthesia

(e) is a technique used to administer noradrenaline in cardiac arrest

Intensive Care Medicine

13.1 Oxygen flux (page 830):
    (a) is defined as the total amount of oxygen delivered to the tissues per unit time
    (b) is independent of the volume of blood flowing through the microcirculation per minute
    (c) is dependent on the arterial oxygen content
    (d) is independent of the oxygen capacity of haemoglobin
    (e) is dependent on the partial pressure of oxygen

13.2 When the heart rate increases (page 830):
    (a) The duration of systole decreases
    (b) The duration of diastole increases
    (c) Stroke volume falls, especially when the heart rate is over 160 bpm
    (d) There is a small increase in myocardial oxygen consumption
    (e) The time available for ventricular filling increases

13.3 Factors determining stroke volume include (page 831):
    (a) The tension of the myocardial fibres at the end of diastole
    (b) Myocardial contractility
    (c) The tension of the myocardial wall during systolic ejection
    (d) Oxyhaemoglobin dissociation curve
    (e) Packed cell volume

13.4 Afterload of the left ventricle is determined by (page 831):
    (a) Stroke volume
    (b) Resistance imposed by the aortic valve
    (c) Peripheral vascular resistance
    (d) Elasticity of the major blood vessels
    (e) Arteriovenous oxygen content difference

13.5 The following statements are correct (page 831):
    (a) The main factor influencing the preload is the venous return.
    (b) Myocardial oxygen consumption increases only slightly with an increase in preload.
    (c) Right ventricular afterload is normally negligible.
    (d) Tachycardia may precipitate ischaemia in areas of the myocardium that had reduced coronary perfusion.
    (e) At any given preload, decreasing the afterload increases the stroke volume.

13.6 The sigmoid shape of the oxyhaemoglobin dissociation curve is important because (page 831):
    (a) Falls in P_aO_2 may be tolerated provided that the percentage saturation remains above 90%.

(b) Increasing the P_aO_2 to above normal has only a minimal effect on oxygen content unless hyperbaric oxygen is administered.

(c) Once the P_aO_2 is on the steep slope of the curve, a small decrease can cause large falls in oxygen content.

(d) Once the P_aO_2 is on the steep slope slight increases can lead to useful increases in oxygen saturation.

(e) It directly influences stroke volume.

13.7 The following statements about inspired alveolar air are correct (page 832):

(a) It is fully devoid of water vapour at body temperature.

(b) The partial pressure of CO_2 is approximately 5.3 kPa.

(c) The partial pressure of oxygen is 13.4 kPa.

(d) Because of the reciprocal relationship between the partial pressures of oxygen and carbon dioxide in the alveoli, a small increase in alveolar oxygen tension can be produced by lowering the alveolar carbon dioxide.

(e) The partial pressure of water is 6.3 kPa at normal body temperature.

13.8 Pathological causes of an alveolar–arterial oxygen difference include (page 832):

(a) Blood bypassing the lungs via the bronchial and thebesian veins

(b) Ventilation/perfusion mismatch

(c) Thinning of the alveolar capillary membrane

(d) Left to right cardiac shunts

(e) Fallot's tetralogy

13.9 Recognized causes of shock include (Table 13.2):

(a) Pulmonary embolus

(b) Restricted cardiac filling

(c) Burns

(d) Sepsis

(e) Coarctation of the aorta

13.10 The sympathoadrenal response to shock results in (Fig 13.8, page 833):

(a) Decrease in heart rate

(b) Decreased systemic resistance

(c) Decreased venous capacitance

(d) Increase in myocardial contractility

(e) Sodium and water excretion

13.11 Endocrine responses to shock include (page 834):

(a) Inhibition of growth hormone release

(b) Release of ACTH

(c) Inhibition of vasopressin release

(d) Release of glucagon

(e) Release of cortisol

13.12 Mediators released in shock include (page 834):
- (a) Prostacyclin
- (b) Thromboxane A_2
- (c) Prostaglandin $F_{2\alpha}$
- (d) Platelet-activating factor
- (e) Tumour necrosis factor

13.13 The following statements are correct (page 835):
- (a) Constitutive nitric oxide synthase is involved in the physiological regulation of vascular tone.
- (b) Inducible nitric oxide synthase is responsible for the sustained vasodilatation that characterizes septic shock.
- (c) Neuronal nitric oxide synthase is an important regulator of myocardial blood flow.
- (d) Selectins are involved in the initiation of leucocyte rolling on vascular endothelium.
- (e) Intercellular adhesion molecules (ICAMs) are involved in the formation of a secular bond which leads to leucocyte migration into tissues.

13.14 Circulatory changes in the early stages of septic shock include (page 835):
- (a) Vasodilatation
- (b) Arteriovenous shunting
- (c) Increased capillary permeability
- (d) Low peripheral resistance
- (e) High cardiac output

13.15 In shock not due to sepsis (pages 835–836):
- (a) There is constriction of the precapillary arterioles in the initial stages.
- (b) There is constriction of the postcapillary venules in the initial stages.
- (c) There is relaxation of the precapillary sphincters when the shock persists.
- (d) There is a relaxation of the postcapillary venules when the shock persists.
- (e) Interstitial oedema occurs when the shock persists.

13.16 Haematological changes in shock include (page 836):
- (a) Increased viscosity
- (b) Activation of the complement cascade
- (c) Platelet aggregation
- (d) Liberation of fibrinogen degradation products
- (e) Conversion of plasmin to plasminogen

13.17 Factors damaging the vascular endothelium in shock include (page 836):
- (a) Microemboli
- (b) Complement activation
- (c) Extravascular leucocyte migration

    (d) Disseminated intravascular coagulation
    (e) Vasoactive compounds

13.18 Metabolic changes in shock include (page 836):
    (a) Fall in blood fatty acids
    (b) Lactic acid enters the Krebs' cycle
    (c) Respiratory acidosis
    (d) Decrease in catecholamine levels
    (e) Fall in blood amino acids

13.19 Shock may result in (page 837):
    (a) Liver failure
    (b) Adult respiratory distress syndrome
    (c) Renal failure
    (d) High cardiac output
    (e) Cardiovascular collapse

13.20 Recognized features of hypovolaemic shock include (page 837):
    (a) Warm peripheries
    (b) Polyuria
    (c) Bradycardia
    (d) Sweating
    (e) Metabolic acidosis

13.21 Typical features of anaphylactic shock include (page 838):
    (a) Warm peripheries
    (b) Urticaria
    (c) Bronchospasm
    (d) Oedema of the face, pharynx and larynx
    (e) Hypovolaemia

13.22 Complications of radial artery cannulation include (Practical box 13.1):
    (a) Hypovolaemia secondary to disconnection
    (b) Vascular occlusion secondary to accidental injection of drugs
    (c) Digital necrosis
    (d) Loss of arterial pulsation
    (e) Thrombosis

13.23 The following statements are correct (pages 839–841).
    (a) Central venous pressure (CVP) measures the patient's circulating volume and the contractile state of the myocardium.
    (b) Fluid challenge to a hypovolaemic patient will result in a fall in CVP.
    (c) Fluid challenge to a normovolaemic patient results in a slight rise in CVP.
    (d) In congestive cardiac failure the central venous pressure is low.
    (e) Fluid challenge in cardiac failure results in a fall in CVP.

13.24 Recognized complications of internal jugular vein occlusion include (Practical box 13.1):
(a) Thrombosis
(b) Pneumothorax
(c) Accidental arterial puncture
(d) Damage to the right thoracic duct
(e) Air embolism

13.25 Complications of Swan–Ganz catheters include (Table 13.3, page 842):
(a) Benign arrhythmias
(b) Endocarditis
(c) Valve trauma
(d) Pulmonary infarction
(e) Pulmonary artery rupture

13.26 The Swan–Ganz catheter measures (page 842):
(a) Pulmonary artery systolic pressures.
(b) Pulmonary artery end-diastolic pressure
(c) Pulmonary capillary wedge pressure
(d) Cardiac output
(e) Aortic diastolic pressure

13.27 Recognized complications of blood transfusion include (page 844):
(a) Hypercalcaemia
(b) Hyperkalaemia
(c) Hypothermia
(d) Decreased oxygen affinity
(e) Impaired coagulation

13.28 Colloidal solutions which have been used for volume expansion include (page 844):
(a) Normal saline
(b) Dextrans
(c) Plasma protein fraction
(d) Gelatin solutions
(e) Hydroxyethyl starch

13.29 The following associations regarding these cardiac inotropes are correct (page 845):
(a) Adrenaline – low doses action on β-adrenergic receptors predominate
(b) Noradrenaline – predominantly an α-adrenergic agonist
(c) Isoprenaline – β-adrenergic antagonist
(d) Dopamine – acts on β-adrenegic and α receptors
(e) Dopexamine – activates DA_1 and DA_2 receptors

13.30 The following statements are correct (page 845):
  (a) When haemodynamic monitoring is not available, adrenaline is the agent of choice in septic shock.
  (b) Bicarbonate should be avoided in extreme persistent metabolic acidosis.
  (c) Isoprenaline is the agent of choice in the management of the critically ill adult.
  (d) Dopexamine causes renal vasoconstriction.
  (e) A combination of dobutamine and noradrenaline should be avoided in patients who are shocked with a low systemic resistance.

13.31 Vasodilator therapy (page 847):
  (a) increases afterload
  (b) reduces systolic ventricular wall tension
  (c) increases myocardial oxygen requirements
  (d) decreases heart size
  (e) improves coronary blood flow

13.32 The following statements are correct (page 848):
  (a) Hydralazine predominantly affects arterial resistance vessels.
  (b) α-Adrenergic antagonists predominantly dilate arterioles.
  (c) Sodium nitroprusside dilates arterioles and venous capacitance vessels.
  (d) Nitrates are predominantly arterial dilators.
  (e) Steroids reduce mortality in septic shock.

13.33 Recognized causes of acute hypoxaemic respiratory (type I) failure include (page 849):
  (a) Guillain–Barré syndrome
  (b) Pulmonary oedema
  (c) Pneumonia
  (d) Fibrosing alveolitis
  (e) Right ventricular failure

13.34 Recognized causes of acid–base balance disturbance are as follows (page 850):
  (a) Respiratory acidosis – following cardiac arrest
  (b) Respiratory alkalosis – high altitudes
  (c) Metabolic acidosis – chronic renal failure
  (d) Metabolic alkalosis – nasogastric suction in pyloric stenosis
  (e) Metabolic acidosis – shock

13.35 The following statements are correct (page 851):
  (a) The concentration of oxygen administered is not important in chronic bronchitis.
  (b) Negative-pressure ventilation is used for long-term ventilation of patients with neuromuscular disease.

(c) Intermittent positive-pressure ventilation (IPPV) decreases carbon dioxide elimination.

(d) IPPV does not require endotracheal intubation.

(e) Oxygen toxicity in humans is well proven.

13.36 Indications for intermittent positive-pressure ventilation include (page 852):

(a) Acute respiratory failure with signs of respiratory distress persisting despite maximal therapy

(b) Acute ventilatory failure due to myasthenia gravis

(c) In head injury to avoid hypoxia and hypercarbia

(d) Severe left ventricular failure with pulmonary oedema

(e) Coma following drug overdose with breathing difficulties

13.37 Complications of endotracheal intubation include (Table 13.7):

(a) Pneumothorax

(b) Subcutaneous emphysema

(c) Tracheal stenosis

(d) Erosion of the innominate artery

(e) Damage to the cricoarytenoid cartilages

13.38 The following statements are correct (pages 853–854):

(a) The primary effect of PEEP is to re-expand underventilated lung units.

(b) The application of CPAP achieves for the spontaneously breathing patient what PEEP does for the ventilated patient.

(c) Synchronized intermittent mandatory ventilation allows the patient to breathe spontaneously between the 'mandatory' tidal volumes delivered by the ventilator.

(d) IPPV with PEEP causes ADH secretion.

(e) IPPV is frequently complicated by a deterioration in gas exchange due to V/Q mismatch and the collapse of peripheral alveoli.

13.39 Positive end-expiratory pressure (PEEP) is useful in severe (page 853):

(a) Emphysema

(b) Asthma

(c) Bacterial pneumonia

(d) Fibrotic lung disease

(e) Unilateral bacterial pneumonia

13.40 Advantages of high-frequency jet ventilation include (page 854):

(a) Cardiac output is maintained

(b) The risk of barotrauma is negligible.

(c) It is useful in ventilating patients with large air leaks.

(d) It is useful in ventilating patients with bronchopleural fistula.

(e) It is useful in ventilating patients with lung lacerations.

13.41 The following statements about weaning and extubation are correct
(page 855):
(a) Weaning is essential even in patients who have received artificial
ventilation for less than 24 hours.
(b) Intermittent mandatory ventilation is a smoother and more controlled
method of weaning than traditional methods of intermittent
spontaneous breathing.
(c) The application of CPAP can prevent alveolar collapse.
(d) Extubation should not be considered until the patient can swallow.
(e) Extubation can be considered even if the patient is unable to cough.

13.42 Recognized clinical features of acute respiratory distress syndrome include
(page 856):
(a) Dyspnoea
(b) Pulmonary capillary wedge pressure more than 16 mmHg
(c) Cyanosis which responds to oxygen therapy
(d) Loss of lung compliance
(e) Diffuse alveolar infiltrates

13.43 Acute respiratory distress syndrome occurs as complication of (Table 13.9):
(a) Trauma
(b) Fat embolism
(c) Systemic hypertension
(d) Left ventricular failure
(e) Sepsis

13.44 The following statements about the management of ARDS are correct
(page 857):
(a) SIMV and pressure-limited ventilation should be avoided.
(b) Repeated position changes between prone and supine may allow
reductions in airway pressures and the inspired oxygen concentration.
(c) The administration of high-dose steroids improves outcome.
(d) Inhaled nitric oxide is contraindicated.
(e) Aerosolized surfactant has recently been clearly seen to reduce
morbidity and mortality.

13.45 A diagnosis of brain death can be considered (page 858):
(a) If the patient is in apnoeic coma secondary to sedatives
(b) If the central body temperature is less than 35°C
(c) If the patient is deep coma and all brain-stem reflexes are absent
(d) If there are profound acid–base abnormalities
(e) If irremediable structural brain damage has been considered with
certainty

Adverse Drug Reactions and Poisoning

14.1 Examples of dose-dependent reactions include (page 862):
- (a) Gout due to thiazides
- (b) Bone marrow suppression due to methotrexate
- (c) Eighth-nerve damage due to aminoglycosides
- (d) Myocardial damage due to doxorubicin therapy
- (e) Aplastic anaemia associated with chloramphenicol

14.2 Examples of dose-independent reactions include (pages 862–863):
- (a) Anaphylaxis due to pencillin
- (b) Coombs'-positive haemolytic anaemia due to methyldopa
- (c) Serum sickness due to carbimazole
- (d) Thrombocytopenic purpura associated with quinine
- (e) Contact dermatitis following topical application of antibiotics

14.3 Clinical features of anaphylaxis include (Emergency box 14.1):
- (a) Bronchodilatation
- (b) Laryngeal spasm
- (c) Hypertension
- (d) Diarrhoea
- (e) Cyanosis

14.4 The following drug-induced adverse effects are correct (Table 14.2):
- (a) Anticonvulsants – megaloblastic anaemia
- (b) Amiodarone – pulmonary fibrosis
- (c) Methysergide – retroperitoneal fibrosis
- (d) Neuroleptics – gout
- (e) Methyldopa – SLE

14.5 Treatment of anaphylaxis includes (Emergency box 14.1):
- (a) Avoid adrenaline
- (b) Oxygen
- (c) Intravenous fluids
- (d) Intravenous hydrocortisone
- (e) Intravenous infusion of chlorpheniramine

14.6 Pseudoallergic reactions (page 863):
- (a) occur on first contact with the drug
- (b) are produced by compounds that are able to prevent the release of histamine
- (c) involve antigen–antibody production
- (d) with intravenous drugs can be avoided by rapid injection
- (e) are never fatal

14.7 The following are examples of pseudoallergic reactions (page 863):
- (a) Morphine-induced bronchospasm
- (b) Morphine-induced itching
- (c) Aspirin-induced urticaria
- (d) *N*-acetylcysteine-induced bronchospasm
- (e) Aspirin-induced bronchospasm

14.8 The following adverse effects of drugs in pregnancy are correct (Table 14.5):
- (a) β-blockers induce growth retardation.
- (b) Carbamezapine-induces neural tube defects
- (c) Antithyroid drugs induce neonatal hypothyroidism.
- (d) Antimalarials cause methaemoglobinaemia in the neonate.
- (e) Stilboesterol causes vaginal carcinoma in the offspring.

14.9 The following drug effects on the fetus are correct (Table 14.5):
- (a) Tetracyclines – eighth-nerve damage
- (b) Aminoglycosides – dental discoloration
- (c) Lithium – neonatal hypothyroidism
- (d) Sulphonamides – kernicterus
- (e) Chloramphenicol – 'grey baby' syndrome

14.10 Drugs whose dosage requires reduction in the elderly due to a fall in GFR include (page 867):
- (a) Digoxin
- (b) Lithium
- (c) Aminoglycosides
- (d) Sedatives
- (e) Tranquillizers

14.11 Drugs known to cause SLE in patients with *N*-acetyltransferase deficiency include (Table 14.2):
- (a) Succinlycholine
- (b) Procainamide
- (c) Phenelzine
- (d) Hydralazine
- (e) Metoprolol

14.12 Drugs known to cause haemolysis in patients with glucose-6-phosphate dehydrogenase deficiency include (Table 6.3):
- (a) Primaquine
- (b) Sulphonamides
- (c) Phenelzine
- (d) Quinine
- (e) Chloramphenicol

14.13 Substances that result in adverse reactions due to MAO inhibition include:
(a) Foods lacking tyramine
(b) Ephedrine
(c) Tricyclic antidepressants
(d) Reserpine
(e) Pethidine

14.14 Drugs known to have 'antabuse' reaction with alcohol include:
(a) Disulphiram
(b) Metronidazole
(c) Cimetidine
(d) Warfarin
(e) Propranolol

14.15 Cimetidine (Table 14.3):
(a) increases the anticoagulant action of warfarin
(b) decreases the sedative effect of diazepam
(c) increases the β-adrenoreceptor blocking action of propranolol
(d) interacts with theophylline to cause arrhythmias
(e) affects isoniazid metabolism

14.16 Cytochrome p450 enzyme-inducing drugs include (Table 14.4):
(a) Phenytoin
(b) Barbiturates
(c) Carbamazepine
(d) Rifampicin
(e) Prednisolone

14.17 Drugs that inhibit liver p450 enzymes include (page 864):
(a) Cimetidine
(b) Erythromycin
(c) Ciprofloxacin
(d) Sodium valproate
(e) Alcohol

14.18 The following statements regarding drug interactions are correct (Table 14.3):
(a) Warfarin interacts with erythromycin to cause uncontrolled bleeding.
(b) Azathioprine interacts with allopurinol to result in bone marrow failure.
(c) Theophylline interacts with cimetidine to cause convulsions.
(d) Lithium interacts with thiazide diuretics to cause ataxia.
(e) β-Blockers interact with verapamil to cause bradycardia.

14.19 Drug-induced changes in cholinergic receptors increase the sensitivity of patients with myasthenia gravis to the following drugs:
(a) Salbutamol
(b) Streptomycin
(c) Neomycin
(d) Kanamycin
(e) Propranolol

14.20 Correct statements regarding enhanced toxicity in inherited diseases include (Table 14.9):
(a) Salicylates reduce bleeding time in haemophilia.
(b) Halothane may induce pyrexia in osteogenesis imperfecta.
(c) Insulin may induce paralysis in periodic paralysis.
(d) Familial dysautonomia patients may show denervation sensitivity with adrenergic agonists.
(e) Succinylcholine may induce malignant hyperthermia in myotonia congenita.

14.21 The following statements are correct (pages 861–884):
(a) Ampicillin may induce rash in glandular fever.
(b) Succinylcholine can induce cardiac arrhythmias in renal failure.
(c) Salicylates induce hepatotoxicity in rheumatoid arthritis.
(d) Theophylline is associated with bronchospasm in cystic fibrosis.
(e) Clofibrate causes myopathy in renal failure.

14.22 Drugs for which therapeutic monitoring is used include (Table 14.8):
(a) Digoxin
(b) Carbamazepine
(c) Gentamicin
(d) Lithium
(e) Phenytoin

14.23 Studies of drug overdoses have revealed that (page 871):
(a) Acute overdoses usually involve only one drug.
(b) Alcohol is the most commonly implicated second drug in mixed self-poisonings.
(c) Patients' statements about the type and amount of drug taken should be relied on.
(d) The use of minor tranquillizers is increasing.
(e) Barbiturates are readily available in the UK.

14.24 Correct statements about acute drug overdose include (page 871):
(a) Most adults are unconscious on arrival at hospital.
(b) Drug overdose should be considered in any patient with an altered conscious level.
(c) Dilated pupils indicate opiate overdose.

    (d) Rectal temperature should be recorded in the unconscious patient.
    (e) Gag reflex should be tested in the conscious patient.

14.25 The physical signs that may aid identification of the agents responsible for poisoning include (Fig 14.6):
    (a) Cherry red colour – opiates
    (b) Constricted pupils – carbon monoxide
    (c) Hypothermia – barbiturates
    (d) Blisters – barbiturates
    (e) Cardiac arrhythmias – tricyclic antidepressants

14.26 In the patient unconcious due to drug overdose (page 872):
    (a) Nursing should be in the supine position.
    (b) Loss of gag reflex is the prime indication for intubation.
    (c) Hypotension is a common feature.
    (d) Catheterization of the bladder is usually unnecessary as it can be emptied by gentle suprapubic pressure.
    (e) Volume expanders such as dextran should be avoided in severe hypotension.

14.27 The following associations regarding drug overdoses are correct (page 872):
    (a) Hypothermia – chlorpromazine
    (b) Rhabdomyolysis – heroin overdose
    (c) Convulsions – tricyclic antidepressants
    (d) Arrhythmias – tricyclic antidepressants
    (e) Convulsions – phenothiazines

14.28 Gastric lavage is indicated with the following poisons (page 873):
    (a) Corrosives
    (b) Paracetamol
    (c) Petrol
    (d) Aspirin
    (e) Paraffin

14.29 Emetics used to induce vomiting in poisoning include (page 873):
    (a) Ipecacuanha
    (b) Apomorphine
    (c) Saline
    (d) Copper sulphate
    (e) Mustard

14.30 The following associations regarding the methods of drug elimination are correct (page 874):
    (a) Forced alkaline diuresis – salicylate poisoning
    (b) Peritoneal dialysis – ethylene glycol
    (c) Haemodialysis – lithium

(d) Haemoperfusion – theophylline

(e) Haemodialysis – ethyl alcohol poisoning

14.31 Salicylates (page 875):

(a) are poorly absorbed from the stomach

(b) delay gastric emptying

(c) at high doses mean that renal excretion becomes important

(d) overdosage produces respiratory alkalosis

(e) overdose results in metabolic acidosis

14.32 Features of salicylate poisoning include (page 875):

(a) Cerebral oedema

(b) Pulmonary oedema

(c) Hyperpyrexia

(d) Tinnitus

(e) Coma

14.33 Correct statements about the treatment of aspirin poisoning include (page 875):

(a) Activated charcoal should not given.

(b) Vitamin K is used to correct hypoprothrombinaemia.

(c) Gastric lavage should be performed in severe cases up to 24 hours after ingestion.

(d) Making the urine acidic is also effective in increasing urine salicylate excretion.

(e) Forced alkaline diuresis is a safe method and does not require supervision.

14.34 Paracetamol poisoning (page 875):

(a) is rare

(b) is never fatal

(c) can cause marked liver necrosis

(d) causes acute renal failure

(e) patients usually recover within 48 hours

14.35 Correct statements about the treatment of paracetamol overdose include (page 876):

(a) Treatment depends on the interval between overdose and presentation.

(b) Blood for paracetamol level measurement should be taken immediately.

(c) Gastric lavage is contraindicated.

(d) The antidote of choice is *N*-acetylcysteine.

(e) Methionine is a reliable antidote.

14.36 In patients who present after 16 hours of paracetamol ingestion (page 876):
    (a) Concentrations of paracetamol are a reliable guide to the value of treatment.
    (b) Glucose levels should be monitored.
    (c) Encephalopathy can be a feature.
    (d) Are treated with fresh frozen plasma for any haemorrhage.
    (e) Cirrhosis is a definite sequela.

14.37 Overdoses of ibuprofen cause (page 877):
    (a) Tinnitus
    (b) Gastrointestinal bleeding
    (c) Headache
    (d) Vomiting
    (e) Renal damage

14.38 Benzodiazepine overdose (page 877):
    (a) causes ataxia
    (b) causes pinpoint pupils
    (c) is treated with naloxone
    (d) causes respiratory depression
    (e) is usually fatal

14.39 Tricyclic antidepressant overdose (page 877):
    (a) usually causes deep coma
    (b) causes urinary retention
    (c) causes ventricular arrhythmias
    (d) causes fixed, dilated pupils
    (e) should never be treated with gastric lavage

14.40 Factors that precipitate lithium poisoning include (page 878):
    (a) Concurrent diuretic therapy
    (b) Increased elimination of the drug by the kidney
    (c) Vomiting
    (d) Diarrhoea
    (e) Exposure to high temperatures

14.41 Correct statements about acute lithium poisoning include (page 878):
    (a) Hypokalaemia is a feature.
    (b) Acute renal failure is a common complication.
    (c) Coma is associated with a poor prognosis.
    (d) Serum lithium concentrations correlate well with the severity.
    (e) Forced diuresis is usually used in treatment.

14.42 The following associations between drugs and antidotes are correct (page 878):
    (a) Digoxin – specific antibody

(b) Phenothiazines – benztropine
(c) Benzodiazepines – flumanezil
(d) Salbutamol – β-blocker
(e) β-Blocker – glucagon

14.43 The following statements are correct (page 879):
(a) Paraquat poisoning is treated with gastric lavage using Fuller's earth.
(b) Hyerbaric oxygen should be considered in unconscious victims of carbon monoxide poisoning.
(c) Most ingested batteries will disintegrate during their passage through the gut.
(d) Organophosphorus poisons can be absorbed through the skin.
(e) Cyanide inhibits cytochrome oxidase.

14.44 Drugs used in cyanide poisoning include (pages 879–880):
(a) Potassium chloride
(b) Sodium nitrite
(c) Sodium chloride
(d) Sodium thiosulphate
(e) Dicobalt edentate

14.45 Correct statements about methanol poisoning include (page 880):
(a) Severe poisoning results in blindness.
(b) Ethanol infusion is useful.
(c) Folinic acid may prevent ocular toxicity.
(d) Haemodialysis should be avoided in severe cases.
(e) It is metabolized by alcohol dehydrogenase.

14.46 Ethanol is used in the treatment of (page 880):
(a) Ethylene glycol poisoning
(b) Chronic mercury poisoning
(c) Methanol poisoning
(d) Chlormethiazole overdose
(e) Acute lead poisoning

14.47 Features of chronic lead poisoning include (page 880):
(a) Blue line on the gums
(b) Abdominal colic
(c) Constipation
(d) Basophil stippling of erythrocytes
(e) Foot drop

14.48 Drugs used in the treatment of lead poisoning include (page 881):
(a) Desferrioxamine
(b) Sodium calcium edetate
(c) D-pencillamine

(d) Dimercaprol
(e) Ethylene glycol

14.49 Features of chronic arsenic poisoning include (page 881):
(a) Raindrop pigmentation of the skin
(b) Excess salivation
(c) Polyneuritis
(d) Anorexia
(e) Weakness

14.50 Poisonous snakes native to the UK include (page 881):
(a) Adder
(b) Russell's viper
(c) Rattlesnakes
(d) Cobras
(e) Kraits

14.51 The following associations are correct (page 881):
(a) Russell's viper – vasculotoxic
(b) Cobra – neurotoxic
(c) Sea snakes – mycotoxic
(d) Viperidae – incoagulable blood
(e) Cobra – local tissue necrosis

14.52 Correct statements about the management of snake bite include (page 881):
(a) An arterial tourniquet should be placed over the bite.
(b) The type of snake should be identified.
(c) Antivenoms must always be given when indicated.
(d) Antivenoms can reverse the effects of venom.
(e) Antitetanus prophylaxis must be given.

14.53 The following statements are correct (page 882):
(a) Scorpion stings are fatal.
(b) Scorpions have a neurotoxic venom.
(c) The black widow spider bite produces muscle spasms.
(d) Death from insect stings is usually due to anaphylaxis.
(e) Hepatitis A can be transmitted by the ingestion of shellfish.

14.54 Poisonous plants commonly ingested include (page 883):
(a) Hemlock
(b) Laburnum
(c) Deadly nightshade
(d) Green potatoes
(e) *Amanita phalloides*

14.55 Features of solvent abuse include (page 884):
  (a) Acute intoxicated state
  (b) Rashes over the face
  (c) Peripheral neuropathy
  (d) Sudden death
  (e) Cardiac arrhythmias

14.56 The following statements are correct (page 884):
  (a) Naloxone is the antidote for cannabis.
  (b) Amphetamine overdose can cause cardiac arrhythmias.
  (c) Tachycardia due to cocaine is usually treated with β-blockers.
  (d) 'Ecstasy' is known to cause rhabdomyolysis.
  (e) 'Ecstasy' is known to result in hyperpyrexia.

Environmental Medicine

15.1 Correct statements about heat and its effects include (page 885):
  (a) The hypothalamus regulates core body temperature.
  (b) The evaporation of sweat is an important mechanism in increasing body temperature.
  (c) Acclimatization to a hotter climate takes at least a year.
  (d) In heat stroke the body temperature exceeds 41°C.
  (e) Heat exhaustion is caused by water and salt depletion.

15.2 Complications of heat injury include (page 886):
  (a) Shock
  (b) Cerebral oedema
  (c) Renal failure
  (d) Hepatic failure
  (e) Coma

15.3 Factors that contribute to hypothermia include (pages 886–887):
  (a) Alcohol
  (b) Hyperthyroidism
  (c) Extremes of heat outside
  (d) Hypnotics
  (e) Following immersion in cold water

15.4 Correct statements about high-altitude illnesses include (pages 888–889):
  (a) The incidence of thromboembolism is increased tenfold compared to that at sea level.
  (b) Acetazolamide aggravates acute mountain sickness.
  (c) High-altitude pulmonary oedema is rarely life-threatening.
  (d) Oxygen should be avoided in acute mountain sickness.
  (e) Chronic mountain sickness is a self-limiting disorder.

15.5 Recognized features of chronic mountain sickness include (page 889):
  (a) Koilonychia
  (b) Polycythaemia
  (c) Right ventricular enlargement
  (d) Cyanosis
  (e) Congested cheeks

15.6 Decompression disorders include (page 889):
  (a) Nitrogen narcosis
  (b) Oxygen narcosis
  (c) Bends
  (d) Chokes
  (e) Pneumothorax

15.7 The delayed effects of radiation include (Table 15.3):
    (a) Dermatitis
    (b) Infertility
    (c) Acute myeloid leukaemia
    (d) Cataract
    (e) Haemopoietic syndrome

15.8 The clinical effects of electric shock include (page 891):
    (a) Ventricular fibrillation
    (b) Muscular contraction
    (c) Spinal cord damage
    (d) Burns
    (e) Dry drowning

15.9 The following statements are correct (pages 891–893):
    (a) Smoke can cause laryngeal stridor.
    (b) Repeated prolonged loud noise can cause permanent hearing loss.
    (c) It has been suggested that excess noise affects the development and reading skills of children.
    (d) The body clock is modulated by various Zeitgebers.
    (e) Legionnaire's disease is frequently due to contamination of air-conditioning systems.

15.10 Correct statements about the management of drowning include (page 892):
    (a) The patient should not be turned to one side.
    (b) The mouth should be cleared of debris.
    (c) Mouth-to-mouth resuscitation is of little use in the presence of fixed dilated pupils.
    (d) Patients are liable to develop acute respiratory distress syndrome.
    (e) The prognosis is poor even if the patient is fully conscious on admission to hospital.

15.11 Ultraviolet (UVA) light causes (page 892):
    (a) Sunburn
    (b) Skin ageing
    (c) Skin cancer
    (d) Snow blindness
    (e) Psoriasis

Endocrinology

16.1 Hormones may be (page 895):
 (a) Polypeptides
 (b) Glycoproteins
 (c) Steroids
 (d) Amines
 (e) Phenols

16.2 The following associations between hormones and second messengers are correct (page 896):
 (a) Cyclic AMP – parathormone
 (b) Cyclic AMP – ACTH
 (c) Calcium phospholipid system – TRH
 (d) Tyrosine kinase – IGF-1
 (e) Tyrosine kinase – insulin

16.3 Hormones act by (page 896):
 (a) Alterations in cell-membrane ion transport
 (b) Alterations in protein synthesis
 (c) Activation of membrane-bound phosphoinositide pathways
 (d) Altering the activity of intracellular enzymes
 (e) Altering binding of the receptor to DNA

16.4 The following types of feedback mechanisms and hormones are correct (page 897):
 (a) Negative feedback – effect of T_3 on the pituitary
 (b) Positive feedback – regulation of menstrual cycle
 (c) Positive feedback – effect of T_4 and T_3 on the pituitary
 (d) Positive feedback – effect of ACTH on the adrenal medulla.
 (e) Positive feedback – effect of T_4 on the pituitary

16.5 The secretions of the following hormones are normally pulsatile (page 898):
 (a) Thyroxine
 (b) Luteinizing hormone
 (c) Follicle-stimulating hormone
 (d) Triiodothyronine
 (e) Cortisol

16.6 Stress can produce rapid increases in the secretion of (page 898):
 (a) ACTH
 (b) Cortisol
 (c) Growth hormone
 (d) Prolactin
 (e) Noradrenaline

16.7 The secretion of the following hormones increases during sleep (page 898):
  (a) Adrenaline
  (b) Growth hormone
  (c) Noradrenaline
  (d) Prolactin
  (e) Thyroxine

16.8 The following statements are correct (page 899):
  (a) When the secretory capacity of a gland is damaged, maximal stimulation by the trophic hormone will give a diminished output.
  (b) In Addison's disease there is a normal response to ACTH.
  (c) A patient with a hormone-producing tumour usually fails to show normal negative feedback.
  (d) In Cushing's disease administration of synthetic steroid causes suppression of ACTH and cortisol production, unlike normal subjects.
  (e) In general stimulation tests are used to confirm suspected excess of hormone.

16.9 Examples of organ-specific autoimmune disease include (Table 16.4):
  (a) Graves' disease
  (b) Myxoedema
  (c) Addison's disease
  (d) Premature ovarian failure
  (e) Vitiligo

16.10 The following associations about the molecular basis of endocrine tumours are correct:
  (a) Abnormal G proteins – prolactinomas
  (b) Chromosome 11 – MEN type 1 tumours
  (c) Chromosome 10 – MEN type 2A
  (d) Chromosome 6 – congenital adrenal hyperplasia
  (e) Mutations of *Ret*-proto-oncogene – MEN 2

16.11 The following associations between endocrine disease and drugs are correct (Table 16.3):
  (a) Metoclopramide – galactorrhoea
  (b) Amiodarone – hyperthyroidism
  (c) Amiodarone – hypothyroidism
  (d) Ketoconazole – hypoadrenalism
  (e) Steroids – diabetes

16.12 Hypothalamic hormones include (page 904):
  (a) Growth hormone
  (b) Luteinzing hormone
  (c) Prolactin
  (d) Thyroid-stimulating hormone
  (e) Adrenocorticotrophic hormone

16.13 The posterior pituitary synthesizes (page 904):
- (a) Antidiuretic hormone
- (b) Vasopressin
- (c) Oxytocin
- (d) Prolactin-inhibiting factor
- (e) Thyrotrophin-releasing hormone

16.14 The hypothalamus contains (page 904):
- (a) Natriuretic factor
- (b) Neuropeptide Y
- (c) Vasoactive intestinal peptide
- (d) Vasopressin
- (e) Oxytocin

16.15 Recognized features of prolactinoma include (Table 16.6):
- (a) Galactorrhoea
- (b) Amenorrhea
- (c) Central obesity
- (d) Gigantism
- (e) Visual field defects

16.16 Pituitary tumours are commonly associated with (page 905):
- (a) Addison's disease
- (b) Nelson's syndrome
- (c) Acromegaly
- (d) Cushing's disease
- (e) Graves' disease

16.17 Recognized causes of hypopituitarism include (Table 16.8):
- (a) Sarcoidosis
- (b) Sheehan's syndrome
- (c) Tuberculosis meningitis
- (d) Craniopharyngioma
- (e) Histiocytosis X

16.18 Clinical features of hypopituitarism include (page 908):
- (a) Hypertension
- (b) Thyrotoxicosis
- (c) 'Alabaster' skin
- (d) Galactorrhoea
- (e) Loss of libido

16.19 The following associations are correct (page 908):
- (a) Kallmann's syndrome – hypogonadism
- (b) Sheehan's syndrome – pituitary hypertrophy
- (c) Pituitary apoplexy – pituitary haemorrhage

(d) Empty sella syndrome – normal pituitary function
(e) Kallmann's syndrome – anosmia

16.20 Tests for hypothalamic–pituitary function include (pages 1206–1208):
(a) Clomiphene test
(b) Insulin tolerance test
(c) TRH test
(d) Short synacthen test
(e) LHRH test

16.21 Correct statements about the therapy of hypopituitarism include (pages 908–909):
(a) Pulsatile LHRH therapy is essential for life.
(b) Thyroid replacement therapy should not commence until replacement steroid therapy has been initiated.
(c) Replacement therapy of thyroid hormones is essential for life.
(d) Diabetes insipidus may be apparent after steroid replacement.
(e) Replacement therapy of glucocorticoids is essential for life.

16.22 The following statements are correct (page 910):
(a) Anorexia nervosa is associated with hypopituitarism.
(b) Heavy training in female athletes is associated with menstrual irregularity.
(c) Stress affects endocrine function.
(d) Emotional deprivation in childhood causes growth retardation.
(e) Up to 8 weeks of gestation the sexes share a common development

16.23 Correct statements about the embryology of the reproductive organs include (page 910):
(a) The epididymis develops from the Wolffian duct.
(b) The vas deferens develops from the Mullerian duct.
(c) Oestrogens induce transformation of the primitive perineum into the testes.
(d) The potential ovary develops in the presence of a Y chromosome.
(e) The development of the Mullerian duct is dependent on testosterone.

16.24 In the male (page 910):
(a) LH inhibits testosterone production from the Leydig cells of the testes.
(b) Testosterone is responsible for the maintenance of libido.
(c) FSH stimulates Sertoli cells in the seminiferous tubules to produce mature sperm.
(d) Testosterone stimulates LHRH secretion.
(e) Inhibin stimulates FSH secretion.

16.25 In the female (page 911):
(a) LH suppresses ovarian androgen production.
(b) FSH inhibits ovarian follicular development.

(c) Oestrogens have a double feedback action on the pituitary.
(d) The corpus luteum develops from the follicle.
(e) Testosterone induces growth and maturation of the uterus.

16.26 In puberty (page 912):
(a) FSH secretion rises last.
(b) Full spermatogenesis occurs comparatively early.
(c) The peak height velocity in boys is reached much earlier than in girls.
(d) Growth in girls is completed earlier than in boys.
(e) The FSH secretion is initially pulsatile.

16.27 Precocious puberty (page 912):
(a) of the idiopathic type is commoner in boys
(b) is that which occurs before the age of 9 years.
(c) is a feature of Forbes–Albright syndrome
(d) of the cerebral type may be the presenting feature of hypothalamic disease
(e) is the same as thelarche

16.28 The following statements are correct (page 913):
(a) Delayed puberty is usually due to hypogonadism.
(b) A rising serum testosterone is an early clue to male puberty.
(c) In boys, testicular volume more than 5 ml indicates the onset of puberty.
(d) In girls the breast bud is the first sign of puberty.
(e) Most children show signs of pubertal development by the age of 14.

16.29 Following menopause (page 913):
(a) FSH levels fall.
(b) LH levels fall.
(c) Oestrogen levels rise.
(d) Bone density increases.
(e) Ischaemic heart disease is less common.

16.30 The effects of HRT in the menopause include (page 913):
(a) Symptomatic improvement in all menopausal symptoms.
(b) A fall in blood pressure in the majority.
(c) Reduction in cerebrovascular disease mortality.
(d) Protection against hip fractures.
(e) An increase in ischaemic heart disease mortality.

16.31 In the ageing male (page 913):
(a) The overall testicular volume increases.
(b) Gonadotrophin levels fall.
(c) Replacement testosterone accelerates osteoporosis.
(d) Finasteride is contraindicated in benign prostatic hypertrophy.
(e) There is a progressive increase in sexual function.

16.32 Prolactin (page 914):
  (a) secretion is inhibited by dopamine
  (b) secretion is reduced by TRH
  (c) stimulates milk secretion
  (d) reduces gonadal activity
  (e) blocks the action of LH on the ovary

16.33 The following statements are correct (page 914):
  (a) A low testosterone with high gonadotrophin rules out primary gonadal disease.
  (b) Low levels of LH and testosterone exclude hypothalamic–pituitary disease.
  (c) Serial ultrasound in the luteal phase is used to demonstrate ovulation.
  (d) Complete demonstration of normal male and female function requires a pregnancy.
  (e) The clomiphene test examines hypothalamic negative feedback.

16.34 Androgens (Table 16.12):
  (a) prevent frontotemporal balding
  (b) maintain the male pattern of pubic hair
  (c) have little effect on testicular size
  (d) prevent pubertal epiphyseal fusion
  (e) maintain libido

16.35 Causes of male hypogonadism include (Table 16.13):
  (a) Hyperprolactinaemia
  (b) Renal failure
  (c) Cirrhosis
  (d) Sickle cell disease
  (e) Hypopituitarism

16.36 Drugs used in androgen replacement therapy include (Table 16.14):
  (a) Mesterolone
  (b) Methyltestosterone
  (c) Tamoxifen
  (d) Testosterone undecanoate
  (e) Testosterone propionate

16.37 Features of Kallman's syndrome include (page 916):
  (a) Isolated deficiency of LHRH
  (b) Anosmia
  (c) Cleft palate
  (d) Colour blindness
  (e) Renal abnormalities

16.38 Features of Klinefelter's syndrome include (page 916):
  (a) Absence of X chromosome

    (b) Seminiferous tubule dysgenesis
    (c) Gynaecomastia
    (d) Mental retardation
    (e) Large testes

16.39 Causes of erectile difficulty include (page 916):
    (a) Autonomic neuropathy
    (b) Hypogonadism
    (c) Psychological
    (d) Vascular disease
    (e) Neurogenic causes

16.40 Drugs causing impotence include (page 916):
    (a) Sildenafil citrate
    (b) β-Blockers
    (c) Diuretics
    (d) Cannabis
    (e) Metoclopramide

16.41 Causes of gynaecomastia include (Table 16.15):
    (a) Hypopituitarism
    (b) Hyperthyroidism
    (c) Digitalis
    (d) Spironolactone
    (e) Cimetidine

16.42 The following statements are correct (page 917):
    (a) Severe illness, even in the absence of weight loss, can lead to amenorrhoea.
    (b) Polycystic ovary syndrome is the most common cause of oligomenorrhoea.
    (c) A minimum body weight is necessary for regular menstruation.
    (d) Hypothyroidism causes amenorrhoea stimulating prolactin secretion.
    (e) Basal levels of FSH, LH, oestrogen and prolactin allow initial distinction between primary gonadal and hypothalmic–pituitary causes of amenorrhoea.

16.43 Features of oestrogen deficiency include (Table 16.16):
    (a) Areolar pigmentation
    (b) Small atrophic breast
    (c) Dry vagina
    (d) Endometrial proliferation
    (e) Osteoporosis

16.44 The following associations between biochemical markers and the causes of amenorrhoea are correct (Table 16.17):
    (a) Hypothyroidism – low prolactin

(b) Severe polycystic ovarian disease – low prolactin
(c) Ovarian dysgenesis – low FSH
(d) Kallman's syndrome – high FSH
(e) Weight loss – high FSH

16.45 Causes of hirsutism include (Table 16.18):
(a) Idiopathic
(b) Polycystic ovarian syndrome
(c) Congenital adrenal hyperplasia
(d) Ovarian neoplasms
(e) Adrenal tumours

16.46 Drugs causing hirsutism include (page 920):
(a) Phenytoin
(b) Diazoxide
(c) Minoxidil
(d) Cyclosporin
(e) Progestogens

16.47 Biochemical features of polycystic ovarian disease include (page 920):
(a) Decreased free androgens
(b) Decreased total testosterone
(c) Increased SHBG
(d) Raised LH:FSH ratio
(e) Marked hyperprolactinaemia

16.48 Recognized features of polycystic ovarian disease include (page 920):
(a) Menstrual disturbance
(b) Hypertension
(c) Hyperlipidaemia
(d) Hirsutism
(e) Amenorrhoea

16.49 Treatment of polycystic ovarian disease includes (page 921):
(a) Reverse circadian rhythm prednisolone therapy
(b) Oral contraceptives
(c) Androgens
(d) Clomiphene
(e) Wedge resection of the adrenals

16.50 Hyperprolactinaemia usually presents with (page 922):
(a) Galactorrhoea
(b) Menorrhagia
(c) Increased libido in both sexes
(d) Subfertility
(e) Osteoporosis in women

16.51 Causes of hyperprolactinaemia include (Table 16.18):
(a) NREM sleep
(b) Stress
(c) Primary hyperthyroidism
(d) Renal failure
(e) Liver failure

16.52 Drugs causing hyperprolactinaemia include (Table 16.18):
(a) Metoclopramide
(b) Methyldopa
(c) Bromocriptine
(d) Cimetidine
(e) Opiates

16.53 Investigations in the management of hyperprolactinaemia include (page 922):
(a) Prolactin levels
(b) Anterior pituitary function
(c) MR scan of the hypothalamus
(d) Visual fields
(e) Thyroid function

16.54 Correct statements about the management of hyperprolactinaemia include (page 922):
(a) Dopamine antagonists are useful.
(b) Trans-sphenoidal surgery often restores normoprolactinaemia in patients with microadenoma, but is rarely completely successful with macroadenomas.
(c) Radiotherapy is rapidly effective.
(d) Small tumours in asymptomatic patients without hypogonadism may need observation only.
(e) Newer agents used include quinagolide.

16.55 Common reasons for stopping oral contraceptives include (Information box 16.6):
(a) Weight loss
(b) Increased libido
(c) Increased blood pressure
(d) Abnormal liver function tests
(e) Migraine

16.56 Drugs known to reduce the contraceptive effect of oral contraceptives include (Information box 16.6):
(a) Antibiotics
(b) Barbiturates
(c) Phenytoin

(d) Carbamazepine
(e) Rifampicin

16.57 Common causes of subfertility include (page 924):
(a) Inadequate intercourse
(b) Hostile cervical mucus
(c) Vaginal factor
(d) Lack of androgen production by adrenals
(e) Ovulatory and tubal problems

16.58 Correct statements about the management of subfertility include (page 924):
(a) The male partner is rarely the cause of infertility.
(b) An early semen analysis is essential.
(c) Examination should include an assessment of secondary sexual characteristics.
(d) Counselling of both partners is essential.
(e) Exclusion of varicocoele is important in women.

16.59 An individual's sex can be defined in the following ways (page 925):
(a) Chromosomal
(b) Gonadal
(c) Phenotypic
(d) Social
(e) Sexual orientation

16.60 Growth hormone release (page 926):
(a) is continuous
(b) is rarely nocturnal
(c) occurs during REM sleep
(d) is increased by acute stress
(e) is decreased by exercise

16.61 Factors involved in linear growth include (page 926):
(a) Emotional deprivation
(b) Intrauterine growth retardation
(c) Thyroid function
(d) Genetics
(e) Renal failure in childhood

16.62 The following statements are correct (page 927):
(a) A child with normal growth velocity is unlikely to have significant endocrine disease.
(b) A sudden cessation of growth suggests major physical disease.
(c) Consistently slow-growing children require full endocrine assessment.

(d) Where constitutional delay is clearly shown and symptoms require intervention, then very low-dose sex steroid courses will usually induce acceleration of growth.

(e) Basal levels of growth hormone are of value in the management of short stature.

16.63 The following associations between puberty and the common causes of short stature are correct (Table 16.20):
(a) Constitutional delay – late puberty
(b) Familial short stature – delayed puberty
(c) GH insufficiency – early puberty
(d) Primary hypothyroidism – delayed puberty
(e) Small-bowel disease – delayed puberty

16.64 The following statements about growth hormone treatment include (page 928):
(a) Treatment with GH derived from human pituitaries is associated with Creutzfeld–Jakob disease.
(b) GH is the drug of choice in the management of 'short normal' children.
(c) GH with oxandrolone is used in Turner's syndrome.
(d) It is useful in Klinefelter's syndrome.
(e) It is useful in Marfan's syndrome.

16.65 Correct statements about investigations in acromegaly include (page 928):
(a) Glucose fails to suppress growth hormone.
(b) MRI scan of the pituitary will almost always reveal the pituitary adenoma.
(c) Visual field defects are common.
(d) IGF-1 level is almost always raised in acromegaly.
(e) Anterior hypopituitarism is common.

16.66 Reduced survival in acromegalics is usually a result of (page 929):
(a) Renal failure
(b) Liver failure
(c) Heart failure
(d) Hypertension
(e) Coronary artery disease

16.67 Correct statements about the treatment of acromegaly include (page 929):
(a) Trans-sphenoidal surgery is generally agreed to be the appropriate first-line therapy.
(b) Transfrontal surgery is usually required except for massive macroadenoma.
(c) External radiotherapy may have to be continued for 1–10 or more years to be effective.

(d) Octreotide is the treatment of choice in resistant cases.
(e) Dopamine agonists used alone are usually reserved for the elderly and frail.

16.68 Features of acromegaly include (Fig 16.18):
(a) Proximal myopathy
(b) Prognathism
(c) Thick greasy skin
(d) Carpal tunnel syndrome
(e) Goitre

16.69 Correct statements about the anatomy of the thyroid include (page 930):
(a) It consists of one median lobe and two lateral lobes.
(b) It is often palpable in normal women.
(c) Embryologically it originates from the base of the tongue.
(d) It consists of follicles lined by cuboidal epithelioid cells.
(e) The gland moves on swallowing.

16.70 Correct statements about the biochemistry of the thyroid include (page 930):
(a) More thyroxine than triiodothyronine is produced.
(b) T_3 is converted into T_4 in peripheral tissues.
(c) Reverse T_3 is the active form of T_3.
(d) Most of T_4 is bound to hormone-binding proteins.
(e) Iodine is essential for thyroid hormone synthesis.

16.71 Factors increasing TBG include (Table 16.21):
(a) Thyrotoxicosis
(b) Nephrotic syndrome
(c) Pregnancy
(d) Hypothyroidism
(e) Phenytoin

16.72 Correct statements about thyroid function tests include (page 931):
(a) TSH levels are useful to discriminate between hyperthyroidism, hypothyroidism and euthyroidism
(b) Thyroid hormone shows significant circadian rhythms.
(c) TRH test is the investigation of choice in thyroid disease.
(d) Total T_3 levels are most useful in hypothyroidism.
(e) TSH assay is useful in 'sick thyroid' syndrome.

16.73 Tests of first choice in the following situations include (page 931):
(a) Total thyroxine – hypothyroidism
(b) Total thyroxine – thyrotoxicosis
(c) Total T_3 – thyrotoxicosis

    (d) TSH – neonatal screening
    (e) TRH test – Graves' disease

16.74 Features of 'sick thyroid' syndrome include (page 931):
    (a) Low total T_4
    (b) High free T_4
    (c) Low total T_3
    (d) High total T_3
    (e) Normal TSH

16.75 Antithyroid antibodies (page 931):
    (a) of the destructive type may affect one-fifth of the normal population
    (b) against TSH receptors are IgM antibodies
    (c) are absent in Graves' disease
    (d) measured by LATS assay bear a close correlation with clinical thyroid disease
    (e) of the destructive and stimulating types usually coexist in most patients

16.76 Causes of hypothyroidism include (Table 16.23):
    (a) Pretibial myxoedema
    (b) Hashimoto's thyroiditis
    (c) Iodine deficiency
    (d) Dyshormogenesis
    (e) Bright's disease

16.77 The clinical features of hypothyroidism include (page 932):
    (a) Tachycardia
    (b) Diarrhoea
    (c) Arrest of pubertal development
    (d) Amenorrhoea in young women
    (e) Cold intolerance

16.78 Correct statements about the investigation of primary hypothyroidism include (page 932):
    (a) TSH is the investigation of choice.
    (b) A high TSH level excludes primary hypothyroidism.
    (c) A low total or free T_4 level confirms the hypothyroid state.
    (d) TSH may be low or normal in pituitary disease.
    (e) Thyroxine tolerance test is diagnostic.

16.79 Recognized features of hypothyroidism include (pages 932–933):
    (a) Anaemia
    (b) Increased aspartate transferase levels
    (c) Increased creatine kinase levels
    (d) Hypercholesterolaemia
    (e) Hyponatraemia

16.80 Correct statements regarding the treatment of hypothyroidism include (page 933):
  (a) Replacement thyroxine therapy is rarely lifelong.
  (b) Patients with ischaemic heart disease require higher initial doses of thyroxine.
  (c) The aim of thyroxine therapy is to restore TSH to the normal range.
  (d) Adequacy of replacement should be assessed after at least 6 weeks on a steady dose.
  (e) Clinical improvement on T_4 may not begin for 2 weeks.

16.81 Features of myxoedema coma include (page 934):
  (a) Hypothermia
  (b) Severe cardiac failure
  (c) Hypoventilation
  (d) Hypoglycaemia
  (e) Hyponatraemia

16.82 Proven measures in the treatment of myxoedema coma include (page 934):
  (a) Large doses of intravenous triiodothyronine
  (b) Intravenous hydrocortisone
  (c) Dextrose infusion
  (d) Thyroxine
  (e) Rapid rewarming

16.83 The following statements are correct (page 934):
  (a) The Guthrie test is used to screen the newborn for primary hyperthyroidism.
  (b) Most elderly patients have unsuspected thyroid disease.
  (c) Goitre is more common in men.
  (d) Goitre is commonly noticed as a cosmetic defect.
  (e) Goitres are usually painless.

16.84 The following associations between the cause and the features of a goitre are correct (page 934):
  (a) Pregnancy – diffuse increase
  (b) Graves' disease – bruit
  (c) de Quervain's thyroiditis – tenderness
  (d) Reidel's thyroiditis – 'woody' gland
  (e) Multinodular goitre – laryngeal palsy

16.85 Causes of goitre include (Table 16.24)
  (a) Lymphomas
  (b) Hashimoto's disease
  (c) Iodine deficiency
  (d) Sulphonylureas
  (e) Sarcoidosis

16.86 The following statements regarding the investigation of a goitre are correct (page 935):
  (a) Thoracic inlet X-rays are done to detect tracheal compression.
  (b) A fine-needle aspiration should be performed in all solitary nodules.
  (c) High-resolution ultrasound is an insensitive method for delineating nodules.
  (d) A cold nodule on the thyroid scan is virtually never malignant.
  (e) Continued observation is required when an isolated thyroid nodule is assumed to be benign without excision.

16.87 Indications for surgery with a goitre include (page 935):
  (a) Pregnancy-induced goitre
  (b) Puberty goitre
  (c) Associated cervical lymphadenopathy
  (d) Pressure symptoms on the trachea
  (e) Cosmetic reasons

16.88 The following associations between cell type and the prognosis of thyroid malignancy include (Table 16.25):
  (a) Papillary – poor, especially in the young
  (b) Follicular – poor even when resected
  (c) Anaplastic – excellent
  (d) Lymphoma – variable
  (e) Medullary cell carcinoma – poor

16.89 The following statements about thyroid carcinoma include (pages 935–936):
  (a) Papillary carcinomas do not take up iodine.
  (b) Anaplastic carcinomas respond to radioactive iodine.
  (c) Plasma thyroglobulin is a sensitive tumour marker.
  (d) Medullary carcinoma is often associated with multiple endocrine neoplasia.
  (e) Medullary carcinoma is usually treated with total thyroidectomy.

16.90 Common causes of hyperthyroidism include (Table 16.26):
  (a) Pituitary-secreting TSH tumours
  (b) hCG-producing tumours
  (c) Graves' disease
  (d) Hyperfunctioning ovarian teratomas
  (e) Struma ovarii

16.91 Graves' disease (page 936):
  (a) is the commonest cause of hyperthyroidism
  (b) is due to an autoimmune process
  (c) is associated with TSH receptor antibodies
  (d) has a natural history of remissions and relapses
  (e) patients may eventually become hypothyroid.

16.92 The following statements are correct (page 937):
- (a) Plummer's disease usually remits after a course of antithyroid drugs.
- (b) Toxic multinodular goitres occur more commonly in men.
- (c) de Quervain's thyroiditis shows transient thyrotoxicosis.
- (d) In the acute phase of de Quervain's thyroiditis thyroid scans show suppression of uptake.
- (e) Toxic multinodular goitres are very sensitive to antithyroid drugs.

16.93 The following statements about thyrotoxicosis are correct (page 937):
- (a) Pretibial myxoedema is seen in every patient.
- (b) Thyroid acropachy is common.
- (c) Thyroid function tests are mandatory in any patient with unexplained atrial fibrillation.
- (d) Children may show weight gain.
- (e) Some elderly patients present with a clinical picture more like hypothyroidism.

16.94 Guidelines for the treatment of thyroid disease include (page 938):
- (a) Large goitres usually remit after a course of antithyroid drugs.
- (b) Radioiodine is rarely used owing to the risk of carcinogenesis.
- (c) Patients with dysthyroid disease may show worsening of eye problems after radioiodine.
- (d) Patients who demonstrate poor compliance with drug therapy should not be offered surgery.
- (e) Patients' preference is not given great weight as they are not aware of all the side effects of treatment.

16.95 Correct statements about β-blockers in hyperthyroidism include (pages 938–939):
- (a) They are used to provide rapid partial symptomatic control.
- (b) They increase the peripheral conversion of T_4 to T_3.
- (c) Those with intrinsic sympathomimetic activity are preferred.
- (d) When patients are clinically and biochemically euthyroid, β-blockers can be stopped.
- (e) They can be used alone in subacute thyroiditis.

16.96 Carbimazole (page 939):
- (a) inhibits the formation of thyroid hormones
- (b) treatment's clinical benefit is apparent within 24 hours
- (c) dose is reviewed every week
- (d) treatment is associated with a 50% relapse rate
- (e) treatment is associated with agranulocytosis

16.97 Subtotal thyroidectomy for thyrotoxicosis (page 939):
- (a) can be performed in patients without previously rendering them euthyroid
- (b) antithyroid drugs are usually stopped at least 3 months before surgery

(c) potassium iodide is administered to reduce the vascularity of the gland
(d) may be associated with early postoperative bleeding
(e) is associated with hypocalcaemia

16.98 Radioactive iodine (page 939):
(a) sometimes causes immediate worsening of hyperthyroidism
(b) causes early discomfort in the neck
(c) should be followed by carbimazole as it will enhance the uptake of radioiodine
(d) treatment is associated with subsequent hypothyroidism
(e) results in euthyroidism within 48 hours after therapy

16.99 The following statements about thyroid crisis are correct (page 939):
(a) Hyperpyrexia is a feature.
(b) Corticosteroids are used to suppress associated hypoadrenalism.
(c) It is a rare condition.
(d) It may be precipitated by stress.
(e) Propranolol is used to control it.

16.100 Correct statements about maternal and fetal hyperthyroidism include (page 940):
(a) Fetal heart rate is a direct biological assay of thyroid status.
(b) Untreated neonatal thyrotoxicosis is associated with hyperactivity in later childhood.
(c) Maternal hyperthyroidism during pregnancy is usually severe.
(d) Radioiodine is useful in maternal hyperthyroidism during pregnancy.
(e) Surgery is usually performed in the second trimester in maternal hyperthyroidism.

16.101 Feature of Graves' eye disease include (page 940):
(a) Unilateral proptosis
(b) Optic atrophy
(c) Lid lag
(d) Corneal scarrring
(e) Conjuctival oedema

16.102 Correct statements about thyroid eye disease include (page 940):
(a) It is always associated with hyperthyroidism.
(b) TSH receptor antibodies are almost invariably found in the serum.
(c) Eye manifestations usually parallel the clinical course of Graves' disease.
(d) Visual impairment from optic nerve pressure may occur.
(e) Cosmetic problems often cause patient anxiety.

16.103 Correct statements about the treatment of thyroid eye disease include (page 941):
(a) Thyrotoxic patients should be made euthyroid.
(b) Hypothyroidism may exacerbate the condition.
(c) Some patients gain relief by sitting upright.
(d) Surgical decompression of the orbits is usually needed.
(e) Irradiation of the orbits should be done before steroid treatment.

16.104 Glucocorticoids inhibit (Table 16.28):
(a) Protein synthesis
(b) Gluconeogenesis
(c) Glycogen deposition
(d) Fat deposition
(e) Sodium retention

16.105 The following statements about mineralocorticoids are correct (page 941):
(a) They act predominantly on the intracellular sodium and potassium balance.
(b) They act predominantly on the proximal tubule of the kidney.
(c) Aldosterone is the predominant mineralocorticoid in humans.
(d) Aldosterone is produced solely in the zona glomerulosa.
(e) The weak mineralocorticoid activity of cortisol is unimportant as it is produced in small quantities.

16.106 The following statements about the physiology of glucocorticoid production are correct (page 942):
(a) It is produced in the adrenal medulla.
(b) Its production is under hypothalamic–pituitary control.
(c) Mineralocorticoid secretion is mainly controlled by the renin–angiotensin system.
(d) The cortisol secreted feeds back on the hypothalamus.
(e) Following adrenalectomy cortisol secretion will be absent.

16.107 The following statements about blood sampling for basal levels of cortisol are correct (page 943):
(a) Time for sampling should be accurately recorded.
(b) Stress need not be minimized.
(c) In suspected Cushing's syndrome sampling should be delayed for at least 48 hours after admission.
(d) Dexamethasone suppression tests are used to assess deficient cortisol production.
(e) ACTH stimulation tests are used to assess excess cortisol production.

16.108 In Addison's disease (page 943):
(a) There is destruction of the entire adrenal cortex.
(b) Glucocorticoid production is reduced.

(c) Mineralocorticoid secretion is intact.
(d) Sex steroid production is excessive.
(e) There is a marked male preponderance.

16.109 Causes of primary hypoadrenalism include (Table 16.31):
(a) Autoimmune disease
(b) Tuberculosis
(c) Phaeochromocytoma
(d) AIDS
(e) Meningococcal septicaemia

16.110 Autoimmune conditions associated with Addison's disease include (page 943):
(a) Pernicious anaemia
(b) Hypoparathyroidism
(c) Premature ovarian failure
(d) Type 2 diabetes
(e) Mucocutaneous candidiasis

16.111 Clinical features of Addison's disease include (Table 16.25):
(a) Pigmentation of flexural regions
(b) Normal supine blood pressure
(c) Postural systolic hypertension
(d) Anorexia
(e) Weight gain

16.112 Correct statements about the investigation of Addison's disease include (page 944):
(a) Once Addison's disease is suspected, investigation is urgent.
(b) Even a single cortisol measurement is of great value.
(c) A short ACTH stimulation test should be performed.
(d) A high plasma ACTH level with low cortisol confirms hypoadrenalism.
(e) Adrenal antibodies indicate tuberculosis.

16.113 Biochemical changes in Addison's disease include (page 944):
(a) Hyponatraemia
(b) Hyperkalaemia
(c) Low urea
(d) Hyperglycaemia
(e) Elevated serum aldosterone

16.114 The adequacy of glucocorticoid dose is judged by (page 945):
(a) Restoration of serum electrolytes to normal
(b) Blood pressure response to posture
(c) Suppression of plasma renin activity to normal

(d) Cortisol levels while on synthetic steroids
(e) Restoration of normal weight

16.115 Causes of ACTH-dependent Cushing's syndrome include (Table 16.33):
(a) Adrenal adenomas
(b) Adrenal carcinomas
(c) Glucocorticoid administration
(d) Alcohol-induced pseudo-Cushing's syndrome
(e) Pituitary-dependent disease

16.116 Clinical features of Cushing's syndrome include (Fig 16.26):
(a) Acne
(b) Frontal balding in females
(c) Hypertension
(d) Proximal myopathy
(e) Purple striae

16.117 Out patient screening methods to confirm the presence of Cushing's syndrome include (page 947):
(a) Overnight dexamethasone test
(b) 24-hour urinary free cortisol test
(c) Insulin tolerance test
(d) 48-hour low-dose dexamethasone test
(e) Circadian rhythm

16.118 Factors that decrease vasopressin include (Table 16.35):
(a) Increased osmolality
(b) Hypovolaemia
(c) Hypothyroidism
(d) Ethanol
(e) Antidepressants

16.119 The usual features of SIADH include (page 952):
(a) Dilutional hypernatraemia due to excessive water excretion
(b) Low plasma osmolality with higher urine osmolality
(c) Continued urinary excretion of sodium > 30 mmol/L
(d) Absence of hypokalaemia
(e) Normal renal and adrenal thyroid function

16.120 Recognized causes of SIADH include (page 953):
(a) Small cell carcinoma of the lung
(b) Alcohol withdrawal
(c) Pneumonia
(d) Meningitis
(e) Carbamazepine

16.121 The following mechanisms regarding the endocrine causes of hypertension are correct (Table 16.38):
(a) Renal artery stenosis – excessive renin production
(b) Phaeochromocytoma – excessive aldosterone production
(c) Acromegaly – excessive mineralocorticoid production
(d) Conn's syndrome – inhibition of 11β-hydroxylase
(e) Liquorice ingestion – exogenous catecholamines

16.122 Features of primary hyperaldosteronism include (page 955):
(a) Hyperkalaemia
(b) Urinary potassium loss
(c) Elevated plasma aldosterone levels suppressed by fludrocortisone administration
(d) Increased plasma renin activity
(e) Elevated plasma aldosterone levels that are not suppressed with normal saline administration

16.123 The following statements about the investigation of phaeochromocytoma are correct (page 956):
(a) Normal levels on three 24-hour collections of metanephrines virtually exclude the diagnosis.
(b) CT scan of the abdomen is of limited use because the tumours are often small.
(c) Scanning with MIBG is of limited use in extra-adrenal tumours.
(d) Simple histological examination will distinguish the benign variants from the malignant ones.
(e) The diagnostic test is an increase in blood pressure with the administration of β-blockers.

16.124 Osteoporosis is a consequence of the following conditions (pages 506–508):
(a) Anorexia nervosa
(b) Hyperthyroidism
(c) Acromegaly
(d) Homocystinuria
(e) Primary biliary cirrhosis

16.125 A 33-year-old woman had a plasma thyroxine level of 38 nm/l. Fasting plasma TSH was not detectable, but these levels were 10 times above control value following intravenous injection of TRH. Clinical features include (pages 930–940):
(a) Excessive axillary hair
(b) Atrophied breasts
(c) History of post partum haemorrhage
(d) Hypopigmentation
(e) Hypertension

16.126 A 25-year-old male presented with excessive sweating, joint pain, difficulty in vision and carpal tunnel syndrome. His investigations revealed a serum calcium of 2.7 mmol/l, urine calcium excretion of 9.8 mmol/day, serum phosphate of 1.7 mmol/l, and plasma creatinine of 45 μmol/l. The following statements are correct (pages 513–516):
(a) This patient has hyperparathyroidism.
(b) Parathormone levels will be appropriate to the calcium levels.
(c) There is shortening of the fourth and fifth metacarpals.
(d) There is increased end-organ sensitivity to parathormone.
(e) The patient has hypopituitarism.

16.127 An 85-year-old man had a 2-year history of back and pelvic pain. Investigations revealed a serum calcium of 2 mmol/l, serum inorganic phosphate of 0.6 mmol/l, serum urate of 0.4 mmol/l, alkaline phosphatase of 130 IU/l, urine calcium of 5.1 mmol/l and a creatinine clearance of 70 ml/min. The following are correct (page 510):
(a) This patient has vitamin A intoxication.
(b) Renal function is abnormal for patients of this age.
(c) The calcium levels can be explained by hyperparathyroidism.
(d) Vitamin D should not be administered.
(e) X-ray of the pelvis will show Looser's zones.

16.128 A 29-year-old male with known complete failure of the anterior pituitary was on replacement cortisol and thyroxine therapy. Following an initial period of improvement he had nocturia. He underwent a fluid deprivation test. Baseline values were: weight 73 kg, urine osmolarity 335 mmol/l, and plasma osmolarity 295 mmol/l. After withholding fluids for 8 hours his weight was 68.9 kg, urine osmolarity 240 mmol/l and plasma osmolarity 303 mmol/l. The following are correct (pages 904–910):
(a) These findings exclude hysterical polydipsia.
(b) The administration of cortisol improved his deficiency.
(c) Antidiuretic hormone has no effect on this patient.
(d) The cortisol should be stopped to improve his symptoms.
(e) All these features can be explained by renal resistance to antidiuretic hormone.

16.129 A 30-year-old female is diagnosed as having thyroid cancer. The following cancers are responsive to ^{131}I therapy (page 935):
(a) Follicular cancer of the thyroid
(b) Medullary cancer of the thyroid
(c) Anaplastic thyroid cancer
(d) Primary lymphoma of the thyroid
(e) Choriocarcinoma of the thyroid

16.130 A 19-year-old female presents with primary amenorrhoea. On examination she has a short stature, webbed neck, lack of breast development, and scanty axillary and pubic hair. Recognized features of this condition include (page 925):
(a) Chromosome 47 XXY
(b) Coarctation of the aorta
(c) Increased carrying angle
(d) Low hairline over the back of the neck
(e) Short fourth metacarpal

16.131 A 38-year-old male has gynaecomastia. There is no other abnormality on examination. He is currently on furosemide, digoxin, spironolactone, cimetidine and ketoconazole. Possible causes for his breast enlargement include (Table 16.15):
(a) Regular use of marijuana
(b) Digoxin therapy for 2 years
(c) Use of cimetidine for the past 8 months
(d) Spiranolactone
(e) Long-term furosemide therapy

Diabetes Mellitus and Other Disorders of Metabolism

17.1 Features of diabetes mellitus include (page 959):
   (a) Chronic hypoglycaemia
   (b) Insulin deficiency
   (c) It is irreversible
   (d) Reduced life expectancy
   (e) Insulin resistance

17.2 Macrovascular features of diabetes mellitus include (page 959):
   (a) Retinopathy
   (b) Nephropathy
   (c) Coronary artery disease
   (d) Peripheral vascular disease
   (e) Stroke

17.3 Insulin (page 959):
   (a) is synthesized in the δ-islet cells of the pancreas
   (b) has an active fragment called C-peptide
   (c) is carried to the liver in the systemic circulation
   (d) is completely degraded in the liver
   (e) is inactivated into proinsulin

17.4 Correct statements about glucose metabolism include (pages 959–960):
   (a) The principal organ of glucose haemostasis is the kidney.
   (b) The liver manufactures the 6-carbon glucose molecule from 3-carbon molecules.
   (c) The brain is the major consumer of glucose.
   (d) Glucose uptake by the brain is dependent on insulin.
   (e) The muscle stores glucose as lactate.

17.5 Correct statements about insulin levels and glucose metabolism include (page 961):
   (a) At low insulin levels glucose production is maximal.
   (b) At low insulin levels glucose utilization is minimal.
   (c) At high insulin levels glucose production is minimal.
   (d) At intermediate plasma insulin levels hepatic glucose production is largely suppressed.
   (e) At intermediate plasma insulin levels peripheral utilization of glucose is low.

17.6 Causes of secondary diabetes include (Table 17.1):
   (a) Friedreich's ataxia

(b) Cushing's syndrome
(c) Cystic fibrosis
(d) Haemochromatosis
(e) Myotonic dystrophy

17.7 Counterregulatory hormones are (page 961):
(a) Erythropoietin
(b) Glucagon
(c) Adrenaline
(d) Cortisol
(e) Growth hormone

17.8 The insulin receptor (page 961):
(a) is a glycoprotein
(b) is a dimer
(c) combines with insulin at the β-subunit
(d) when activated causes the migration of the GLUT-4 glucose transporter to the cell surface
(e) DNA sequence coding has been located on the short arm of chromosome 19.

17.9 Hereditary features of NIDDM include (page 964):
(a) HLA linkage
(b) High degree of concordance in identical twins
(c) Glucokinase gene abnormalities
(d) Presents more commonly in those of European extraction than those with south Asian ancestry
(e) It is twice as prevalent in people of African and Caribbean ancestry than in white Europeans.

17.10 Evidence for the autoimmune nature of IDDM includes (pages 963–964):
(a) Islet cell antibodies
(b) Insulin antibodies
(c) Antibodies to glutamic acid decarboxylase
(d) Treatment with cyclosporine prolongs β-cell survival
(e) Antibodies to the intracellular portion of two islet peptides derived from the tyrosine phosphatase family

17.11 Autoimmune diseases associated with IDDM include (page 964):
(a) Autoimmune thyroid disease
(b) Addison's disease
(c) Pernicious anaemia
(d) Hypertension
(e) Maturity-onset diabetes of the young (MODY)

17.12 Correct statements about insulin secretion include (page 965):
(a) Normal subjects have a biphasic response to intravenous glucose.

(b) In NIDDM the first-phase insulin response to intravenous glucose is exaggerated.
(c) In NIDDM insulin secretion in response to oral glucose is delayed.
(d) In NIDDM the insulin response to oral glucose is exaggerated.
(e) Abnormalities of insulin secretion in NIDDM develop early in the course of the disease.

17.13 Features of NIDDM include (page 965):
(a) Progressive β-cell loss
(b) Amyloid deposits in the β-cells of the pancreas
(c) Obesity
(d) Insulin resistance
(e) Non-ketotic hyperosmolar state

17.14 Impaired glucose tolerance (pages 965–966):
(a) in an obese individual makes progression to diabetes more likely
(b) is associated with liver disease
(c) exists in about a fifth of the normal population
(d) is associated with the development of specific microvascular complications of diabetes
(e) is associated with a risk of cardiovascular disease that is twice that of people with normal GTT.

17.15 Features of tropical diabetes include:
(a) Onset after the fourth decade
(b) History of severe malnutrition
(c) Fluctuating insulin resistance
(d) Absence of ketoacidosis when insulin is withdrawn
(e) Insulin dependence

17.16 Recognized features of subacute-presentation diabetes include (page 966):
(a) Thirst
(b) Polyuria
(c) Weight loss
(d) Balanitis
(e) Visual blurring

17.17 Complications of diabetes which may be a presenting feature include (page 966):
(a) Impotence
(b) Retinopathy
(c) Staphylococcal skin infections
(d) Polyneuropathy
(e) Peripheral gangrene

17.18 Correct statements about investigations in diabetes include (page 966):
- (a) In symptomatic patients a single elevated blood glucose ≥ 11.1 mmol/L^{-1} indicates diabetes.
- (b) In asymptomatic patients the diagnosis is made on fasting venous blood glucose levels above 6.7 mmol/L^{-1}.
- (c) A glucose tolerance test is essential before making a diagnosis in all patients.
- (d) Glycosuria is diagnostic of diabetes.
- (e) Fasting lipid levels to exclude hyperlipidaemia should be measured only after the blood glucose is brought under control.

17.19 Correct statements about drugs used in the treatment of diabetes include (page 969):
- (a) Troglitazone has been withdrawn in the UK because of hepatotoxicity.
- (b) Acarbose inhibits the absorption of dietary carbohydrates.
- (c) Repaglinide stimulates insulin production at meal times.
- (d) Troglitazone reduces insulin resistance.
- (e) Insulin sensitizers interact with peroxisome proliferator-activated receptor-γ, a nuclear receptor which regulates genes involved in lipid metabolism.

17.20 Correct statements about therapy in diabetes include (pages 967–968):
- (a) All patients with diabetes require diet therapy.
- (b) Insulin is always indicated in a patient with ketoacidosis.
- (c) Oral hypoglycaemics should be avoided in pregnancy.
- (d) When diet fails in NIDDM, obese patients are usually treated with a biguanide.
- (e) When diet fails in NIDDM, thin patients are usually treated with a sulphonylurea.

17.21 Correct statements about therapy in diabetes include (page 968):
- (a) The diet is no different from a diet considered healthy for the population as a whole.
- (b) Unrefined carbohydrates should be avoided.
- (c) Underweight patients should be given a high-calorie diet.
- (d) Alcohol is forbidden.
- (e) Patients on insulin should avoid snacks between meals.

17.22 Sulphonylureas (page 968):
- (a) promote insulin secretion in response to glucose
- (b) close ATP-sensitive channels on β-cell membrane
- (c) should be avoided in ketotic patients
- (d) are the drugs of choice in pregnant diabetics
- (e) is useful substitute to insulin during major surgery

17.23 Sulphonylureas (page 968):
- (a) bind to circulating albumin

(b) should be used with care in liver disease
(c) cause hypoglycaemia
(d) may cause cholestatic jaundice
(e) particularly chlorpropamide, are associated with a facial flush when alcohol is taken

17.24 Sulphonylureas best avoided in renal impairment include (Table 17.4):
(a) Tolbutamide
(b) Chlopropamide
(c) Glipizide
(d) Gliclazide
(e) Glibenclamide

17.25 Biguanides (page 968):
(a) induce hypoglycaemia in normal volunteers
(b) reduce gluconeogenesis
(c) increase insulin sensitivity
(d) suppress hepatic glucose output
(e) can cause lactic acidosis

17.26 The advantages of pen injection devices to administer insulin include (pages 969–970):
(a) Zinc insulin can be used
(b) Useful in the visually impaired
(c) Pen needles are available on prescription
(d) Convenient to carry around
(e) Can be used discreetly in public places

17.27 Factors that can affect insulin absorption include (page 969):
(a) Site of injection, with absorption being more rapid from the abdomen than from the arm
(b) Local subcutaneous blood flow
(c) Exercise
(d) Warm environment
(e) Local massage

17.28 Correct statements about insulin include (page 969):
(a) Human insulin is produced by DNA coding of cultured yeast or bacterial cells.
(b) Insulin prepared in a clear solution is short acting.
(c) Human insulin may result in antibody formation.
(d) Insulin lispro (Humalog) is an analogue in which reversal of the sequence of two amino acids on the β chain has produced an insulin which dissociates more rapidly from hexamers.
(e) The injection site should be changed regularly to prevent lipohypertrophy.

17.29 Ideal control with insulin therapy is often hard to achieve because (page 970):
  (a) The insulin injected passes into the systemic circulation before passing to the liver.
  (b) The onset and offset of action of subcutaneous soluble insulin are too slow.
  (c) The subcutaneous absorption of longer-acting insulin preparations can be erratic.
  (d) The levels of injected insulin invariably peak and decline, unlike constant basal levels seen in the normal state.
  (e) 50% of insulin produced by the pancreas is cleared by the liver.

17.30 Types of work unsuitable for insulin-treated diabetics include (page 971):
  (a) The medical profession
  (b) Driving heavy goods vehicles
  (c) Journalism
  (d) Piloting an aircraft
  (e) Working close to dangerous machinery in motion

17.31 Complications of insulin therapy include (page 971):
  (a) Injection site abscesses
  (b) Lipoatrophy
  (c) Lipohypertrophy
  (d) Hypoglycaemia
  (e) Insulin resistance

17.32 Features of dawn phenomenon include (page 972):
  (a) Fasting hyperglycaemia
  (b) Nocturnal hypoglycaemia
  (c) Nocturnal peak of growth hormone secretion
  (d) Insulin resistance
  (e) Somogyi effect

17.33 Recognized clinical features of hypoglycaemia include (page 972):
  (a) Sweating
  (b) Pounding of the heart
  (c) Cold sweat
  (d) Aggressive behaviour
  (e) Convulsions

17.34 Correct statements about the treatment of hypoglycaemia include (page 972):
  (a) Intravenous insulin is the drug of choice.
  (b) Milk should be avoided.
  (c) Unconscious patients should be given intravenous glucose.

(d) Unconscious patients should be given intramuscular glucagon.

(e) Any form of rapidly absorbed carbohydrate will relieve early symptoms.

17.35 Correct statements about measuring control of diabetes include (pages 972–973):

(a) The urine dipstick test for glucose is a simple and accurate method.

(b) Fasting blood glucose concentration is a useful guide to therapy with NIDDM.

(c) The dipstick test for urinary ketones is usually useful in routine outpatient management.

(d) A random blood glucose test is of limited value.

(e) Home blood glucose monitoring is essential for good diabetic control.

17.36 Glycosylated (page 973):

(a) haemoglobin provides an index of average blood glucose concentration over the preceding 6 weeks

(b) plasma proteins reflect glycaemic control over the preceding 3 weeks

(c) haemoglobin is a more useful test than glycosylated plasma proteins

(d) plasma proteins are useful in pregnancy

(e) plasma proteins are useful in patients with haemoglobinopathy

17.37 Correct statements about intensive insulin therapy include (page 973):

(a) Early retinopathy may benefit from 2–3 years of intensive therapy.

(b) Retinopathy may show transient deterioration when strict control is first established.

(c) Advanced retinal changes do not benefit from intensive therapy.

(d) Proteinuria benefits from intensive therapy.

(e) Hypoglycaemia is rare with this treatment.

17.38 The main causes of diabetic ketoacidosis include (page 974):

(a) Ketonuria

(b) Metabolic acidosis

(c) Previously undiagnosed diabetes

(d) Interruption of insulin therapy

(e) Stress of intercurrent illness

17.39 Correct statements about diabetic ketoacidosis include (page 974):

(a) Insulin deficiency is a prerequisite.

(b) Stable patients do not readily develop ketoacidosis when insulin is withdrawn.

(c) There is an excess of counterregulatory hormones.

(d) Fluid depletion rarely occurs.

(e) Hepatic ketogenesis is inhibited.

17.40 Recognized biochemical changes in diabetic ketoacidosis include (page 974):
(a) Hepatic glucose production is reduced.
(b) Peripheral uptake by muscle is accelerated.
(c) Osmotic diuresis.
(d) Plasma osmolality falls.
(e) Respiratory acidosis.

17.41 Clinical features of diabetic ketoacidosis include (page 975):
(a) Hyperventilation
(b) Vomiting
(c) The breath smells of ketone
(d) Abdominal pain
(e) Coma

17.42 Complications of diabetic ketoacidosis include (page 976):
(a) Hypotension
(b) Coma
(c) Cerebral oedema
(d) Hypothermia
(e) Deep vein thrombosis

17.43 Recognized features of non-ketotic hyperosmolar state include (page 977):
(a) Significant ketosis
(b) Severe hyperglycaemia
(c) Severe dehydration
(d) It is characteristic of uncontrolled insulin-dependent diabetes mellitus
(e) Impairment of consciousness

17.44 Hyperosmolar state may predispose to (page 977):
(a) Pneumonia
(b) Pyelonephritis
(c) Stroke
(d) Myocardial infarction
(e) Arterial insufficiency in the lower limbs

17.45 Correct statements about non-ketotic hyperosmolar state include (page 978):
(a) Many patients are extremely sensitive to insulin.
(b) Normal saline is the standard of fluid replacement.
(c) Half-normal saline is the treatment of choice, when available.
(d) Survivors will need insulin therapy for the rest of their life.
(e) Reported mortality is around one-third of those afflicted.

17.46 Lactic acidosis in diabetics (page 978):
(a) may occur with biguanide therapy
(b) was usually associated with phenformin therapy

(c) is extremely uncommon in patients taking metformin
(d) is evidenced by severe respiratory acidosis
(e) is associated with a low mortality

17.47 The major causes of death in diabetics include (pages 959–985):
(a) Splenic infarction
(b) Infective endocarditis
(c) Nephropathy
(d) Stroke
(e) Heart disease

17.48 Recognized features of 'syndrome X' include (page 978):
(a) Central obesity
(b) Hypertension
(c) Dyslipoproteinaemia
(d) Hypoinsulinaemia
(e) High risk of coronary artery disease

17.49 Recognized features of diabetic eye disease include (page 979):
(a) It is the commonest cause of blindness in the population as a whole up to the age of 65.
(b) Cataracts
(c) Rubeotic glaucoma
(d) Sixth cranial nerve palsy
(e) Rubeosis iridis

17.50 Correct statements about diabetic retinopathy include (pages 979–980):
(a) After 20 years of IDDM almost all patients have some retinopathy.
(b) Background retinopathy constitutes a serious threat to vision.
(c) Maculopathy does not lead to blindness in the absence of proliferation.
(d) The earliest sign of preproliferative retinopathy is the appearance of 'hard exudates'.
(e) Proliferative retinopathy is associated with the formation of new vessels.

17.51 Correct statements about the management of diabetic eye disease include (pages 980–981):
(a) There is no specific medical treatment for background retinopathy.
(b) Rapid progression may occur in pregnant patients.
(c) The progress is slow in those with nephropathy.
(d) Proliferative retinopathy is treated by laser photocoagulation.
(e) Fluorescein angiography is used to define the extent of rubeosis.

17.52 Early referral of diabetics to an ophthalmologist is essential when (page 980):
(a) Background retinopathy is recognized

    (b) Visual acuity is deteriorating
    (c) Hard exudates encroach the macula
    (d) Cottonwool spots appear
    (e) New vessel formation occurs

17.53 The kidney may be damaged by diabetes in the following ways (page 981):
    (a) Interstitial nephritis
    (b) Tubular necrosis
    (c) Glomerular damage
    (d) Ischaemia due to hypertrophy of afferent and efferent arterioles
    (e) Ascending infection

17.54 Correct statements about diabetic glomerular sclerosis include (page 981):
    (a) Microalbuminuria is a predictive marker of increased cardiovascular risk in NIDDM.
    (b) The earliest functional abnormality is renal hypertrophy with raised glomerular filtration.
    (c) The initial structural lesion in the glomerulus is thickening of the basement membrane.
    (d) A rise in plasma creatinine is an early feature.
    (e) The earliest evidence of glomerular involvement is microalbuminuria.

17.55 Correct statements about the management of diabetic nephropathy include (page 982):
    (a) ACE inhibitors and calcium channel blockers are the drugs of choice for the control of hypertension.
    (b) Chlorpropamide is the drug of choice in such patients.
    (c) Insulin requirements increase.
    (d) Diabetic retinopathy in such patients tends to progress rapidly and frequent ophthalmic supervision is essential.
    (e) Aggressive treatment of blood pressure has been shown to slow the rate of deterioration in renal failure.

17.56 Correct statements about diabetic neuropathy include (pages 982–983):
    (a) Occlusion of the vasa nervosum is the prime cause in the symmetrical type.
    (b) Accumulation of sorbitol and fructose in the Schwann cells has been implicated.
    (c) The earliest functional stage is an increase in nerve conduction velocity.
    (d) The earliest histological change is segmental demyelination.
    (e) In the early stages the axons are damaged.

17.57 Correct statements about diabetic neuropathy include (page 983):
    (a) Third cranial nerve lesions have intact pupillary reflexes.
    (b) Amyotrophy often resolves with careful control of blood glucose.
    (c) Vagal neuropathy results in tachycardia.

    (d) Vagal damage can lead to gastroparesis.
    (e) Impotence is common.

17.58 Factors that produce tissue necrosis in the diabetic foot include
(page 984):
    (a) Ischaemia
    (b) Infection
    (c) Neuropathy
    (d) Hypothermia
    (e) Hypotension

17.59 Correct statements about the management of diabetics during surgery
include (page 985):
    (a) Insulin should not be injected into glucose solution.
    (b) Long-acting insulin should be stopped the day before surgery and
        soluble insulin substituted.
    (c) Diabetic patients should be last on the theatre list.
    (d) Postoperatively insulin is maintained until the patient is able to eat.
    (e) Non-insulin-treated patients should stop medications 2 days before
        the operation.

17.60 Correct statements about pregnancy in diabetics include (page 985):
    (a) Urinary glucose is valuable in the control of diabetes.
    (b) Insulin requirements rise in pregnancy.
    (c) Retinopathy may deteriorate during pregnancy.
    (d) Poorly controlled diabetes is associated with fetal macrosomia.
    (e) The infant is more susceptible to hyaline membrane disease than
        infants of non-diabetics of similar maturity.

17.61 Factors that predispose to recurrent severe hypoglycaemia in diabetics
include (page 986):
    (a) Overtreatment with insulin
    (b) Pituitary insufficiency
    (c) Renal failure
    (d) Diabetic gastroparesis
    (e) Exocrine pancreatic failure

17.62 Factors that predispose to recurrent ketoacidosis include (page 987):
    (a) Inappropriate insulin combination
    (b) Urinary tract infection
    (c) Thyrotoxicosis
    (d) Psychosocial causes
    (e) Tuberculosis

17.63 Causes of hypoglycaemia include (page 987):
    (a) Hereditary fructose intolerance
    (b) Advanced liver disease

(c) Insulinoma
(d) Excessive alcohol ingestion
(e) Large sarcomas

17.64 Recognized presenting features of insulinomas include (Table 17.8):
(a) Abnormal behaviour
(b) Grand mal seizures
(c) Palpitations
(d) Sweating
(e) Dyspnoea

17.65 Whipple's triad includes (page 987):
(a) Demonstration of inappropriately high insulin levels during hypoglycaemia
(b) Symptoms associated with fasting
(c) Hyperglycaemia during symptomatic episodes
(d) Glucose aggravates the symptoms
(e) Abnormal (diabetic) glucose tolerance

17.66 Correct statements about the management of insulinoma include (page 988):
(a) Diazoxide is useful when the insulinoma is malignant.
(b) Symptoms may remit with octreotide.
(c) Blind laparotomy is the surgical procedure of choice.
(d) Localization is possible using a rapid insulin assay on blood sampled at different levels from the pancreatic vein.
(e) The most effective treatment is surgical excision of the tumour.

17.67 Endocrine causes of hypoglycaemia include (page 988):
(a) Thyrotoxicosis
(b) Addison's disease
(c) Isolated ACTH deficiency
(d) Hypopituitarism
(e) Cushing's syndrome

17.68 Causes of drug-induced hypoglycaemia include (page 989):
(a) Propranolol
(b) Biguanide therapy for diabetes
(c) Pentamidine
(d) Salicylates
(e) Quinine

17.69 Chylomicrons (page 989):
(a) are synthesized in the small intestine postprandially
(b) contain a large amount of cholesterol
(c) transport digested fat to the liver

(d) when newly formed contain several apoproteins

(e) are devoid of triglyceride

17.70 Very low-density lipoprotein particles (page 989):

(a) are synthesized in the liver

(b) contain most of the endogenously synthesized cholesterol

(c) lack apoprotein B 100

(d) contain apoprotein C

(e) are the precursors of intermediate low-density lipoprotein molecules

17.71 Correct statements about low-density lipoprotein include (page 990):

(a) It is the main carrier of cholesterol.

(b) It has a single apoprotein B100 on the surface.

(c) The number of hepatic LDL receptors regulates circulating LDL concentration.

(d) HMG CoA reductase regulates circulating LDL concentration.

(e) LDL is converted into bile salts.

17.72 High-density lipoprotein particles (page 990):

(a) are produced in the kidney

(b) are produced in the intestine

(c) carry about one-third of the total circulating cholesterol in the blood

(d) are capable of transporting cholesterol from the periphery to the liver

(e) take up cholesterol from cell membranes in the peripheral tissues

17.73 Correct statements about serum lipid levels include (page 991):

(a) The total cholesterol from a fasting sample consists mainly of LDL.

(b) The triglyceride concentrations in a fasting sample reflect VLDL particles.

(c) Chylomicrons are normally increased in the fasting state.

(d) Serum cholesterol does not change significantly after a meal.

(e) Plasma lipid concentrations can be deranged for up to 3 months following a myocardial infarction.

17.74 Correct statements about lipoprotein concentration and cardiovascular risk include (page 991):

(a) There is a strong association between both total and LDL cholesterol concentrations and coronary heart risk.

(b) Young men with the monogenic disorder familial hypercholesterolaemia rarely die of premature cardiac disease.

(c) There is an increasing improvement in cardiovascular risk with increasing duration of treatment for hyperlipidaemia.

(d) HDL particles appear to protect against atheroma.

(e) Raised total cholesterol concentration predisposes to a serious risk despite the absence of other cardiovascular risk factors.

17.75 Indications for measuring serum lipid levels include (page 991):
(a) Family history of premature coronary heart disease
(b) Presence of xanthoma
(c) Presence of corneal arcus before the age of 40
(d) Hypertension
(e) Acute pancreatitis

17.76 Causes of secondary hyperlipidaemia include (Table 17.9):
(a) Nephrotic syndrome
(b) Hyperthyroidism
(c) Poorly controlled diabetes mellitus
(d) Thiazides
(e) Hepatic dysfunction

17.77 Features of heterozygous familial hypercholesterolaemia include (pages 992–993):
(a) The average general practitioner would have about four patients on his list.
(b) Patients may have no physical signs.
(c) Xanthelasma are diagnostic of familial hypercholesterolaemia.
(d) Affected children have no LDL receptors in the liver.
(e) The diagnosis is made on the presence of very high plasma cholesterol concentrations unresponsive to dietary modification.

17.78 Hypertriglyceridaemia is associated with an increased risk of (page 994):
(a) Pancreatitis
(b) Retinal vein thrombosis
(c) Cardiovascular events
(d) Hepatoma
(e) Gastric cancer

17.79 Drugs that cause hypertriglyceridaemia include (page 994):
(a) Thiazides
(b) Nicotinic acid
(c) Alcohol
(d) Fish oil
(e) Glucocorticoids

17.80 Correct statements about the management of hypercholesterolaemia include (pages 989–997):
(a) Most patients with polygenic hypercholesterolaemia will require drug therapy.
(b) Perimenopausal women with hypercholesterolaemia should not be offered hormone replacement therapy because they respond adversely to exogenous oestrogens with a rise in lipids.
(c) Individuals with familial hypercholesterolaemia will require both diet and drugs.

(d) A reduction of body weight is not recommended in polygenic hypercholesterolaemia.
(e) Statins should be avoided in survivors of myocardial infarction when the cholesterol level is below 6 mmol/l.

17.81 Correct statements about drugs used in hyperlipidaemia include (pages 989–997):
(a) Probucol is a first-line agent.
(b) Fibrates reduce HDL cholesterol concentration.
(c) Bile acid-binding resins reduce LDL cholesterol concentration.
(d) HMG CoA reductase inhibitors reduce HDL cholesterol.
(e) Concurrent therapy with HMG CoA reductase inhibitors and fibrates is usually avoided.

17.82 The main elements of a lipid-lowering diet are (page 997):
(a) Reduction of total fat intake
(b) Increase in saturated fat intake
(c) Reduction of dietary cholesterol intake
(d) Increase fibre content
(e) Achieve ideal body weight

17.83 Causes of hypolipidaemia include (page 997):
(a) Tangier's disease
(b) Severe protein – energy malnutrition
(c) Severe malabsorption
(d) Intestinal lymphangiectasia
(e) Galactosaemia

17.84 Recognized features of galactosaemia include (page 999):
(a) Cataracts
(b) Renal tubular defects
(c) Hepatosplenomegaly
(d) Mental retardation
(e) Deficiency of galactose-1-phosphate uridyl transferase

17.85 In Fanconi's syndrome there is defective tubular reabsorption of (page 999):
(a) Amino acids
(b) Phosphate
(c) Bicarbonate
(d) Glucose
(e) Urate

17.86 Features of Lowe's syndrome include (page 999):
(a) Aminoaciduria
(b) Abnormal skull shape
(c) Mental retardation

    (d) Cataracts
    (e) Hypotonia

17.87 In cystinuria there is defective tubular reabsorption and jejunal absorption of (page 1000):
    (a) Cystine
    (b) Lysine
    (c) Ornithine
    (d) Arginine
    (e) Fatty acids

17.88 Malabsorption of tryptophan occurs in (page 1001):
    (a) Blue diaper syndrome
    (b) Hartnup's disease
    (c) Familial iminoglycinuria
    (d) Cystinosis
    (e) Methionine malabsorption syndrome

17.89 Gaucher's disease (page 1001):
    (a) is due to accumulation of glucosylceramide in the lysosomes
    (b) is due to a deficiency in glucocerebrosidase
    (c) involves the spleen
    (d) is common in Ashkenazi Jews
    (e) of the non-neuropathic type may show improvement with alglucerase infusion

17.90 Niemann–Pick disease (page 1001):
    (a) is due to a deficiency of lysosomal sphingomyelinase
    (b) results in accumulation of sphingomyelin and glycosphingolipids in the macrophages
    (c) results in foam cells in the marrow
    (d) causes mental retardation
    (e) causes hepatosplenomegaly

17.91 Recognized features of mucopolysaccharidoses include (page 1001):
    (a) Accumulation of glycosaminoglycans in the lysosomes
    (b) Hypermobile joints
    (c) Dysostosis
    (d) Poor vision
    (e) Mental retardation

17.92 Recognized features of Tay–Sachs disease include (page 1001):
    (a) Epilepsy
    (b) Dementia
    (c) Blindness
    (d) Cherry red spot-like macula
    (e) Common in Ashkenazi Jews

17.93 Fabry's disease (page 1002):
  (a) is inherited in an autosomal dominant manner
  (b) is due to a deficiency of lysosome hydrolase α-galactosidase
  (c) causes accumulation of glycosphingolipids with terminal α-galactosyl moieties
  (d) results in renal problems in adult life
  (e) patients present with peripheral nerve involvement

17.94 Cystinosis (page 1002):
  (a) is inherited in an autosomal dominant manner
  (b) is characterized by the accumulation of cystine in the reticuloendothelial cells
  (c) in infants is usually fatal in the first year due to renal failure
  (d) in adults is benign
  (e) results in corneal deposits of cystine

17.95 The following associations in amyloidosis are correct (page 1002):
  (a) Portugese type – neuropathic amyloidosis
  (b) Familial Mediterranean fever – renal amyloidosis
  (c) Chronic haemodialysis – carpal tunnel syndrome
  (d) Down's syndrome – cerebral deposits
  (e) Immunocyte-related amyloidosis – macroglossia

17.96 The following associations in amyloidosis are correct (page 1002):
  (a) Portugese type – prealbumin in β sheets
  (b) Familial Mediterranean fever – AA fibrils
  (c) Chronic haemodialysis – β-microglobulin
  (d) Down's syndrome – A4 protein
  (e) Immunocyte-related amyloidosis – amyloid light (AL) chains

17.97 Reactive systemic amyloidosis is associated with (page 1003):
  (a) Overproduction of serum amyloid A (SAA)
  (b) Tuberculosis
  (c) Rheumatoid arthritis
  (d) Malignancy
  (e) Nephrotic syndrome

17.98 Correct statements about porphyrin metabolism include (pages 1003–1004):
  (a) Porphyrins consists of four pyrrole rings.
  (b) The chief rate-limiting step in the production of haem is δ-ALA synthetase.
  (c) Porphobilinogen deaminase is raised in acute porphyrias.
  (d) In porphyria excess production of porphyrins occurs in the liver.
  (e) In porphyria excess production of porphyrins occurs in the bone marrow.

17.99 Features of acute intermittent porphyria include (page 1004):
    (a) Abdominal pain
    (b) Polyneuropathy
    (c) Bullous eruption
    (d) Family history
    (e) The urine turns red-brown on standing

17.100 Correct statements about the investigation and management of acute intermittent porphyria include (page 1004):
    (a) Ehrlich's aldehyde test is performed on the urine.
    (b) Erythrocyte PBG deaminase should be measured in family members.
    (c) High carbohydrate intake is beneficial.
    (d) Intravenous haematin infusion is beneficial.
    (e) Liver function tests are abnormal.

17.101 Features of porphyria cutanea tarda include (page 1005):
    (a) Bullous eruption on exposure to sunlight
    (b) Alcohol is an aetiological agent
    (c) Abnormality of hepatic uroporphyrinogen decarboxylase
    (d) Decreased urinary uroporphyrin
    (e) Exacerbations can be induced by venesection

17.102 Features of erythropoietic protoporphyria include (page 1005):
    (a) Inherited as an autosomal recessive trait.
    (b) Presents with irritation of the skin on exposure to sunlight.
    (c) Increased protoporphyrin in red cells.
    (d) Oral β-carotene is useful in alleviating symptoms.
    (e) Renal involvement may occur.

Neurological Disease

18.1 Common neurological conditions in developing countries include (page 1007):
(a) Leprosy
(b) Tuberculous meningitis
(c) Tetanus
(d) Cerebral malaria
(e) Cysticercosis

18.2 Common neurological conditions in the UK include (Table 18.1):
(a) Herpes zoster
(b) Stroke
(c) Sciatica
(d) Epilepsy
(e) Dementia

18.3 Pain receptors responsible for headache are present in (page 1008):
(a) Brain substance
(b) Extra cranial vessels
(c) Muscles of the neck
(d) Paranasal sinuses
(e) Teeth

18.4 Recognized features of 'headache of intracranial pressure' include (page 1008):
(a) It is typically worse after lying down for some hours.
(b) It is present on waking.
(c) It is accompanied by vomiting.
(d) It is made worse by sneezing.
(e) It is made worse by coughing.

18.5 Mechanisms for pressure headache include (page 1008):
(a) Displacement of meninges by intracranial mass lesions
(b) Displacement of basal vessels by intracranial mass lesions
(c) Shift of meninges and basal vessels by cerebral oedema
(d) Cough-induced changes in cerebrospinal fluid
(e) Irritation of the scalp by tumour

18.6 Conditions that are suspected with headaches of subacute onset include (page 1009):
(a) Myasthenia gravis
(b) Intracranial mass lesion
(c) Encephalitis
(d) Viral meningitis
(e) Giant cell arteritis

18.7 Causes of a single episode of severe headache include (page 1009):
    (a) Parkinson's disease
    (b) Migraine
    (c) Subarachnoid haemorrhage
    (d) Meningitis
    (e) Hypotension

18.8 Causes of recurrent headache include (page 1008):
    (a) Hypertension without affecting the brain
    (b) Migraine
    (c) Tension
    (d) Glaucoma
    (e) Sinusitis

18.9 The following assocations are correct (page 1009):
    (a) Hemiplegia – festinant gait
    (b) Parkinson's disease – spastic gait
    (c) Diseases of cerebellar vermis – truncal ataxia
    (d) Tabes dorsalis – high-stepping or stamping gait
    (e) Frontal lobe lesions – gait apraxia

18.10 Conditions that should be considered when patients describe blackouts include (page 1010):
    (a) Epilepsy
    (b) Syncope
    (c) Hypoglycaemia
    (d) Heart blocks
    (e) Panic attacks

18.11 Recognized neurotransmitters include (page 1011):
    (a) L-dopa
    (b) Noradrenaline
    (c) Adrenaline
    (d) Carbidopa
    (e) Opioid peptides

18.12 Destructive lesions within the left fronto-temporo-parietal region in right-handed people cause (page 1013):
    (a) Dressing apraxia
    (b) Dysphasia
    (c) Constructional apraxia
    (d) Agraphia
    (e) Alexia

18.13 The following statements are correct (page 1013):
    (a) Almost all right-handed people have language function in the right hemisphere.

(b) Most left-handed people have language function in the left hemisphere.
(c) Many aphasic patients are somewhat dysarthric.
(d) Naming difficulty is an early sign in all types of aphasia.
(e) Disorders in right-handed patients with right hemisphere lesions are more difficult to define but comprise abnormalities of perception of internal and external space.

18.14 Causes of dysarthria include (page 1013):
(a) Local lesions of the tongue
(b) Cerebellar disease
(c) Parkinson's disease
(d) Lower motor lesions of the lower cranial nerves
(e) Upper motor lesions of the lower cranial nerves

18.15 In Broca's aphasia (page 1013):
(a) The lesion is in the left parietal lobe.
(b) There is reduced fluency of speech.
(c) Comprehension is preserved.
(d) The patient is mute.
(e) There is a failure to construct speech.

18.16 In Wernicke's aphasia (page 1013):
(a) The lesion is in the left temporoparietal region.
(b) Language is fluent.
(c) The words are incorrect.
(d) There may be outpouring of jargon.
(e) There is memory loss.

18.17 Destructive lesions of the temporal region cause (Table 18.6, 18.7):
(a) *Déjà vu* phenomenon
(b) Complex partial seizures
(c) Formed visual hallucinations
(d) Conjugate deviation of head and eyes away from the lesion
(e) Hemiparesis

18.18 Correct statements about memory and its disorders include (page 1013):
(a) Disorders of memory follow damage to the medial surface of the temporal lobe.
(b) Bilateral lesions are usually necessary to cause amnesia.
(c) In organic disorders of memory the more remote events are recalled poorly, with intact memory of more recent events.
(d) Memory loss is a part of dementia of any cause.
(e) Lesions of the occipital lobe can cause memory loss.

18.19 Causes of amnestic syndrome include (Table 18.4):
(a) Following hypoglycaemia

    (b) Herpes simplex encephalitis
    (c) Severe head injury
    (d) Posterior cerebral artery occlusion
    (e) Wernicke–Korsakoff syndrome

18.20 The sense of smell (page 1014):
    (a) may be lost with head injury
    (b) may be lost in meningiomas of the olfactory groove
    (c) may be permanently lost after upper respiratory viral infection
    (d) is diminished in nasal obstruction
    (e) is carried by the second cranial nerve

18.21 Causes of papilloedema include (Table 18.7):
    (a) Accelerated hypertension
    (b) Subarachnoid haemorrhage
    (c) Intracranial mass lesion
    (d) Hypocalcaemia
    (e) Severe anaemia

18.22 Visual acuity (page 1015):
    (a) is tested with a Snellen chart
    (b) when impaired due to refractive errors cannot be corrected with lenses
    (c) when impaired due to refractive errors can be corrected with a pinhole
    (d) can be tested with a white hatpin
    (e) means impaired colour vision

18.23 The following associations are correct (pages 1015–1016):
    (a) Scotoma – glaucoma
    (b) Tunnel vision – retinitis pigmentosa
    (c) Paracentral scotoma – optic nerve lesion
    (d) Total unilateral visual loss with loss of pupillary light reflex – complete optic nerve lesions
    (e) No visual impairment – retrobulbar neuritis

18.24 In papilloedema (page 1015):
    (a) the earliest ophthalmological sign is redness of the disc
    (b) spontaneous retinal venous pulsation is clearly seen
    (c) the physiological cup is obliterated
    (d) there is a diminution of the blind spot
    (e) small haemorrhages may surround the disc

18.25 Conditions that may simulate papilloedema include (page 1015):
    (a) Optic atrophy
    (b) Drusen
    (c) Myelinated nerve fibres

(d) Hypermetropia
(e) Retrobulbar neuritis

18.26 Causes of optic atrophy include (page 1016):
(a) Infarction of the nerve
(b) Multiple sclerosis
(c) Syphilis
(d) Vitamin D deficiency
(e) Methyl alcohol poisoning

18.27 Causes of bitemporal hemianopia include (page 1016):
(a) Tumour of the occipital cortex
(b) Pituitary neoplasm
(c) Craniopharyngioma
(d) Secondary neoplasm
(e) Temporal lobe lesions

18.28 Correct statements about the occipital cortex include (page 1016):
(a) Homonymous hemianopic defects occur as a result of lesions in the occipital cortex.
(b) The occipital pole is supplied by the middle cerebral artery.
(c) The macular region of the retina is at the occipital pole.
(d) It is supplied by the anterior cerebral artery.
(e) Absent pupillary responses are a characteristic feature of cortical blindness.

18.29 Sympathetic fibres to the eye (page 1016):
(a) constrict the pupil
(b) originate in the hypothalamus
(c) emerge from the spinal cord close to the lung apex
(d) when affected cause Horner's syndrome
(e) of the postganglionic type arise in the ciliary ganglion

18.30 Correct statements about the light reflex include (page 1016):
(a) The afferent fibres do not cross in chiasm.
(b) It is the same as the convergence reflex.
(c) The efferent fibres pass to both lateral geniculate bodies.
(d) The efferent fibres are parasympathetic fibres.
(e) The contralateral pupil constricts during a consensual reflex.

18.31 Pupillary constriction is a feature of (page 1017):
(a) Old age
(b) Argyll–Robertson pupil
(c) Holmes–Adie syndrome
(d) Horner's syndrome
(e) Third cranial nerve palsy

18.32 Causes of Horner's syndrome include (Table 18.8):
(a) Massive cerebral infarction
(b) Lateral medullary syndrome
(c) Syringomyelia
(d) Cervical rib
(e) Migraine

18.33 Correct statements about Horner's syndrome include (page 1018):
(a) It is due to interruption of the parasympathetic fibres to one eye.
(b) Lesions distal to the superior cervical ganglion do not affect sweating at all.
(c) Proptosis is a prominent feature.
(d) There is slight ptosis.
(e) A lesion distal to the superior cervical ganglion causes denervation hypersensitivity of the pupil.

18.34 Correct statements about conjugate gaze palsy include (page 1018):
(a) Conjugate gaze palsy is due to oculomotor nerve palsy.
(b) A destructive frontal-lobe lesion causes failure of conjugate lateral gaze to the side opposite to the lesion.
(c) A unilateral destructive brain-stem lesion involving the parapontine reticular formation causes failure of horizontal gaze towards the side of the lesion.
(d) Squint is a prominent feature.
(e) Ptosis is a prominent feature.

18.35 Internuclear ophthalmoplegia (page 1019):
(a) is due to a lesion within the medial longitudinal fasciculus
(b) when bilateral is almost pathognomonic of multiple sclerosis
(c) of the right side causes nystagmus on abduction of the left eye
(d) on the right side causes failure of adduction of the right eye
(e) is a common feature of normal ageing

18.36 Impaired vertical upward gaze is a recognized feature of (page 1019):
(a) Lower brain-stem tumours
(b) Parinaud's syndrome
(c) Progressive supranuclear palsy
(d) Normal ageing
(e) Sixth cranial nerve palsy

18.37 Squint (page 1019):
(a) of the concomitant type is usually associated with diplopia
(b) of the paralytic type is maximal in the direction of the action of the weak muscle
(c) of the concomitant type is associated with defective vision in the deviating eye

(d) when latent is assessed with the *cover test*
(e) may be a feature of myasthenia gravis

18.38 Common causes of an oculomotor nerve lesion include (Table 18.19):
(a) Aneurysm of anterior communicating artery
(b) 'Coning' of the temporal lobe
(c) Diabetes mellitus
(d) Infarction of the medulla
(e) Midbrain tumour

18.39 The following statements are correct (page 1020):
(a) In diabetes, infarction of the third nerve usually spares the pupil.
(b) In a third-nerve palsy the eye can still abduct.
(c) In a third-nerve palsy the eye can rotate inwards or intort.
(d) In an isolated third-nerve palsy the patient complains of diplopia when attempting to look down and away from the affected side.
(e) In a sixth-nerve lesion there is a convergent squint with diplopia maximal on looking to the side of the lesion.

18.40 Causes of abducent nerve lesions include (page 1020):
(a) Multiple sclerosis
(b) Raised intracranial pressure
(c) Nasopharyngeal carcinoma
(d) Diabetes mellitus
(e) As a sequel of head injury

18.41 Correct statements about the trigeminal nerve include (page 1020):
(a) It is mainly a motor nerve.
(b) Sensory fibres from its divisions pass to the trigeminal ganglion at the apex of the petrous temporal bone.
(c) Ascending fibres transmitting the sensation of light touch enter the nucleus in the upper midbrain.
(d) Motor fibres arise in the upper pons.
(e) Descending fibres carry pain and temperature sensation from the spinal tract of the fifth nerve.

18.42 The following statements regarding the signs of a trigeminal nerve lesion are correct (page 1021):
(a) Diminution of the corneal reflex is often the last sign of a fifth-nerve lesion.
(b) A complete fifth-nerve lesion causes contralateral sensory loss to the face.
(c) A complete fifth-nerve lesion causes the jaw to deviate to the side opposite to the lesion when the mouth is opened.

    (d) Brain-stem lesions of the lower trigeminal nuclei produce circumoral sensory loss.

    (e) When the spinal tract alone is involved, the sensory loss is restricted to pain and temperature sensation.

18.43 Causes of trigeminal nerve lesions include (page 1021):
    (a) Multiple sclerosis
    (b) Syringobulbia
    (c) Acoustic neuroma
    (d) Aneurysm of the external carotid artery
    (e) Cavernous sinus thrombosis

18.44 Clinical features of trigeminal neuralgia (tic douloureux) include (page 1021):
    (a) It is seen most commonly in young adults.
    (b) It is almost always bilateral.
    (c) The pain characteristically occurs at night.
    (d) Spontaneous remissions last for months or years before recurrence.
    (e) The corneal reflex is preserved.

18.45 The facial nerve (page 1022):
    (a) arises from its nucleus in the medulla oblongata
    (b) supplies the muscles of facial expression
    (c) carries sensory taste fibres from the posterior third of the tongue via the chorda tympani
    (d) leaves the skull through the stylomastoid foramen
    (e) supplies sensory fibres to the cornea

18.46 Features of unilateral lower motor neurone lesion of the face include (page 1022):
    (a) Weakness of the lower part of the face on the side opposite the lesion.
    (b) The frontalis muscle is spared.
    (c) Eye closure and blinking are not affected.
    (d) The platysma muscle is weak.
    (e) There is relative preservaton of spontaneous 'emotional' movement compared to voluntary movement.

18.47 Causes of facial nerve involvement include (page 1023):
    (a) Sarcoidosis
    (b) Myasthenia gravis
    (c) Ramsay Hunt syndrome
    (d) Dystrophia myotonica
    (e) Guillain–Barré syndrome

18.48 Features of Bell's palsy include (page 1023):
    (a) Associated fifth cranial nerve involvement
    (b) Pain behind the ear is common at the onset

(c) Marked unilateral facial weakness
(d) Most of the patients are left with a severe, unsightly, residual weakness
(e) The condition is usually bilateral

18.49 Causes of hemifacial spasm include (page 1023):
(a) Idiopathic
(b) Acoustic neuroma
(c) Paget's disease of the skull
(d) Following Bell's palsy
(e) Pressure from aberrant vessels in the cerebellopontine angle

18.50 Cochlear nerve (page 1024):
(a) Auditory fibres from the cochlea pass to nuclei in the medulla.
(b) Fibres from the cochlear nuclei pass upwards through the lateral lemnisci.
(c) Fibres from the cochlear nuclei pass upwards to the lateral geniculate bodies.
(d) Fibres from the cochlear nuclei pass upwards to the temporal gyri.
(e) Auditory fibres arise from the spiral organ of Corti.

18.51 The vestibular nuclei are connected to the (page 1024):
(a) Spinal cord
(b) Cerebellum
(c) Nuclei of ocular muscles
(d) Parapontine reticular formation
(e) Temporal lobe

18.52 Correct statements about the clinical features of the vestibulocochlear nerve include (page 1024):
(a) Deafness indicates a vestibular lesion.
(b) The main symptom of a vestibular nerve lesion is vertigo.
(c) In cochlear nerve lesions both bone and air conduction are decreased.
(d) Nystagmus is the principal sign of a cochlear nerve lesion.
(e) Vomiting frequently accompanies acute vertigo of any cause.

18.53 Causes of vertigo include (Table 18.11):
(a) Ethyl alcohol
(b) Multiple sclerosis
(c) Gentamicin toxicity
(d) Ménière's disease
(e) Cerebellopontine angle lesion

18.54 Correct statements about nystagmus include (pages 1024–1025):
(a) True nystagmus is sustained and demonstrable within binocular gaze.
(b) Pendular nystagmus is characteristic of 'acquired' neurological diseases.

(c) Horizontal nystagmus due to central lesions is usually transient.
(d) Vertical nystagmus is caused only by central lesions.
(e) Downbeat nystagmus is caused by lesions around the foramen magnum.

18.55 Correct statements about the investigations of vestibulocochlear nerve lesions include (page 1025):
  (a) Audiometry is of value in distinguishing sensorineural deafness from conductive deafness.
  (b) Ice-cold water in the left ear causes nystagmus, with the fast movement to the right.
  (c) Warm water in the left ear causes nystagmus with the fast movement to the left.
  (d) Auditory evoked potentials record the response from a repetitive click stimulus.
  (e) The level of lesion may be detected by abnormalities in response to auditory evoked potentials.

18.56 Features of cerebellopontine angle lesions include (page 1025):
  (a) Perceptive deafness
  (b) Contralateral cerebellar signs
  (c) Ipsilateral pyramidal signs
  (d) Sixth cranial nerve lesion
  (e) Seventh cranial nerve lesion

18.57 Causes of cerebellopontine angle lesions include (page 1025):
  (a) Temporal lobe infarction
  (b) Acoustic neuroma
  (c) Meningioma
  (d) Secondary neoplasm
  (e) Gentamicin toxicity

18.58 The glossopharyngeal nerve (page 1026):
  (a) arises in the pons
  (b) leaves the skull through the jugular foramen
  (c) is the efferent pathway of the gag reflex
  (d) supplies taste fibres to the anterior two-thirds of the tongue
  (e) supplies the stylopharyngeus muscle

18.59 The vagus nerve (page 1026):
  (a) is the afferent pathway for the gag reflex
  (b) supplies the larynx
  (c) supplies the upper oesophagus
  (d) supplies the sympathetic fibres of the heart
  (e) supplies the parasympathetic fibres to abdominal viscera

18.60 Causes of recurrent laryngeal nerve lesion include (page 1027):
(a) Mediastinal tumours
(b) Cortical infarcts
(c) Aneurysm of the aorta
(d) Secondary spread from carcinoma of the bronchus
(e) Trauma to the neck

18.61 Causes of hypoglossal nerve palsy include (page 1027):
(a) Syringobulbia
(b) Motor neurone disease
(c) Poliomyelitis
(d) Carcinoma of the nasopharynx
(e) Glomus tumour of the jugular foramen

18.62 In pseudobulbar palsy (page 1027):
(a) There is marked wasting of the tongue.
(b) The gag reflex is absent.
(c) Jaw jerk is exaggerated.
(d) Emotional lability is a feature.
(e) Palatal reflexes are preserved.

18.63 Causes of pseudobulbar palsy include (page 1027):
(a) Parkinson's disease
(b) Motor neurone lesions
(c) Multiple sclerosis
(d) Cerebrovascular disease
(e) Lower motor neurone hypoglossal nerve palsy.

18.64 The corticospinal tracts (page 1027):
(a) originate from the neurones of fifth layer of the cortex
(b) terminate on sensory nuclei of the cranial nerves
(c) terminate in the anterior horn cells of the spinal cord
(d) decussate in the upper midbrain
(e) fibres in the anterior corticospinal tracts carry crossed fibres

18.65 Signs of an upper motor neurone lesion include (Table 18.13):
(a) Marked muscle wasting
(b) Exaggerated tendon reflexes
(c) Loss of abdominal reflexes
(d) Cogwheel rigidity
(e) Normal electrical excitability of muscle

18.66 Causes of a spastic paraparesis include (Table 18.14):
(a) Spinal cord compression
(b) Parasagittal cortical meningoma
(c) Middle cerebral artery occlusion

(d) Multiple sclerosis
(e) Motor neurone disease

18.67 The features of extrapyramidal system involvement include (page 1030):
(a) Tremor
(b) Spasticity
(c) Bradykinesia
(d) Muscle wasting
(e) An extensor plantar response

18.68 The extrapyramidal system consists of (page 1030):
(a) Internal capsule
(b) Caudate nucleus
(c) Globus pallidus
(d) Putamen
(e) Substantia nigra

18.69 In Parkinson's disease there is a reduction in (Table 18.15):
(a) cholinergic activity
(b) dopamine in the putamen
(c) noradrenaline in the putamen
(d) glutamic acid decarboxylase in the substantia nigra
(e) 5-hydroxytryptamine in the putamen.

18.70 Causes of cerebellar syndrome include (Table 18.16):
(a) Medulloblastoma
(b) Anticonvulsant drugs
(c) Hypothyroidism
(d) Chronic alcohol abuse
(e) Multiple sclerosis

18.71 The following associations are correct (page 1031):
(a) Lesion in one cerebellar lobe – dyssynergia on the side opposite to the lesion
(b) Cerebellar lobar lesion – nystagmus
(c) Cerebellar connections – titubation
(d) Cerebellar vermis – truncal ataxia
(e) Flocculonodular lobe – hypotonia

18.72 Postural tremor is exaggerated in (page 1031):
(a) Cerebellar disease
(b) Anxiety
(c) Hyperthyroidism
(d) Parkinson's disease
(e) Lithium poisoning

18.73 Causes of lower motor neurone lesion include (page 1032):
- (a) Poliomyelitis
- (b) Occlusion of the middle cerebral artery
- (c) Motor neurone disease
- (d) Polyneuropathy
- (e) Myasthenia gravis

18.74 Sensory modalities which travel uncrossed in the posterior columns to the gracile and cuneate nuclei include (pages 1032–1033):
- (a) Pain
- (b) Light touch
- (c) Temperature
- (d) Vibration sense
- (e) Two-point discrimination

18.75 The following statements are correct (page 1033):
- (a) The sensory cortex is the prefrontal region.
- (b) Tinel's sign is another term for causalgia.
- (c) Neuralgia means local pain in the distribution of a damaged nerve.
- (d) Lightning pains are a feature of tabes dorsalis.
- (e) Lhermitte's sign indicates a cervical cord lesion.

18.76 Lhermitte's phenomenon occurs in (page 1034):
- (a) Multiple sclerosis
- (b) Glossopharyngeal neuralgia
- (c) Subacute combined degeneration of the cord
- (d) Radiation myelopathy
- (e) Trigeminal neuralgia

18.77 Pain (page 1035):
- (a) may be spontaneous in thalamic lesions
- (b) is a prominent feature of destructive cortical lesions
- (c) sensation may be modulated by other sensory modalities
- (d) when chronic may be accompanied by depression
- (e) in postherpetic neuralgia is caused by transcutaneous electric nerve stimulation

18.78 The parasympathetic efferent nerve supply to the bladder and genitalia causes (Table 18.19):
- (a) Detrusor muscle contraction
- (b) Penile erection
- (c) Engorgement of the clitoris
- (d) Orgasm
- (e) Ejaculation

18.79 The following statements are correct:
- (a) Frontal lesions cause socially inappropriate micturition.

(b) Precentral lesions cause difficulty in initiating micturition.
(c) Postcentral lesions cause loss of sensation of bladder fullness.
(d) Bilateral pyramidal tract lesions cause frequency of micturition and incontinence.
(e) Conus medullaris lesions cause a flaccid atonic bladder which overflows without warning.

18.80 Correct statements about sensory ataxia include:
(a) It is due to a diminution of the sense of touch.
(b) The gait is narrow-based.
(c) Romberg's test is positive.
(d) The patient cannot accurately perceive the position of the legs.
(e) The gait is high-stepping.

18.81 Plain X-ray of the skull will show intracranial calcification in (page 1037):
(a) Tuberculoma
(b) Oligodendroglioma
(c) Cysticercosis
(d) The wall of an aneurysm
(e) Pineal calcification

18.82 Investigations in neurological disease include (Table 18.20):
(a) Urinary ketones – coma
(b) Macrocytosis – vitamin B_{12} deficiency
(c) Bence–Jones proteins – cord compression
(d) High ESR – giant cell arteritis
(e) Glycosuria – polyneuropathy

18.83 CT scanning is used for the diagnosis of (Table 1037):
(a) Cerebral tumours
(b) Intracerebral infarction
(c) Cerebral atrophy
(d) Subarachnoid haemorrhage
(e) Subdural haematoma

18.84 The advantages of MRI over CT include (page 1038):
(a) MRI images distinguish clearly between white matter and grey matter in the brain.
(b) Spinal cord and nerve roots are imaged directly.
(c) The resolution of MRI is greater than CT.
(d) MRI does not involve radiation.
(e) Magnetic resonance angiography images blood vessels without the need for contrast.

18.85 MRI is used in the diagnosis of (page 1038):
(a) Brain tumours
(b) Syringomyelia

(c) Lesions of multiple sclerosis
(d) Lesions at the foramen magnum
(e) Cord compression

18.86 Slow-wave EEG abnormalities are seen in (pages 1039–1040):
(a) Brain death
(b) Epilepsy
(c) Encephalitis
(d) Dementia
(e) Hypoglycaemia

18.87 Lumbar puncture for examination of the CSF is performed for the diagnosis of (page 1040):
(a) A suspected mass lesion in the brain
(b) Any cause of raised intracranial pressure
(c) Encephalitis
(d) Meningitis
(e) Meninogomyelocoele in the lumbosacral region

18.88 The following associations are correct (page 1042):
(a) Elevated creatine phosphokinase – primary muscle disease
(b) Low serum caeruloplasmin – Wilson's disease
(c) Antibodies to acetylcholine receptor protein – myasthenia gravis
(d) Oligoclonal bands in the CSF – multiple sclerosis
(e) Delay in latency of visual evoked potentials despite clinical recovery of vision – retrobulbar neuritis

18.89 Correct statements about psychometric assessment include (page 1042):
(a) It is used to assess cognitive function.
(b) Preservation of performance IQ in the presence of a deterioration of verbal IQ indicates dementia.
(c) It is particularly useful in depression.
(d) Lack of concentration can impair scores.
(e) Low subtest scores indicate impaired function of specific regions of the brain.

18.90 The following statements are correct (page 1043):
(a) Confusion is the state of altered consciousness in which the patient is bewildered and misinterprets the world around them.
(b) Delirium is a state of high arousal in which there is confusion.
(c) Coma is a state of arousable unresponsiveness.
(d) Stupor is an abnormal sleepy state from which the patient can be aroused by stimuli that may need to be repeated or vigorously applied.
(e) Sleep is a state of mental and physical inactivity from which the subject cannot be aroused.

18.91 Causes of coma include (page 1043):
- (a) A single focal lesion of the cerebral hemisphere not compressing the brain stem
- (b) Uraemia
- (c) Septicaemia
- (d) Brain-stem haemorrhage
- (e) Porphyria

18.92 The following statements about respiration in coma are correct (page 1045):
- (a) Kussmaul's respiration is alternating hyperpnoea and apnoea.
- (b) Cheyne–Stokes respiration is deep sighing respiration.
- (c) Central neurogenic hyperventilation is seen in patients with pontine lesions.
- (d) Ataxic respiration occurs when the medullary respiratory centre is damaged.
- (e) Excessive yawning in a stuporose patient indicates lower brain-stem damage.

18.93 The following statements about the pupils in coma are correct (page 1045):
- (a) Unilateral fixed and dilated pupils indicates Horner's syndrome.
- (b) Pinpoint pupils are a feature of pontine haemorrhage.
- (c) Horner's syndrome is a feature of 'coning'.
- (d) Fixed and dilated pupils are a cardinal sign of brain death.
- (e) Midpoint pupils that react to light are characteristic of coma of metabolic origin.

18.94 Correct statements about abnormalities of conjugate gaze include (page 1045):
- (a) Sustained conjugate lateral gaze occurs opposite to the side of a destructive hemisphere lesion.
- (b) In pontine brain-stem lesions sustained conjugate lateral gaze occurs towards the side of the lesion.
- (c) In an irritative lesion in the frontal region conjugate deviation may occur away from the side of the lesion.
- (d) Skew deviation of the eye indicates a lesion of the cerebral hemispheres.
- (e) Abnormalities of conjugate gaze may cause hemianopia.

18.95 The following statements are correct (page 1046):
- (a) Stroke is a focal neurological deficit caused by demyelination.
- (b) A stroke is said to be completed when the deficit has reached maximum.
- (c) Transient ischaemic attack is a focal deficit lasting less than a week.
- (d) Transient ischaemic attacks have a tendency to recur.
- (e) The clinical picture of stroke may be caused by cerebral tumours.

18.96 Risk factors for stroke include (Table 18.26):
(a) Diabetes mellitus
(b) Berry aneurysms
(c) Polycythaemia
(d) Cigarette smoking
(e) Hypertension

18.97 The circle of Willis is supplied by (page 1048):
(a) External carotid arteries
(b) Basilar arteries
(c) Union of vertebral arteries
(d) Brachial artery
(e) Axillary artery

18.98 Atheromatous plaques are common at the following sites (page 1048):
(a) The origins of the common carotid arteries
(b) The origins of the internal carotid arteries
(c) Within the carotid syphon
(d) Within the subclavian vessels
(e) The origins of vertebral arteries

18.99 Cerebral autoregulation is impaired by (page 1048):
(a) Severe hypotension
(b) Severe hypertension
(c) Polycythaemia
(d) Raised intracranial pressure
(e) Change in arterial $P\text{co}_2$

18.100 The following statements about TIAs are correct (page 1049):
(a) Amaurosis fugax is a sudden transient loss of vision in one eye due to the passage of emboli through retinal arteries.
(b) Amaurosis fugax is suggestive of a TIA in the posterior circulation.
(c) Five years after a TIA 40% of patients will have suffered a stroke.
(d) Headache usually precedes a TIA.
(e) A TIA in the posterior circulation is generally of more serious prognosis than a TIA in the anterior circulation.

18.101 Cerebral infarction causes (page 1049):
(a) Lateral medullary syndrome
(b) Hemiplegia
(c) Pseudobulbar palsy
(d) The 'locked in' syndrome
(e) Aphasia when the non-dominant lobe is affected

18.102 The following statements are correct (page 1050):
(a) Lacunar infarctions are usually not associated with hypertension.
(b) Pure motor strokes are caused by lacunar infarcts.

(c) Multi-infarct dementia shows a stepwise deterioration with each subsequent infarct.
(d) Cortical blindness follows infarction of the anterior cerebral arteries.
(e) Sudden dysarthria with a clumsy hand is caused by a single lacunar infarct.

18.103 Recognized features of lateral medullary syndrome include (Table 18.29):
(a) Ipsilateral hemiparesis
(b) Contralateral nystagmus
(c) Contralateral ataxia
(d) Ipsilateral spinothalamic sensory loss
(e) Contralateral Horner's syndrome

18.104 Correct statements about the investigation of cerebrovascular disease include (page 1051):
(a) Lumbar puncture should be routinely done in stroke.
(b) CT scanning is more sensitive in detecting infarction than CT.
(c) Carotid Doppler and duplex scanning is of little value in demonstrating stenosis of the internal carotid arteries.
(d) Angiography is valuable in anterior circulation TIAs.
(e) Vertebral angiography should be performed in all patients with posterior circulation TIAs.

18.105 The following statements about the management of cerebrovascular disease are correct (page 1052):
(a) Internal carotid endarterectomy is considered in those who have internal carotid artery stenosis that narrows the arterial lumen by more than 70%.
(b) The control of high blood pressure is the single most important factor in the prevention of stroke.
(c) Soluble aspirin has been shown to reduce substantially the incidence of further events in patients who have TIA or cerebral infarction.
(d) Anticoagulants are potentially dangerous in the 2 weeks following cerebral infarction.
(e) Baclofen is sometimes useful in the management of flaccidity following a stroke.

18.106 Correct statements about the prognosis of stroke include (page 1052):
(a) Between one-third and one-half of patients will die in the first month following a stroke.
(b) Early mortality is lower for strokes due to intracerebral haemorrhage than those due to thromboembolic infarction.
(c) A poor outcome is likely when there is a defect in conjugate gaze.
(d) Recurrent strokes are rare.
(e) Many patients die subsequently of a myocardial infarction.

18.107 Causes of intracerebral haemorrhage include (page 1053):
  (a) Charcot–Bouchard aneurysms
  (b) Aortic aneurysms
  (c) 'Berry' aneurysms
  (d) Arteriovenous malformations
  (e) Hypertension

18.108 Typical sites of intracerebral haemorrhage include (page 1053):
  (a) Basal ganglia
  (b) Pons
  (c) Cerebellum
  (d) Subcortical white matter
  (e) Subdural haematoma

18.109 Correct statements about the management of intracerebral haemorrhage include (page 1053):
  (a) CT scanning is reliable in differentiating it from cerebral infarction.
  (b) The general management is as for cerebral infarction.
  (c) Surgical removal should be considered in deepening coma.
  (d) Anticoagulant drugs prevent recurrent episodes when given acutely.
  (e) The immediate prognosis is excellent.

18.110 Recognized features of subarachnoid haemorrhage include (page 1053):
  (a) Occipital headache
  (b) Coma
  (c) Neck stiffness
  (d) Subhyaloid haemorrhage
  (e) Painful third-nerve palsy

18.111 Causes of subarachnoid haemorrhage include (Table 18.31):
  (a) Arteriovenous malformations
  (b) Berry malformations
  (c) Mitral stenosis
  (d) Coarctation of the aorta
  (e) Polycystic kidneys

18.112 Common sites of saccular aneurysms include (page 1053):
  (a) The junction of the posterior communicating artery and the internal carotid artery
  (b) The junction of the anterior communicating artery and the anterior cerebral artery
  (c) The bifurcation of the middle cerebral artery
  (d) The basilar artery
  (e) The opthalmic artery

18.113 Correct statements about the investigation of subarachnoid haemorrhage include (page 1054):
(a) The CSF is xanthochromic several hours before the haemorrhage.
(b) Lumbar puncture is essential before CT scan.
(c) CT scanning is useful for very small bleeds.
(d) Carotid and vertebral angiography is usually performed in all fit patients.
(e) Lumbar puncture is useful in differentiating the main causes of SAH.

18.114 Correct statements about the management of subarachnoid haemorrhage include (page 1054):
(a) Nearly half the patients with SAH are either dead or moribund before they reach hospital.
(b) Once in hospital rebleeds are rare.
(c) Nimodipine has been shown to reduce mortality.
(d) Dexamethasone has been shown to be very effective in reducing morbidity and mortality.
(e) Severe spasm of the intracranial arteries is a good prognostic sign.

18.115 Subdural haemorrhage is (page 1054):
(a) caused by a tear in a branch of a middle meningeal artery
(b) almost always due to head injury
(c) common in the elderly
(d) seen in patients with alcohol abuse
(e) common following cortical venous thrombosis

18.116 Epilepsy (page 1055):
(a) is due to paroxysmal discharge of cerebral neurones
(b) is not recurrent
(c) when arising from the temporal lobe is associated with '*déjà vu*' phenomenon
(d) may be preceded by Todd's paralysis
(e) is rare in Africa

18.117 Petit mal epilepsy:
(a) is almost invariably a disorder of the elderly
(b) is accompanied by a spike-and-wave pattern of the EEG
(c) is used to describe the absence attacks of partial seizures
(d) is the same as Jacksonian seizures
(e) is usually associated with a focal lesion

18.118 The following statements are correct:
(a) Generalized seizure implies abnormal electrical activity which is widespread in the brain.
(b) A simple partial seizure describes a seizure without loss of awareness.
(c) A complex partial seizure describes a seizure with loss of awareness.

(d) Myoclonic seizures are events where there is isolated muscle jerking.

(e) Petit mal describes only 3 Hz seizures, rather than clinically similar absence attacks with partial seizures.

18.119 Aetiological factors precipitating seizures include (Table 18.33):

(a) Perinatal trauma

(b) Cerebral infarction

(c) Multiple sclerosis

(d) Flickering television screen

(e) Pyrexia

18.120 Seizures may occur with the following metabolic abnormalities (pages 1056–1057):

(a) Hypoglycaemia

(b) Porphyria

(c) Hyponatraemia

(d) Hypocalcaemia

(e) Uraemia

18.121 Correct statements about the electroencephalogram (EEG) in epilepsy include (page 1057):

(a) The EEG is the single most useful investigation in the study of a seizure.

(b) During a seizure the EEG is abnormal in less than half the cases.

(c) A cortical spike focus is associated with seizure activity.

(d) A normal EEG between attacks excludes epilepsy.

(e) An abnormal interictal EEG proves that an attack was epileptic.

18.122 Anticonvulsant drugs (page 1058):

(a) are indicated following a single seizure

(b) must be given in combination for effective control of epilepsy

(c) withdrawal should not be considered until the patient has been free of all fits for at least 2 years

(d) intoxication causes a syndrome of ataxia, nystagmus and dysarthria

(e) must be avoided if the patient is mentally retarded

18.123 Chronic administration of phenytoin can cause (page 1058):

(a) Gum hypertrophy

(b) Osteomalacia

(c) Folate deficiency

(d) Polyneuropathy

(e) Encephalopathy

18.124 Correct statements about driving and epilepsy include (page 1059):

(a) A person who has suffered an epileptic attack while awake must refrain from driving for 1 year from the date of attack before a Group 1 driving licence may be issued.

    (b) Truck drivers must have been free of epileptic attacks for at least the last 10 years on anticonvulsant medications.

    (c) Attacks occurring exclusively in sleep must be shown to have occurred over a 3-year period before a Group 1 driving licence may be issued.

    (d) It is the duty of the doctor to inform the licensing authorities regarding epilepsy patients

    (e) Patients should not drive during reduction of doses of antiepileptics and for 6 months following stopping anticonvulsants.

18.125 Syncope is a feature of (page 1060):
  (a) Aortic stenosis
  (b) Hypertrophic cardiomyopathy
  (c) Drop attacks
  (d) Night terrors
  (e) Excess sensitivity of the carotid sinus

18.126 Sleep apnoea (page 1061):
  (a) is associated with shortened periods of apnoea during REM sleep
  (b) occurs with brain-stem lesions
  (c) is associated with airway obstruction
  (d) may be accompanied by snoring
  (e) is associated with syncope

18.127 Correct statements about the aetiology of idiopathic Parkinson's disease include (page 1062):
  (a) There is a lower prevalence in smokers.
  (b) They die less frequently from lung cancer than the normal population.
  (c) Minute doses of methyl-phenyl tetrahydropyridine may cause irreversible Parkinson's syndrome.
  (d) The condition is usually inherited.
  (e) Survivors of encephalitis lethargica develop parkinsonism.

18.128 Recognized features of Parkinson's disease include (page 1063):
  (a) Micrographia
  (b) Intention tremor
  (c) Clasp-knife spasticity
  (d) Greasy skin
  (e) Dementia

18.129 Correct statements about the natural history of Parkinson's disease include (page 1063):
  (a) Remissions are common.
  (b) The rate of progression is very variable.
  (c) Death usually results from bronchopneumonia.

(d) During great emotion the patient is released for seconds and is able to move quickly.

(e) Benign forms can run over several decades.

18.130 Slowing of movement is a feature of (page 1063):
  (a) Parkinson's disease
  (b) Hypothyroidism
  (c) Depression
  (d) Hyperthyroidism
  (e) Cushing's disease

18.131 Some features of parkinsonism are seen in (page 1063):
  (a) Alzheimer's disease
  (b) Multi-infarct dementia
  (c) As a sequela to repeated head injury
  (d) Hypoxia
  (e) Atherosclerosis

18.132 The following statements about the management of idiopathic Parkinson's disease are correct (page 1064):
  (a) Levodopa should not be given in combination with benserazide.
  (b) The great majority of patients improve initially with levodopa.
  (c) Depression is treated with type A monoamine oxidase inhibitors in patients on levodopa.
  (d) Sterotactic surgery of the thalamus is used to reduce akinesia.
  (e) Fetal transplants of adrenal medulla produce major clinical improvement.

18.133 Unwanted effects of levodopa include (page 1064):
  (a) Nausea
  (b) Chorea
  (c) Confusion
  (d) On–off syndrome
  (e) Episodes of 'freezing'

18.134 Approaches to the treatment of complications of levodopa include (page 1064):
  (a) Reduced doses, with the interval between doses being lengthened.
  (b) Selegiline is used to smooth out the response to levodopa.
  (c) Apomorphine is the best method of smoothing out the fluctuations in response.
  (d) Periods of drug withdrawal are sometimes helpful.
  (e) The doses are increased.

18.135 Examples of 'parkinsonism plus' syndromes include (page 1065):
  (a) Chronic tardive dyskinesia
  (b) Acute dystonic reactions

(c) Olivopontocerebellar degeneration
(d) Shy–Drager syndrome
(e) Progressive supranuclear palsy

18.136 Features of benign essential tremor include (page 1065):
(a) Autosomal recessive trait.
(b) Pathologically there is patchy neuronal loss in the cerebellum.
(c) The tremor is usually worse in the upper limbs.
(d) Salbutamol reduces the tremor.
(e) It is a forerunner of Parkinson's disease.

18.137 Features of Wilson's disease include (page 1065):
(a) Autosomal dominant trait
(b) Deposition of copper in the cornea
(c) Progressive intellectual impairment
(d) Cirrhosis
(e) Akinetic–rigid syndrome

18.138 Causes of chorea include (Table 18.39):
(a) Alcohol
(b) Phenytoin
(c) Thyrotoxicosis
(d) Systemic lupus erythematosus
(e) Stroke

18.139 Features of Huntington's disease include (page 1066):
(a) Mutation analysis allows the identification of presymptomatic individuals
(b) Progressive dementia
(c) Autosomal dominant trait with full penetrance
(d) History of rheumatic fever
(e) Tetrabenazine has been shown to reduce the progression of the disease

18.140 Examples of generalized dystonia include (Table 18.40):
(a) Spasmodic torticollis
(b) Writer's cramp
(c) Dystonia musculorum deformans
(d) Oromandibular dystonia
(e) Blepharospasm

18.141 The following statements regarding multiple sclerosis are correct (page 1068):
(a) The onset is usually in the third and fourth decades.
(b) The prevalence is directly proportional to the distance from the equator.
(c) The inheritance is autosomal dominant.

(d) In Norway it is distinctly uncommon in coastal fishing communities compared to agricultural areas.
(e) It has been suggested that it is related to the consumption of large quantities of animal fat.

18.142 Clinical features of multiple sclerosis include (page 1068):
(a) It shows remissions and exacerbations.
(b) It may be a progressive condition.
(c) Lesions can occur at different parts of the CNS.
(d) CNS lesions almost always occur at the same time.
(e) No single group of symptoms or signs is diagnostic of this condition.

18.143 Recognized features of multiple sclerosis include (page 1069):
(a) Optic neuritis
(b) Retrobulbar neuritis
(c) Internuclear ophthalmoplegia
(d) Spastic paraparesis
(e) Dementia

18.144 Conditions with a relapsing pattern include (page 1069):
(a) Friedreich's ataxia
(b) CNS sarcoidosis
(c) Systemic lupus erythematosus
(d) Behçet's syndrome
(e) Motor neurone disease

18.145 The following investigations are useful in the diagnosis of multiple sclerosis (page 1069):
(a) Peripheral nerve studies
(b) Examination of the cerebrospinal fluid
(c) EEG
(d) Visual evoked responses
(e) MRI scan

18.146 Correct statements about the management of multiple sclerosis include (page 1070):
(a) Patients should not be informed of the diagnosis unless they demand it.
(b) Corticosteroids are known to improve the outlook in the long term.
(c) Urinary tract infections frequently exacerbate the symptoms.
(d) Baclofen is useful when there are flexor spasms in the lower limbs.
(e) β-Interferon reduces the relapse rate by a third.

18.147 Infective causes of meningitis in the UK include (Table 18.41):
(a) *Coccidiodes immitis*
(b) *Mycobacterium tuberculosis*
(c) *Haemophilus influenzae*

(d) *Histoplasma capsulatum*
(e) *Cryptococcus neoformans*

18.148 The following associations in meningitis are correct (page 1071):
(a) Petechial rash – meningococcal infection
(b) Ear disease – pneumococcal infection
(c) Working with drains – leptospirosis
(d) Immunocompromised patients – HIV infection
(e) Pleurodynia – enterovirus

18.149 Typical CSF changes in bacterial meningitis include (Table 18.44):
(a) Elevated glucose
(b) Elevated protein
(c) Increased polymorphs
(d) Crystal-clear appearance
(e) Absence of mononuclear cells

18.150 Impairment of consciousness in uncomplicated meningitis indicates (page 1071):
(a) Venous sinus thrombosis
(b) Severe cerebral oedema
(c) Hydrocephalus
(d) Cerebral abscess
(e) Encephalitis

18.151 Correct statements about the management of meningitis include (page 1072):
(a) Meningitis is an emergency that has a high mortality even in countries with highly developed systems of health care.
(b) Meningococcal meningitis should be treated with penicillin within minutes of clinical diagnosis.
(c) Oral penicillin is the drug of choice in meningococcal infection.
(d) Viral meningitis is a self-limiting condition.
(e) Gram staining of the CSF may demonstrate the organism.

18.152 Causes of CSF pleocytosis include (Table 18.45):
(a) Intracranial abscess
(b) Syphilis
(c) Encephalitis
(d) Neoplastic meningitis
(e) Following subarachnoid haemorrhage

18.153 Causes of encephalitis include (page 1073):
(a) Mumps virus
(b) Coxsackie virus
(c) Influenza virus

(d) Hepatitis A virus
(e) Adenovirus

18.154 The differential diagnosis of encephalitis include (page 1073):
  (a) Bacterial meningitis with cerebral oedema
  (b) Cerebral abscess
  (c) Acute disseminated encephalomyelitis
  (d) Toxic confusional states in febrile illnesses
  (e) Cerebral malaria

18.155 Correct statements about the management of encephalitis include (page 1073):
  (a) EEG shows slow-wave changes.
  (b) Brain biopsy is routinely performed in all cases.
  (c) Suspected herpes simplex encephalitis is treated with acyclovir.
  (d) If the patient is in coma the outlook is poor.
  (e) Prophylactic immunization is possible against Japanese B encephalitis.

18.156 Varicella zoster causes (page 1074):
  (a) Myelitis
  (b) Meningoencephalitis
  (c) Motor radiculopathy
  (d) Ramsay Hunt syndrome
  (e) Post herpetic neuralgia

18.157 Features of tabes dorsalis include (page 1074):
  (a) Lightning pains
  (b) Ataxia
  (c) Charcot's joints
  (d) Argyll Robertson pupils
  (e) Ptosis

18.158 Neurological manifestations of AIDS include (page 1075):
  (a) Aseptic meningitis
  (b) Kuru
  (c) Paraparesis
  (d) Mononeuritis multiplex
  (e) Progressive multifocal leucoencephalopathy

18.159 The following associations are correct (page 1075):
  (a) Rabies – encephalitis
  (b) Tetanus – spasms
  (c) Lyme disease – chronic radiculopathy
  (d) Tuberculoid leprosy – bulbar palsy
  (e) Poliomyelitis – mononeuritis multiplex

18.160 Correct statements about gliomas include (page 1078):
    (a) They are malignant.
    (b) They originate in the neurons.
    (c) They may be associated with neurofibromatosis.
    (d) They usually metastasize outside the CNS.
    (e) Their cause is unknown.

18.161 The following associations are correct (page 1078):
    (a) Astrocytoma – arise within the cerebellum
    (b) Oligodendroglioma – calcification is common
    (c) Meningioma – arises from the arachnoid matter
    (d) Neurofibroma – arises from Schwann cells
    (e) Primary intracranial tumours – almost always metasize to the liver

18.162 Examples of false localizing signs in mass lesions include (page 1079):
    (a) A left frontal meningioma causing disturbances of personality
    (b) A sixth-nerve lesion due to compression during its long intracranial course
    (c) A right parietal glioma of optic radiation causing a left homonymous field defect
    (d) A third-nerve lesion due to the uncus of the temporal lobe herniating caudally and compressing the nerve
    (e) Hemiparesis on the same side as a hemisphere tumour

18.163 Correct statements about the investigation of intracranial tumours include (page 1080):
    (a) CT scan is useful in determining the nature of the lesion.
    (b) Contrast enhancement adds to the discriminating ability of CT.
    (c) Lumbar puncture is useful when the differential diagnosis includes a mass lesion.
    (d) EEG shows marked focal slow-wave changes over the region of a cerebral abscess.
    (e) A technetium brain scan is very discriminatory and shows lesions missed by CT.

18.164 Recognized clinical features of pseudotumour cerebri include (page 1080):
    (a) An increase in size of the cerebral ventricles
    (b) Papilloedema
    (c) Sixth-nerve palsy
    (d) Elevated CSF pressure
    (e) Sagittal sinus thrombosis

18.165 Causes of hydrocephalus include (page 1081):
    (a) Subarachnoid haemorrhage
    (b) Arnold–Chiari malformation
    (c) Stenosis of the aqueduct of Sylvius

(d) The Dandy–Walker syndrome

(e) Tuberculous meningitis

18.166 Migraine (page 1081):
  (a) invariably means unilateral headache
  (b) is associated with visual disturbance
  (c) is associated with gastrointestinal disturbance
  (d) is associated with aphasia
  (e) may be associated with hemiplegia

18.167 Migraine is associated with (page 1082):
  (a) the ingestion of chocolate
  (b) the ingestion of cheese
  (c) the menopause
  (d) the contraceptive pill
  (e) the development of hypertension

18.168 Drugs used in the prophylaxis of migraine include (page 1083):
  (a) Paracetamol
  (b) Propranolol
  (c) Ergotamine tartrate
  (d) Pizotifen
  (e) Amitryptiline

18.169 Features of giant cell arteritis include (page 1083):
  (a) Headache
  (b) Jaw claudication
  (c) Proximal limb girdle pain
  (d) Visual loss
  (e) Amaurosis fugax

18.170 Rare complications of giant cell arteritis include (page 1084):
  (a) Brain-stem ischaemia
  (b) Cortical blindness
  (c) Ischaemic neuropathy of the peripheral nerves
  (d) Cranial nerve lesions
  (e) Aortic involvement

18.171 Correct statements about the investigation of temporal arteritis include (page 1084):
  (a) The ESR is usually normal
  (b) Plasma α_2-globulins are depressed.
  (c) Plasma albumin is raised.
  (d) Normochromic normocytic anaemia occurs.
  (e) Biopsy of the temporal artery may be normal.

18.172 In head injury (page 1084):
- (a) Linear fracture of the skull base is almost always associated with neurological sequelae.
- (b) Depressed fracture of the skull vault is followed by a high incidence of post-traumatic epilepsy.
- (c) Loss of conciousness over several hours indicates severe brain injury.
- (d) Benign positional vertigo is a transient sequela.
- (e) Post-traumatic amnesia over 24 hours indicates severe brain injury.

18.173 Causes of spinal cord compression include (Table 18.48):
- (a) Transverse myelitis
- (b) Spinal tuberculosis
- (c) Lathyrism
- (d) Metastases
- (e) Epidural haematoma

18.174 Recognized features of syringomyelia include (page 1086):
- (a) Dissociated sensory loss
- (b) Loss of upper limb reflexes
- (c) Wasting of the hand muscles
- (d) Spastic paraparesis
- (e) Horner's syndrome

18.175 Features of motor neurone disease include (page 1088):
- (a) Pseudobulbar palsy
- (b) Cerebellar signs
- (c) Spastic paraparesis
- (d) Glove and stocking anaesthesia
- (e) Survival in most patients is for two decades following diagnosis

18.176 Features of Alzheimer's disease include (page 1114):
- (a) It is usually seen below the age of 40
- (b) A familial tendency is usually the case
- (c) Severe depression
- (d) Memory loss
- (e) Cortical atrophy on CT scan

18.177 Causes of cerebral palsy include (page 1089):
- (a) Kernicterus
- (b) Hypoxia in utero
- (c) Trauma during parturition
- (d) Neonatal cerebral haemorrhage
- (e) Febrile convulsions

18.178 Features of cerebral palsy include (page 1089):
- (a) Failure to achieve normal developmental milestones
- (b) Spastic diplegia

(c) Infantile hemiparesis
(d) Spina bifida
(e) Anencephaly

18.179 Features of von Recklinghausen's disease include (page 1090):
(a) Café-au-lait patches
(b) Meningioma
(c) Plexiform neuroma
(d) Phaeochromocytoma
(e) Scoliosis

18.180 Neuroectodermal syndromes include (page 1090):
(a) Spina bifida
(b) Neurofibromatosis
(c) Tuberous sclerosis
(d) Sturge–Weber syndrome
(e) Friedreich's ataxia

18.181 Features of Friedreich's ataxia include (pages 1090–1091):
(a) Nystagmus
(b) Abnormal sequence of DNA triple nucleotide repeats in the gene for fraxatin
(c) Absent reflexes in lower limbs
(d) Cardiomyopathy
(e) Pes cavus

18.182 Recognized features of peroneal muscular atrophy include (page 1096):
(a) Mononeuritis multiplex
(b) The legs resemble inverted champagne bottles
(c) Pes cavus
(d) Retinitis pigmentosa
(e) Optic atrophy

18.183 Causes of carpal tunnel syndrome include (page 1092):
(a) Hyperthyroidism
(b) Diabetes mellitus
(c) Pregnancy
(d) Acromegaly
(e) Rheumatoid arthritis

18.184 Causes of mononeuritis multiplex include (page 1093):
(a) Sarcoidosis
(b) Diabetes mellitus
(c) Rheumatoid arthritis
(d) Leprosy
(e) AIDS

18.185 Features of Guillain–Barré syndrome include (page 1093):
 (a) Severe myopathy
 (b) Weakness of distal limb muscles
 (c) Sensory loss
 (d) Ataxia
 (e) Autonomic changes

18.186 Varieties of diabetic neuropathy include (page 1094):
 (a) Symmetrical sensory polyneuropathy
 (b) Multiple cranial nerve lesions
 (c) Amyotrophy
 (d) Autonomic neuropathy
 (e) Mononeuropathy

18.187 Deficiency of the following vitamins causes neuropathy (Table 18.53):
 (a) Vitamin D
 (b) Thiamin
 (c) Pyridoxine
 (d) Nicotinic acid
 (e) Ascorbic acid

18.188 Drugs causing pure motor neuropathy include (Table 18.54):
 (a) Phenytoin
 (b) Isoniazid
 (c) Gold
 (d) Dapsone
 (e) Nitrofurantoin

18.189 Features of Wernicke–Korsakoff syndrome include (page 1095):
 (a) Spastic paraplegia
 (b) Bilateral lateral rectus palsies
 (c) Amnesia
 (d) Ataxia
 (e) Vestibular paralysis

18.190 The effects of ethyl alcohol include (Table 18.55):
 (a) Delirium tremens
 (b) Cerebellar degeneration
 (c) Central pontine myelinolysis
 (d) Degeneration of corpus callosum
 (e) Polyneuropathy

18.191 Features of subacute degeneration of the cord include (page 1096):
 (a) It is caused by pyridoxine deficiency
 (b) Exaggerated knee jerks
 (c) Absent ankle jerks

(d) Megaloblastic changes in bone marrow
(e) The spinal cord signs are immediately reversed by parenteral vitamin B_{12}

18.192 Autonomic neuropathy causes (page 1096):
(a) Glove and stocking anaesthesia
(b) Postural hypotension
(c) Impotence
(d) Dissociated sensory loss
(e) Cardiac arrhythmias

18.193 Causes of spondylosis include (page 1097):
(a) Ageing
(b) Trauma
(c) Rheumatoid arthritis
(d) Epidural abscess
(e) Cervical rib

18.194 The following associations are correct (page 1097):
(a) Protrusion of the seventh cervical disc – loss of triceps jerk
(b) Posterior cervical disc protrusion – difficulty in walking
(c) Central thoracic disc protrusion – quadriparesis
(d) Lateral lumbar disc protrusion – straight-leg raising is limited
(e) Spinal stenosis – buttock claudication

18.195 Non-metastatic manifestations of malignancy include (pages 1098–1099):
(a) Eaton–Lambert syndrome
(b) Dementia
(c) Cerebellar syndrome
(d) Mononeuritis multiplex
(e) Spinal cord compression

18.196 Metabolic causes of myopathy include (Table 18.57):
(a) Cushing's syndrome
(b) Polymyositis
(c) Duchenne muscular dystrophy
(d) Myasthenia gravis
(e) Thyroid disease

18.197 Features of polymyositis include (page 1100):
(a) Pseudohypertrophy
(b) Muscle weakness is typically distal
(c) Dysphagia
(d) Serum creatinine phosphokinase is always elevated
(e) Raised ESR

18.198 A subacute proximal myopathy is caused by (Table 18.59):
(a) General anaesthesia
(b) Diamorphine
(c) Acute alcohol excess
(d) Clofibrate
(e) Lithium

18.199 Myasthenia gravis is associated with (page 1101):
(a) Thyrotoxicosis
(b) Rheumatoid arthritis
(c) Cardiomyopathy
(d) Pernicious anaemia
(e) Systemic lupus erythematosus

18.200 Features of myasthenia gravis include (pages 1101–1102):
(a) Peripheral neuropathy
(b) Fatiguability
(c) Thymic aplasia
(d) Serum acetylcholine receptor antibodies
(e) Respiratory difficulty

18.201 Drugs to be avoided in myasthenia gravis include (page 1102):
(a) Pyridostigmine
(b) Aminoglycosides
(c) Oral atropine
(d) Magnesium sulphate enemas
(e) Azathioprine

18.202 Features of Duchenne muscular dystrophy include (page 1103):
(a) Absence of dystrophin
(b) Atrophy of calf muscles
(c) X-linked dominant inheritance
(d) Gross elevation of creatine phosphokinase
(e) Cardiac involvement

18.203 Features of myotonia congenita include (pages 1103–1104):
(a) Cataracts
(b) Frontal baldness
(c) Cardiomyopathy
(d) Intellectual impairment
(e) Glucose intolerance

18.204 Features of facioscapulohumeral dystrophy include (page 1103):
(a) Autosomal recessive inheritance
(b) Normal life expectancy
(c) Grossly elevated serum creatine phosphokinase

(d) Pseudohypertrophy is common

(e) Onset in the seventh decade

18.205 The following associations are correct (pages 1099–1104):

(a) Myasthenia gravis – reduction in the number of acetylcholine receptor antibodies

(b) Myotonias – defective chloride ion membrane conductance

(c) McArdle's syndrome – enzyme defect in the glycolytic pathway

(d) Malignant hyperpyrexia – muscle membrane defect

(e) Eaton–Lambert syndrome – defective acetylcholine release at neuromuscular junctions

Psychological Medicine

19.1 The following statements about psychiatric morbidity among adults in the UK are correct (Information box 19.1):
- (a) Less than 15% of adults have a neurotic health problem.
- (b) The most prevalent neurotic disorder is mixed anxiety and depressive disorder followed by generalized anxiety disorder.
- (c) Women are more likely to have a neurotic health problem than men.
- (d) Women are three times more likely than men to have alcohol dependence.
- (e) Alcohol and drug dependence are more prevalent in young adults, particularly young men aged 16–24.

19.2 The psychiatric interview is of prime importance because it (page 1106):
- (a) is a technique for obtaining information
- (b) is during this interview that the patient is treated
- (c) allows assessment of the patient's emotions
- (d) allows rapport with the patient
- (e) is used to obtain a concise assessment of the case

19.3 The following statements about behaviour are correct (pages 1106–1107):
- (a) Stereotypy is repetition of movements that appear to have a purpose.
- (b) Mannerisms are a repetition of movements that do not appear to have functional significance.
- (c) Negativism is when patients do the opposite of what is asked.
- (d) Echopraxia is when the patient automatically imitates the interviewer's movements, despite being asked not to do this.
- (e) Patients with retarded depression are often tremulous and restless, adjusting their clothing and pacing up and down.

19.4 The following statements are correct (page 1107):
- (a) Pressure of thought occurs in depression.
- (b) Poverty of thought occurs in mania.
- (c) Thought blocking suggests schizophrenia.
- (d) Flight of ideas is characteristic of mania.
- (e) Perseveration is associated with dementia.

19.5 The following statements are correct (page 1108):
- (a) Claustrophobia is the fear of open spaces.
- (b) Agoraphobia is the fear of spiders.
- (c) An obsession is a recurrent, persistent thought that enters the mind despite the individual's effort to resist it.
- (d) A compulsion is a repetitive and seemingly purposeful action performed in a sterotyped way.
- (e) Emotions that are changeable in a rapid, abrupt and excessive way are termed labile emotions.

19.6 A delusion is an abnormal belief arising from disordered judgement and which is (Information box 19.2):
(a) held with absolute conviction
(b) amenable to reason
(c) not shared by those of a common cultural background
(d) modifiable by experience
(e) false

19.7 Examples of delusions include (pages 1108–1109):
(a) Thought insertion
(b) Over valued ideas
(c) Thought broadcasting
(d) Ideas of reference
(e) Passivity

19.8 Hallucinations are (page 1109):
(a) Misperceptions of external stimuli
(b) Most likely to occur when the general level of sensory stimulation is reduced
(c) Independent of the individual's will
(d) Perceived alongside normal perceptions
(e) Perceived as having qualities of normal perception

19.9 The following statements are correct (page 1109):
(a) Ideas of reference are held by people who are particulary self-conscious.
(b) Registration is the ability to add new material to existing memory stores.
(c) Retention is the ability to retain the memory.
(d) Recall is the ability to bring back memory into awareness.
(e) Recognition is the feeling of familiarity indicating that a particular person, event or object has been encountered before.

19.10 The following statements about defence mechanisms include (page 1110):
(a) Repression is the exclusion from awareness of memories that would cause anxiety if allowed to enter consciousness.
(b) Regression is the unconscious adoption of patterns of behaviour appropriate to an earlier stage of development.
(c) Rationalization refers to the unconscious process whereby a false but acceptable explanation is provided for behaviour that in fact has other, much less acceptable, origins.
(d) Sublimation refers to the unconscious diversion of unacceptable outlets into acceptable outlets.
(e) Reaction formation refers to the unconscious adoption of behaviour opposite to that which reflect the individual's true feelings and intentions.

19.11 Anxiety is associated with the following physical diseases:
  (a) Hyperthyroidism
  (b) Phaeochromocytoma
  (c) Hypoglycaemia
  (d) Partial seizures
  (e) Alcohol withdrawal

19.12 Causes of delirium include (Table 19.6):
  (a) Thiamin deficiency
  (b) Hepatic failure
  (c) Hypoglycaemia
  (d) Anticonvulsant intoxication
  (e) Alcohol withdrawal

19.13 The following statements are correct (pages 1113–1116):
  (a) Delirium is an acute or subacute condition in which impairment of consciousness is accompanied by abnormalities of perception and mood.
  (b) Dementia is an acquired global impairment of intellect, memory and personality without impairment of consciousness.
  (c) The amnestic syndrome is characterized by a marked impairment of memory occurring in clear consciousness, and not as a part of a delirium or a dementia.
  (d) The organic delusional syndrome is characterized by marked mood changes that result from organic brain damage.
  (e) In severe delirium haloperidol should be avoided.

19.14 Recognized clinical features of Alzheimer's disease include:
  (a) Impaired ability to learn new information
  (b) A decline in language function
  (c) Apraxia
  (d) Agnosia
  (e) Paranoia

19.15 Recognized pathological features of Alzheimer's disease include (pages 1114–1115):
  (a) Ubiquitin is found in association with neurofibrillary tangles.
  (b) The hippocampus is characteristically spared.
  (c) Aggregation of β-amyloid protein is a central event.
  (d) There is an increase in the enzyme superoxide dismutase in the frontal cortex.
  (e) The ε_{-2} allele of the apolipoprotein E gene is over-represented in Alzheimer's disease.

19.16 Correct statements about dementia include (page 1115):
  (a) Vascular dementia is the second most common cause of dementia.
  (b) Vessel occlusion is the most common cause of vascular dementia.

(c) Typically in vascular dementia there are no signs of cortical dysfunction.

(d) In Pick's disease there is selective atrophy of the temporal lobes.

(e) Multi-infarct dementia results from involvement of several vessels supplying the cerebral cortex and subcortical structures.

19.17 Correct statements about the management of dementia include (page 1116):

(a) Vascular dementia is usually treated with aspirin.

(b) Patient's with Parkinson's disease and dementia usually show marked cognitive improvement with selegiline and dopaminergic drugs.

(c) Tacrine has been shown to improve cognitive defect of Alzheimer's disease.

(d) Donepezil is contraindicated in Alzheimer's disease.

(e) HRT in postmenopausal women has been shown to have protective effects against developing Alzheimer's disease.

19.18 First-rank symptoms of schizophrenia include (page 1117):

(a) Visual hallucinations

(b) Auditory hallucinations

(c) Thought insertion

(d) Thought broadcasting

(e) Mania

19.19 The following statements about schizophrenia are correct (page 1118):

(a) Positive schizophrenia responds poorly to neuroleptics.

(b) Paranoid schizophrenia is the most common presentation of schizophrenia throughout the world.

(c) In hebephrenic schizophrenia the clinical picture is dominated by a markedly shallow and inappropriate mood.

(d) Catatonic schizophrenia is common in developed countries.

(e) Delusions in chronic schizophrenia are often held with little emotional response.

19.20 Drugs causing psychosis include (Table 19.10):

(a) Diazepam

(b) Glucocorticoids

(c) Digitalis

(d) Phenytoin

(e) Amantadine

19.21 Unwanted anticholinergic effects of neuroleptic drugs include (Table 19.12):

(a) Tardive dyskinesia

(b) Akathisia

(c) Dry mouth

(d) Blurred vision
(e) Cholestatic jaundice

19.22 Correct statements about neuroleptic drugs in schizophrenia include (page 1119):
(a) They reduce psychomotor excitement.
(b) They affect sleep.
(c) They are most effective in the management of chronic, negative symptoms.
(d) Complete control of positive symptoms can take up to 3 months.
(e) They act by stimulating dopamine receptors D_1 and D_2.

19.23 The following statements about antipsychotics are correct (page 1120):
(a) Clozapine has been shown to have a dramatic therapeutic effect on positive and negative symptoms, cognitive function and quality of life.
(b) Olanzepine has affinity for 5-HT_2, D_1, D_2 and muscarinic receptors.
(c) Sertindole is associated with QT interval prolongation.
(d) Sulpiride is used to control florid positive symptoms.
(e) Butyrophenones are powerful antipsychotics used in the treatment of acute schizophrenia and mania.

19.24 Criteria for endogenous depression include (page 1121):
(a) A fluctuating depression responsive to environmental change.
(b) Self-pity rather than self-blame.
(c) A clear precipitating cause.
(d) A vulnerable personality.
(e) Early-morning waking.

19.25 Features of minor depression include (Table 19.15):
(a) Mood persistently low
(b) Persistent suicidal feelings
(c) Delusions usually present
(d) Hallucinations usually present
(e) Patient capable of being lifted out of gloom and sadness

19.26 Unwanted anticholinergic effects of tricyclic antidepressants include (Table 19.19):
(a) Arrhythmias
(b) Lowered seizure threshold
(c) Weight gain
(d) Blurred vision
(e) Tremor

19.27 The following statements are correct (page 1125):
(a) In patients with cardiac disease mianserin is preferred over nortriptyline.

(b) Fluoxetine acts by way of selective inhibition of serotonin uptake only within the synaptic cleft.

(c) Venlafaxine is a potent inhibitor of both 5-HT and noradrenaline uptake.

(d) MAOIs are safely administered with foods containing tyramine.

(e) MAOs are used in depressions that present with marked anxiety and obsessional features, and which lack marked biological symptoms characteristic of severe depression.

19.28 Electroconvulsive therapy is the treatment of first choice in depression when (page 1126):

(a) The patient is dangerously suicidal.

(b) A delay in treatment represents a serious risk to health.

(c) There is marked anxiety.

(d) The patient is refusing food and drink.

(e) The patient is in a depressive stupor.

19.29 Correct statements about the treatment of mania include (page 1126):

(a) First attacks of mania usually require treatment for up to 3 months.

(b) Lithium is used as a prophylactic agent in patients with repeated episodes.

(c) Carbamazepine is used in both the prophylaxis and treatment of manic states.

(d) Lithium carbonate can take 10 days to take effect.

(e) On treatment with neuroleptics symptoms such as grandiosity respond quicker than excitement and overactivity.

19.30 Correct statements about the course and prognosis of manic–depressive disorder include (page 1127):

(a) Between two-thirds and three-quarters of patients admitted with a major depressive illness will suffer at least one relapse requiring hospital admission.

(b) It has been estimated that about one-fifth of depressives never fully recover.

(c) Virtually all manic patients recover.

(d) Subsequent depressive disorder is common in manic patients who relapse.

(e) The continuation of antidepressant therapy for up to 6 months after recovery from a depressive episode does reduce the probability of recurrence.

19.31 Unwanted effects of lithium therapy include (page 1126):

(a) Weight gain

(b) Non-toxic goitre

(c) Hypothyroidism

(d) Nephrogenic diabetes insipidus

(e) Ataxia

19.32 The following statements are correct (pages 1127–1128):
(a) Suicide is commoner in women.
(b) Deliberate self-harm (DSH) is commoner in men.
(c) The majority of DSH occurs in people over the age of 65.
(d) The majority of suicides occur in people under the age of 35.
(e) A formal psychiatric disorder is common in DSH.

19.33 Factors that increase the risk of suicide include (Table 19.20):
(a) Previous suicide attempt
(b) Early dementia
(c) Family history of suicide
(d) Recent loss of job
(e) Living alone

19.34 The following statements are correct:
(a) The psychopath is a person who manifests a persistent disorder or disability of mind which results in abnormally aggressive or seriously irresponsible conduct.
(b) An anxiety neurosis is a condition in which anxiety dominates the clinical symptoms.
(c) Panic attacks are sudden and unpredictable attacks of anxiety usually accompanied by severe physical symptoms.
(d) Phobic anxiety is where anxiety is triggered by a single stimulus or a set of stimuli that are predictable and that normally cause no particular concern to others.
(e) An anxious personality is an individual who has a lifelong tendency to experience tension and anxiety.

19.35 Features of anxiety disorder include (page 1129, Table 19.21):
(a) Auditory hallucinations
(b) Disturbed sleep
(c) Thought insertion
(d) Hyperventilation syndrome
(e) Increased libido

19.36 Correct statements about the psychological treatment of neurosis include (page 1130):
(a) Relaxation training can be as effective as drugs in relieving mild anxiety.
(b) The term behaviour therapy is applied to psychological treatments derived from experimental psychology and intended to change behaviour.
(c) Flooding treatment is based on the finding that conditioned fear responses dissipate when experimental animals are prevented from running away from fear-provoking situations.

(d) The treatment of choice for agoraphobia is programmed practice.
(e) A form of behaviour therapy that is particularly effective treatment for obsessional rituals is response prevention.

19.37 Withdrawal syndrome with benzodiazepines includes (Table 19.23):
(a) Akathisia
(b) Insomnia
(c) Convulsions
(d) Anxiety
(e) Tardive dyskinesia

19.38 Obsessional symptoms are a feature of (page 1130):
(a) Anxiety neurosis
(b) Depression
(c) Schizophrenia
(d) Parkinson's disease
(e) Huntington's chorea

19.39 Correct statements about the management of obsessive–compulsive disorder include (page 1131):
(a) Response prevention is particularly effective.
(b) Modelling involves demonstrating to the patient what is required and encouraging them to follow this example.
(c) When obsessional thoughts accompany rituals, thought stopping is advocated.
(d) Anxiolytic drugs provide long-lasting symptomatic relief.
(e) Clomipramine is useful against obsessional symptoms accompanied by depression.

19.40 Symptoms of dissociative (conversion) disorders (page 1132):
(a) occur in the absence of physical pathology
(b) are produced consciously
(c) are caused by the overactivity of the parasympathetic system
(d) are associated with vagal overactivity
(e) are more common in men than in women

19.41 Examples of dissociative hysterical symptoms include (Table 19.24):
(a) Paralysis
(b) Tremor
(c) Repeated vomiting
(d) Mutism
(e) Somnambulism

19.42 The following statements are correct (page 1132):
(a) Dissociative amnesia commences suddenly.
(b) Dissociative pseudodementia involves memory loss and behaviour that initially suggests severe and generalized intellectual deterioration.

(c) In multiple personality there are rapid alterations between two patterns of behaviour, each of which is forgotten by the patient when the other is present.
(d) In mass hysteria the combined effects of suggestion and shared anxiety produces explosive outbreaks of sickness or other disturbed behaviour.
(e) Briquet's syndrome usually occurs in men.

19.43 Typical symptoms of post-traumatic stress disorder include (page 1134):
(a) Flashbacks
(b) Emotional blunting
(c) A sense of detachment from people
(d) Autonomic hyperarousal with hypervigilance
(e) Marked anxiety and depression

19.44 Features of alcohol dependence syndrome include (Table 19.28):
(a) Morning drinking
(b) Unable to keep to a drink limit
(c) Trembling after drinking the day before
(d) Morning retching and vomiting
(e) Tolerance to alcohol is altered

19.45 Risk factors for alcohol dependence syndrome include (page 1136):
(a) Marital difficulties
(b) Work problems
(c) An affected relative
(d) In doctors
(e) In journalists

19.46 Withdrawal symptoms from alcohol include (Table 11.38):
(a) Tremor of outstretched hands
(b) Insomnia
(c) Agitation
(d) Fits
(e) Delirium tremens

19.47 Management of delirium tremens includes (Table 19.30):
(a) Patients are treated on an outpatient basis.
(b) Intravenous chlormethiazole is the drug of choice.
(c) Thiamine should be avoided.
(d) Any dehydration should be corrected.
(e) Oral disulfiram.

19.48 The following statements are correct (page 1140):
(a) Glue sniffing can cause death.
(b) Amphetamine causes physical rather than psychological dependence.
(c) Cannabis causes a severe withdrawal syndrome.

(d) LSD is hallucinogenic.
(e) Physical dependence occurs with morphine.

19.49 Conditions associated with narcotic addicts include (page 1141):
(a) Infective endocarditis
(b) Tuberculosis
(c) Glomerulonephritis
(d) Tetanus
(e) Viral hepatitis B

19.50 Aetiological factors implicated in anorexia nervosa include
(pages 1142–1143):
(a) Disturbance of hypothalamic function
(b) A disturbance in body image
(c) Dietary problems in early life
(d) Overprotective relationships
(e) Lack of conflict resolution

19.51 Indicators of a poor outcome in anorexia nervosa include (page 1143):
(a) A long initial illness
(b) Severe weight loss
(c) Bulimia
(d) Vomiting
(e) Difficulties in relationships

19.52 Disorders of adult personality and behaviour include (page 1144):
(a) A paranoid personality is characterized by a preoccupation with
unsubstantiated conspiratorial explanations of events.
(b) A schizoid personality has a limited capacity to express emotions.
(c) A dissocial personality is characterized by a callous unconcern for the
feelings of others.
(d) A histrionic personality is characterized by self-dramatization.
(e) An anankastic personality is the same as obsessive–complusive
personality.

19.53 Complications of vomiting include:
(a) Cardiac arrhythmias
(b) Renal impairment
(c) Tetany
(d) Muscular paralysis
(e) Eroded dental enamel

19.54 Medical conditions affecting sexual performance include (Table 19.35):
(a) Angina pectoris
(b) Alcoholic cirrhosis
(c) Asthma

(d) Renal failure
(e) Neuropathy

19.55 Drugs adversely affecting sexual arousal include (Table 19.36):
(a) Cimetidine
(b) Alcohol
(c) Methyldopa
(d) Clonidine
(e) Benzodiazepines

19.56 Features of transsexualism include (page 1146):
(a) A sense of belonging to the opposite sex
(b) A sense of estrangement from one's own body
(c) A strong desire to resemble physically the opposite sex
(d) A wish to be accepted in the community as belonging to the opposite sex
(e) A sense of having been born into the wrong sex

19.57 The conditions to be met before an appropriate compulsory section form is signed include (page 1146):
(a) The patient must be suffering from a defined mental disorder.
(b) The patient must be at risk to his health.
(c) The patient must be a risk to other people's safety.
(d) The patient must be unwilling to accept hospitalization voluntarily.
(e) The patient's written consent is required.

Dermatology

20.1 Correct statements about the epidermis include (pages 1149–1150):
 (a) It consists of stratified epithelium.
 (b) The stratum corneum contains nucleate cornified cells.
 (c) Keratinocytes form the major cells in the epidermis.
 (d) Langerhans' cells derive from the bone marrow.
 (e) Merkel cells are involved in sensation.

20.2 The following statements about skin structure are correct (page 1151):
 (a) The epidermojunctional area is highly antigenic.
 (b) The eccrine sweat glands produce wax in the ears.
 (c) The Meibomian glands on the eyelids are modified sweat glands.
 (d) The apocrine sweat glands are present particularly in the palms.
 (e) The eccrine sweat glands do not function until puberty.

20.3 Cutaneous manifestations of staphylococcal infection include (page 1152):
 (a) Furuncles
 (b) Follicular impetigo
 (c) Erysipelas
 (d) Toxic shock syndrome
 (e) Toxic epidermal necrolysis

20.4 Recognized features of erysipeloid include (page 1154):
 (a) It is caused by contact with the carcases of pigs.
 (b) It is caused by streptococci.
 (c) It is self-limiting.
 (d) Systemic features are common.
 (e) The skin lesions heal with permanent and disfiguring scars.

20.5 Recognized features of erythrasma include (page 1153):
 (a) It occurs over skin flexures.
 (b) It is associated with *Cornyebacterium minutissimum.*
 (c) There is excessive sweating.
 (d) Poor hygiene.
 (e) Oral erythromycin will eradicate extensive disease.

20.6 Cutaneous manifestations of *Mycobacterium tuberculosis* include (page 1154):
 (a) Lupus vulgaris
 (b) Verrucosa cutis
 (c) Bazin's disease
 (d) Erythema induratum
 (e) Scrofuloderma

20.7 Correct statements about leprosy include (page 1154):
   (a) Biopsy in tuberculoid leprosy shows multiple bacilli.
   (b) Peripheral nerves may be enlarged.
   (c) In untreated tuberculoid leprosy the facial skin may become thickened.
   (d) It is caused by *Mycobacterium leprae*.
   (e) Nerve damage in leprosy leads to loss of sensation.

20.8 Recognized clinical manifestations of herpes simplex include (page 1154):
   (a) Primary herpes simplex I infection in children may be asymptomatic
   (b) Herpetic whitlow is common in nursing personnel
   (c) Erythema multiforme
   (d) Keratitis
   (e) Eczema herpeticum

20.9 Drugs used in the management of herpes simplex include (page 1155):
   (a) Penciclovir
   (b) Idoxuridine
   (c) Acyclovir
   (d) Ampicillin
   (e) Erythromycin

20.10 Factors predisposing to candidiasis include (page 1158):
   (a) Corticosteroids
   (b) Cytotoxics
   (c) Antibiotics
   (d) Oral contraceptives
   (e) AIDS

20.11 Ringworm fungi include (page 1156):
   (a) *Candida* spp.
   (b) Scabies
   (c) *Epidermophyton*
   (d) *Microsporum*
   (e) *Trichophyton*

20.12 Scabies (page 1159):
   (a) is caused by the male mite of *Sarcoptes scabei*
   (b) is transmitted by skin-to-skin contact
   (c) rarely causes itching
   (d) is treated with malathion
   (e) management includes treatment of close contacts

20.13 Correct statements about atopic eczema include (page 1160):
   (a) Genetic studies in atopy have shown linkage to three different loci.
   (b) Serum IgE levels are depressed in this condition.
   (c) Dietary factors may exacerbate it.

(d) In these patients *Staphylococcus aureus* is found less frequently on normal skin than expected.

(e) Herpes simplex may become disseminated on atopic skin.

20.14 Correct statements about the prognosis and treatment of atopic eczema include (page 1161):

(a) With a typical pattern on involvement and an early onset the prognosis is poor.

(b) About a third of atopic children have a dry skin in addition to eczema.

(c) The use of perfumed soaps should be encouraged.

(d) Steroids are used as an emollient.

(e) The reduction of exposure to house dust mite may improve facial eczema.

20.15 Recognized features of discoid or nummular eczema include (page 1162):

(a) It rarely occurs in the middle-aged or elderly.

(b) A previous history of skin disease is common.

(c) The skin lesions are coin-shaped.

(d) It tends to follow a chronic course rather than an acute/subacute pattern.

(e) There is often an infective aetiology.

20.16 Correct statements about seborrhoeic eczema include (page 1163):

(a) It affects areas of skin that lack sebaceous glands.

(b) It is common in patients with AIDS.

(c) It is a recognized feature of Parkinson's disease.

(d) In the elderly it can cause erythroderma.

(e) Ketoconazole shampoo and arachis oil are useful for scalp involvement.

20.17 Recognized features of irritant or allergic contact dermatitis include (page 1163):

(a) Type IV delayed hypersensitivity is a pathogenetic mechanism.

(b) Sensitivity to the antigen rarely lasts lifelong.

(c) An unusual pattern of the rash should arouse suspicion.

(d) Contact eczema occurs after repeated exposure to a chemical substance, but only in those people who are susceptible to develop an allergic reaction.

(e) Irritant eczema can occur in any individual.

20.18 Recognized features of psoriasis include (page 1165):

(a) It affects males more than females.

(b) Red, scaly well-demarcated plaques.

(c) It is common before 15 years of age.

(d) Arthropathy.

(e) It is often associated with a family history.

20.19 Recognized precipitating factors for psoriasis include (page 1165):
(a) Infection
(b) Emotional trauma
(c) Mechanical trauma
(d) Lithium carbonate
(e) Propranolol

20.20 Correct statements regarding the clinical features of psoriasis include (page 1165):
(a) Scalp involvement is common in plaque psoriasis.
(b) Köbner phenomenon is the occurrence of new plaques of psoriasis at sites of skin trauma.
(c) In pustular psoriasis the pustules are infected.
(d) Nail involvement can occur in isolation with no evidence of psoriasis elsewhere.
(e) Onycholysis is a recognized feature.

20.21 Drugs used in the management of psoriasis include (page 1166):
(a) Dithranol
(b) Coal tar
(c) Tetracycline
(d) Calcipotriol
(e) Methotrexate

20.22 Biopsies in urticaria should be obtained when (page 1167):
(a) The weals last longer than 2 months.
(b) Weals lack purpuric staining.
(c) Circulating immune complexes are absent in the sera.
(d) The attacks are not accompanied by arthralgia.
(e) Antibiotics are absent in the sera.

20.23 Common trigger factors for urticaria include (page 1167):
(a) Terfenadine
(b) Seafood
(c) Salicylates
(d) Strawberries
(e) Penicillin allergy

20.24 Causes of physical urticaria include (page 1167):
(a) Hot baths
(b) Pressure
(c) Cold
(d) Ultraviolet light
(e) Sweating

20.25 Recognized features of hereditary angio-oedema include (page 1168):
(a) Autosomal recessive pattern

(b) Excessive C_1 esterase inhibitor
(c) Lymphoproliferative disorders
(d) Airway obstruction
(e) Erythema marginatum

20.26 Drugs effective in the management of hereditary angio-oedema include (page 1168):
(a) C_1 esterase inhibitor concentrates
(b) Stanozolol
(c) Danozol
(d) Fresh frozen plasma
(e) Adrenaline

20.27 A lichen planus-like rash can be caused by (page 1168):
(a) Levamisole
(b) Penicillamine
(c) Antimalarials
(d) Gold
(e) Graft-versus-host disease

20.28 Recognized features of lichen planus include (page 1168):
(a) Köbner phenomenon
(b) Purplish planar papules
(c) Wickham's striae
(d) Dysformic nails.
(e) Postinflammatory hyperpigmentation

20.29 Pathogenetic factors implicated in acne vulgaris include (Fig 20.19):
(a) Altered sweat gland activity
(b) Alteration of sebaceous glands
(c) *Propionibacterium acnes*
(d) Androgen effect
(e) Genetic susceptibility

20.30 Recognized features of rosacea include (page 1171):
(a) Comedones
(b) Infected pustules
(c) Telangiectasia
(d) Males have more severe disease
(e) Rhinopyma

20.31 Drugs used in the treatment of rosacea include (page 1171):
(a) PUVA
(b) Tetracycline
(c) Metronidazole
(d) Isotretinoin
(e) Topical steroids

20.32 Conditions that benefit from ultraviolet light include (pages 1171–1172):
  (a) Hyperkeratosis
  (b) Epidermal dysplasia
  (c) Acne
  (d) Eczema
  (e) Psoriasis

20.33 Photosensitive skin conditions include (Table 20.5):
  (a) Ehlers–Danlos syndrome
  (b) Hutchson's summer pellagra
  (c) Actinic reticuloid
  (d) Solar elastosis
  (e) Pseudoxanthoma elasticum

20.34 Drugs associated with photosensitivity include (Table 20.5):
  (a) Tetracyclines
  (b) Thiazides
  (c) Frusemide
  (d) Phenothiazines
  (e) Retinoids

20.35 Causes of erythroderma include (Table 20.6):
  (a) Psoriasis
  (b) Gold therapy
  (c) Sulphonamide therapy
  (d) HIV infection
  (e) Toxic shock syndrome

20.36 Causes of erythema nodosum include (Table 20.7):
  (a) Oral contraceptive pill
  (b) Inflammatory disease
  (c) Sarcoidosis
  (d) Tuberculosis
  (e) Histoplasmosis

20.37 Causes of erythema multiforme include (page 1174):
  (a) Herpes simplex
  (b) *Mycoplasma pneumoniae*
  (c) Sulphonamide
  (d) Tuberculosis
  (e) Connective tissue disease

20.38 Recognized features of erythema multiforme include (page 1174):
  (a) Erythematous papules
  (b) Frank bullae
  (c) Mucosal disease

(d) Stevens–Johnson syndrome
(e) Panophthalmitis

20.39 Conditions associated with pyoderma gangrenosum include (page 1175):
(a) Seropositive arthropathy
(b) Multiple myeloma
(c) Inflammatory bowel disease
(d) Seronegative arthropathy
(e) Polycythaemia vera

20.40 Acanthosis nigricans is seen in (page 1175):
(a) Systemic sclerosis
(b) Gastrointestinal malignancy
(c) Juvenile obesity with insulin resistance
(d) Polycystic ovarian disease
(e) Endocrine diseases

20.41 Recognized clinical features of dermatomyositis include (page 1175):
(a) Proximal myopathy
(b) Photosensitive rash
(c) Nailfold capillary changes
(d) Dysphagia
(e) Respiratory muscle involvement

20.42 Recognized clinical features of scleroderma include (page 1175):
(a) Raynaud's phenomenon
(b) Loss of digits
(c) Acrosclerosis
(d) Telangiectasia
(e) Ischaemia

20.43 Recognized clinical features of morphoea include (page 1175):
(a) Systemic features are common.
(b) Males are more frequently affected.
(c) Facial hemiatrophy.
(d) Plaques.
(e) Hyperpigmentation.

20.44 Sclerodermatous skin changes may be seen in (page 1176):
(a) Chronic Lyme disease
(b) Chronic graft-versus-host disease
(c) Vinyl chloride disease
(d) Eosinophilic myalgia
(e) Bleomycin therapy

20.45 Recognized features of discoid lupus erythematosus include (page 1176):
    (a) Serum antinuclear factor is positive in one-third of cases
    (b) Follicular plugging
    (c) Alopecia
    (d) Scarring of skin
    (e) Erythematous scaled plaques

20.46 Recognized cutaneous features of systemic lupus erythematosus include (page 1176):
    (a) Photosensitivity
    (b) Butterfly rash on the cheeks
    (c) Nailfold capillary dilatation
    (d) Purpura
    (e) Urticaria

20.47 Cutaneous manifestations of sarcoidosis include (page 1177):
    (a) Erythema nodosum
    (b) Macular lesions with central depigmentation
    (c) Lupus pernio
    (d) Micropapular lesions
    (e) Subcutaneous nodules

20.48 Cutaneous features of neurofibromatosis include (page 1177):
    (a) Café-au-lait spots
    (b) *Molluscum fibrosum*
    (c) Plexiform neuromas
    (d) Elephantiasis neuromatosa
    (e) Axillary freckling

20.49 Skin conditions that cause pruritus include (page 1177):
    (a) Scabies
    (b) Atopic eczema
    (c) Candidiasis
    (d) Urticaria
    (e) Pityriasis versicolor

20.50 Systemic conditions that cause pruritus include (Table 20.8):
    (a) Hyperthyroidism
    (b) Lymphoma
    (c) Polycythaemia vera
    (d) Uraemia
    (e) Primary biliary cirrhosis

20.51 Clinical features of tuberous sclerosis include (page 1178):
    (a) Adenoma sebaceum
    (b) Periungual fibromas
    (c) Shagreen patches

    (d) Mental retardation
    (e) Café-au-lait spots

20.52 Cutaneous manifestations of diabetes include (page 1178):
    (a) Pretibial myxoedema
    (b) Necrobiosis lipodica
    (c) Cheiroarthropathy
    (d) Granuloma annulare
    (e) Blisters

20.53 The following associations regarding bullous disease and direct immunofluorescence are correct (pages 1179–1180):
    (a) Pemphigus vulgaris – antigen–antibody complexes localize within the intercellular substance of the epidermis
    (b) Bullous pemphigoid – IgG and C_3 staining of the basement membrane
    (c) Epidermolysis bullosa acquisita – IgG deposition at the epidermodermal junction
    (d) Dermatitis herpetiformis – IgA deposits in unaffected skin
    (e) Pemphigus vulgaris – IgG within the epidermis

20.54 The following associations are correct (page 1180):
    (a) Pemphigus vulgaris – mucosa rarely affected
    (b) Bullous pemphigoid – mucosa is commonly affected
    (c) Dermatitis herpetiformis – gliadin antibodies in the serum
    (d) Bullous pemphigoid – skin lesions on the flexural aspect of limbs
    (e) Dermatitis herpetiformis – skin lesions on the extensor surfaces of the body

20.55 Primary tumours from the following sites can metastasize to the skin (page 1183):
    (a) Breast
    (b) Stomach
    (c) Lung
    (d) Kidney
    (e) Heart

20.56 Correct statements about malignant skin tumours include (page 1183):
    (a) Basal cell carcinoma is the most common cancer of the skin.
    (b) Basal cell carcinoma usually metastasizes to distant sites.
    (c) A single episode of severe sunburn is a significant risk factor for malignant melanoma.
    (d) Lentigo maligna is a lymphomatous invasion of the skin by T lymphocytes.
    (e) Kaposi's sarcoma is a vascular, multifocal, malignant tumour.

20.57 There is an increased frequency of squamous carcinomas in (page 1183):
    (a) Albinos

    (b) Xeroderma pigmentosum
    (c) Human papilloma virus warts
    (d) Those protected from sunlight
    (e) Those with ionizing radiation for ankylosing spondylitis

20.58 Kaposi's sarcoma is seen in (page 1185):
    (a) Patients with AIDS
    (b) Immunosuppressed patients secondary to chemotherapy
    (c) Elderly males of Jewish origin
    (d) Africans
    (e) *Pityrosporum ovale* infection

20.59 A pemphigus-like eruption has been seen with drugs such as
(Table 20.12):
    (a) Penicillin
    (b) Captopril
    (c) Rifampicin
    (d) Prednisolone
    (e) Methotrexate

20.60 Causes of leg ulceration include (Table 20.10):
    (a) Kaposi's sarcoma
    (b) Basal cell carcinoma
    (c) Tuberculosis
    (d) Pyoderma gangrenosum
    (e) Rheumatoid vasculitis

20.61 Venous ulcers are often accompanied by (page 1185):
    (a) Absent peripheral pulses
    (b) Hyperpigmentation
    (c) A history of claudication
    (d) Cellulitis
    (e) Systolic hypertension

20.62 Correct statements about pressure sores include (page 1186):
    (a) They are due to skin hyperaemia from sustained pressure over a bony
        point.
    (b) The majority of pressure sores occur in hospital.
    (c) Most patients with ulcers involving the subcutaneous tissue die in the
        first 4 months.
    (d) At-risk patients should be regularly turned to allow even pressure on
        the hips.
    (e) Red/blue discoloration of the skin can lead to ulcers in 1–2 hours.

20.63 Predisposing factors for pressure sores include (page 1186):
    (a) Rheumatoid arthritis
    (b) Diabetes mellitus

(c) Peripheral vascular disease
(d) Anaemia
(e) Malnutrition

20.64 Causes of necrotizing venulitis include (Table 20.11):
(a) Henoch–Schönlein purpura
(b) SLE
(c) Rheumatoid arthritis
(d) Hepatitis B
(e) Dental abscess

20.65 Recognized causes of lymphoedema include (page 1187):
(a) Recurrent cellulitis
(b) Yellow nail syndrome
(c) Infiltration due to malignant disease
(d) Following radiotherapy
(e) Filariasis

20.66 Recognized manifestations of Ehlers–Danlos syndrome include
(page 1187):
(a) Joint hypermobility
(b) Aortic rupture
(c) Hyperextensible skin
(d) Pulmonary stenosis
(e) Tricuspid stenosis

20.67 Recognized manifestations of Marfan's syndrome include (page 1188):
(a) Mitral valve prolapse
(b) Short stature
(c) Upper segment of the body smaller than the lower segment of the
body
(d) Arm span is less than the height of the patient
(e) Dislocation of the lens of the eye

20.68 Recognized examples of hypopigmentation include (page 1188):
(a) Mongolian blue spot
(b) Pityriasis versicolor
(c) Vitiligo
(d) Pityriasis alba
(e) Naevus of Ito

20.69 Causes of generalized hypermelanosis include (page 1188):
(a) Neurofibromatosis
(b) Haemochromatosis
(c) Addison's disease
(d) Albright's syndrome
(e) Cushing's syndrome

20.70 The following associations for nail changes are correct (page 1190):
   (a) Half-and-half nails – renal failure
   (b) Koilonychia – iron-deficiency anaemia
   (c) Onycholysis – thyrotoxicosis
   (d) White bands – hypoalbuminaemia
   (e) Splinter haemorrhages – infective endocarditis

20.71 Drugs associated with urticaria include (Table 20.12):
   (a) Codeine
   (b) Opiates
   (c) Aspirin
   (d) Captopril
   (e) Indomethacin

20.72 Drugs associated with allergic vasculitis and purpura include (Table 20.12):
   (a) Allopurinol
   (b) Amiodarone
   (c) Captopril
   (d) Gold
   (e) Sulphonamides

20.73 Drugs associated with LE-like syndrome include (Table 20.12):
   (a) Isoniazid
   (b) β-Blockers
   (c) Penicillamine
   (d) Lithium
   (e) Steroids

20.74 Drugs associated with erythematous morbilliform eruptions include (Table 20.12):
   (a) Ampicillin
   (b) Sulphonamides
   (c) Phenytoin
   (d) Gold
   (e) Gentamicin

20.75 Drugs associated with toxic epidermal necrolysis include (Table 20.12):
   (a) NSAIDs
   (b) Penicillins
   (c) Sulphonamides
   (d) Allopurinol
   (e) Barbiturates

20.76 Drugs associated with fixed drug eruptions include (Table 20.12):
   (a) Tetracycline
   (b) Sulphonamides

(c) Oral contraceptives
(d) Salicylates
(e) Phenolphthalein

20.77 Drugs associated with lupus erythematosus-like rash include
(Table 20.12):
(a) Hydralazine
(b) Procainamide
(c) Phenytoin
(d) Penicillamine
(e) Isoniazid

20.78 Drugs causing acneform eruptions include (Table 20.12):
(a) Corticosteroids
(b) Androgens
(c) Oral contraceptives
(d) Anticonvulsants
(e) Iodides

20.79 Drugs that cause hypertrichosis include (page 1192):
(a) Cortisone
(b) Minoxidil
(c) Hydantoins
(d) Cyclosporin A
(e) Cyclophosphamide

20.80 Causes of diffuse hair loss include (page 1191):
(a) Hyperthyroidism
(b) Hypothyroidism
(c) Iron deficiency
(d) Lithium
(e) Vitamin A

20.81 Alopecia areata occurs in association with (page 1191):
(a) Thyrotoxicosis
(b) Addison's disease
(c) Pernicious anaemia
(d) Vitiligo
(e) Down's syndrome

20.82 Examples of haemangiomas include (page 1192):
(a) Keratoacanthoma
(b) Capillary naevus
(c) Port-wine stain
(d) Strawberry naevus
(e) Epidermal naevus

Infectious Diseases, Tropical Medicine and Sexually Transmitted Diseases
Answers

1.1 (a) F	**1.7** (a) T	**1.13** (a) T	**1.19** (a) T
(b) T	(b) F	(b) T	(b) T
(c) T	(c) F	(c) T	(c) T
(d) T	(d) T	(d) F	(d) T
(e) T	(e) T	(e) F	(e) F
1.2 (a) F	**1.8** (a) T	**1.14** (a) T	**1.20** (a) T
(b) T	(b) T	(b) T	(b) T
(c) T	(c) F	(c) T	(c) T
(d) T	(d) T	(d) T	(d) T
(e) T	(e) T	(e) T	(e) T
1.3 (a) T	**1.9** (a) T	**1.15** (a) T	**1.21** (a) F
(b) T	(b) T	(b) T	(b) T
(c) T	(c) T	(c) T	(c) T
(d) T	(d) T	(d) T	(d) T
(e) T	(e) T	(e) T	(e) T
1.4 (a) F	**1.10** (a) T	**1.16** (a) T	**1.22** (a) T
(b) T	(b) T	(b) F	(b) T
(c) T	(c) T	(c) F	(c) T
(d) T	(d) T	(d) T	(d) T
(e) T	(e) T	(e) T	(e) T
1.5 (a) T	**1.11** (a) F	**1.17** (a) T	**1.23** (a) F
(b) T	(b) F	(b) T	(b) T
(c) T	(c) T	(c) F	(c) T
(d) T	(d) F	(d) T	(d) T
(e) T	(e) T	(e) T	(e) T
1.6 (a) T	**1.12** (a) T	**1.18** (a) T	**1.24** (a) F
(b) F	(b) T	(b) T	(b) F
(c) T	(c) F	(c) T	(c) F
(d) F	(d) F	(d) T	(d) F
(e) F	(e) T	(e) T	(e) F

1.25	(a) T	1.33	(a) T	1.41	(a) T	1.49	(a) F
	(b) T		(b) T		(b) T		(b) T
	(c) T		(c) T		(c) F		(c) T
	(d) F		(d) F		(d) T		(d) T
	(e) F		(e) T		(e) T		(e) T
1.26	(a) F	1.34	(a) F	1.42	(a) T	1.50	(a) F
	(b) T		(b) F		(b) T		(b) T
	(c) T		(c) F		(c) F		(c) T
	(d) T		(d) F		(d) T		(d) T
	(e) T		(e) F		(e) T		(e) T
1.27	(a) T	1.35	(a) T	1.43	(a) F	1.51	(a) T
	(b) T		(b) F		(b) F		(b) T
	(c) F		(c) T		(c) T		(c) T
	(d) T		(d) T		(d) T		(d) F
	(e) T		(e) T		(e) T		(e) F
1.28	(a) T	1.36	(a) F	1.44	(a) F	1.52	(a) T
	(b) T		(b) T		(b) T		(b) T
	(c) T		(c) F		(c) T		(c) T
	(d) T		(d) T		(d) T		(d) T
	(e) F		(e) F		(e) F		(e) T
1.29	(a) T	1.37	(a) T	1.45	(a) T	1.53	(a) T
	(b) T		(b) T		(b) T		(b) T
	(c) T		(c) T		(c) F		(c) T
	(d) T		(d) T		(d) T		(d) T
	(e) T		(e) T		(e) F		(e) F
1.30	(a) T	1.38	(a) T	1.46	(a) T	1.54	(a) T
	(b) F		(b) F		(b) F		(b) T
	(c) F		(c) T		(c) F		(c) F
	(d) T		(d) F		(d) T		(d) F
	(e) T		(e) T		(e) T		(e) T
1.31	(a) T	1.39	(a) T	1.47	(a) F	1.55	(a) T
	(b) T		(b) T		(b) F		(b) T
	(c) T		(c) T		(c) F		(c) T
	(d) T		(d) T		(d) T		(d) T
	(e) T		(e) F		(e) T		(e) T
1.32	(a) F	1.40	(a) F	1.48	(a) T	1.56	(a) F
	(b) T		(b) T		(b) T		(b) T
	(c) T		(c) T		(c) T		(c) F
	(d) T		(d) F		(d) T		(d) T
	(e) F		(e) T		(e) T		(e) T

1.57	(a)	T	**1.65**	(a)	T	**1.73**	(a)	T	**1.81**	(a) F

1.57
(a) T
(b) T
(c) T
(d) T
(e) F

1.58
(a) T
(b) T
(c) T
(d) T
(e) T

1.59
(a) T
(b) T
(c) F
(d) F
(e) T

1.60
(a) F
(b) T
(c) T
(d) T
(e) T

1.61
(a) T
(b) F
(c) T
(d) T
(e) T

1.62
(a) F
(b) T
(c) T
(d) T
(e) T

1.63
(a) T
(b) T
(c) T
(d) T
(e) T

1.64
(a) F
(b) F
(c) T
(d) T
(e) T

1.65
(a) T
(b) T
(c) F
(d) T
(e) T

1.66
(a) T
(b) T
(c) T
(d) T
(e) T

1.67
(a) F
(b) T
(c) T
(d) T
(e) T

1.68
(a) T
(b) T
(c) T
(d) T
(e) T

1.69
(a) T
(b) T
(c) T
(d) T
(e) F

1.70
(a) T
(b) T
(c) T
(d) T
(e) F

1.71
(a) T
(b) T
(c) T
(d) F
(e) F

1.72
(a) F
(b) F
(c) T
(d) T
(e) T

1.73
(a) T
(b) T
(c) T
(d) T
(e) T

1.74
(a) F
(b) T
(c) F
(d) T
(e) F

1.75
(a) T
(b) T
(c) T
(d) F
(e) T

1.76
(a) T
(b) F
(c) T
(d) F
(e) T

1.77
(a) T
(b) T
(c) T
(d) T
(e) T

1.78
(a) F
(b) T
(c) T
(d) T
(e) T

1.79
(a) T
(b) T
(c) T
(d) T
(e) T

1.80
(a) F
(b) T
(c) T
(d) F
(e) T

1.81
(a) F
(b) T
(c) T
(d) T
(e) T

1.82
(a) T
(b) T
(c) T
(d) T
(e) T

1.83
(a) F
(b) F
(c) T
(d) F
(e) T

1.84
(a) T
(b) T
(c) T
(d) T
(e) T

1.85
(a) T
(b) T
(c) T
(d) T
(e) T

1.86
(a) T
(b) T
(c) F
(d) F
(e) T

1.87
(a) T
(b) F
(c) F
(d) T
(e) T

1.88
(a) T
(b) T
(c) T
(d) T
(e) T

1.89	(a) T	**1.97**	(a) T	**1.105**	(a) T	**1.113**	(a) T
	(b F		(b) F		(b) T		(b) T
	(c) F		(c) T		(c) T		(c) F
	(d) F		(d) T		(d) T		(d) T
	(e) F		(e) T		(e) F		(e) F
1.90	(a) T	**1.98**	(a) F	**1.106**	(a) F	**1.114**	(a) F
	(b) T		(b) F		(b) F		(b) F
	(c) T		(c) F		(c) T		(c) T
	(d) T		(d) F		(d) T		(d) T
	(e) T		(e) F		(e) T		(e) T
1.91	(a) T	**1.99**	(a) T	**1.107**	(a) T	**1.115**	(a) F
	(b) T		(b) T		(b) T		(b) T
	(c) T		(c) T		(c) T		(c) T
	(d) T		(d) T		(d) T		(d) F
	(e) T		(e) T		(e) F		(e) T
1.92	(a) T	**1.100**	(a) T	**1.108**	(a) T	**1.116**	(a) T
	(b) T		(b) T		(b) T		(b) T
	(c) T		(c) T		(c) T		(c) T
	(d) T		(d) T		(d) T		(d) T
	(e) F		(e) F		(e) T		(e) T
1.93	(a) F	**1.101**	(a) T	**1.109**	(a) F	**1.117**	(a) F
	(b) T		(b) T		(b) T		(b) T
	(c) T		(c) T		(c) F		(c) T
	(d) T		(d) T		(d) T		(d) F
	(e) T		(e) T		(e) T		(e) T
1.94	(a) T	**1.102**	(a) T	**1.110**	(a) F	**1.118**	(a) F
	(b) T		(b) T		(b) T		(b) F
	(c) T		(c) F		(c) T		(c) T
	(d) T		(d) F		(d) T		(d) T
	(e) T		(e) F		(e) T		(e) F
1.95	(a) T	**1.103**	(a) T	**1.111**	(a) T	**1.119**	(a) T
	(b) T		(b) T		(b) T		(b) F
	(c) T		(c) T		(c) T		(c) T
	(d) T		(d) T		(d) T		(d) T
	(e) T		(e) T		(e) F		(e) F
1.96	(a) T	**1.104**	(a) T	**1.112**	(a) F	**1.120**	(a) F
	(b) T		(b) F		(b) F		(b) F
	(c) T		(c) T		(c) T		(c) T
	(d) F		(d) T		(d) T		(d) T
	(e) T		(e) T		(e) F		(e) T

1.121 (a) T
(b) F
(c) F
(d) T
(e) T

1.122 (a) F
(b) T
(c) F
(d) F
(e) T

1.123 (a) T
(b) F
(c) T
(d) F
(e) T

1.124 (a) T
(b) T
(c) T
(d) F
(e) F

1.125 (a) F
(b) F
(c) T
(d) F
(e) T

1.126 (a) T
(b) T
(c) F
(d) T
(e) T

1.127 (a) T
(b) T
(c) F
(d) T
(e) T

1.128 (a) F
(b) T
(c) T
(d) T
(e) T

1.129 (a) T
(b) T
(c) T
(d) F
(e) F

1.130 (a) T
(b) T
(c) T
(d) T
(e) T

1.131 (a) T
(b) T
(c) F
(d) T
(e) T

1.132 (a) T
(b) T
(c) T
(d) T
(e) F

1.133 (a) T
(b) T
(c) F
(d) T
(e) T

1.134 (a) T
(b) T
(c) T
(d) T
(e) F

1.135 (a) F
(b) T
(c) T
(d) F
(e) T

1.136 (a) F
(b) F
(c) T
(d) T
(e) T

1.137 (a) T
(b) T
(c) T
(d) T
(e) T

1.138 (a) F
(b) T
(c) T
(d) F
(e) T

1.139 (a) F
(b) F
(c) T
(d) T
(e) F

1.140 (a) T
(b) T
(c) T
(d) T
(e) T

1.141 (a) F
(b) F
(c) F
(d) T
(e) T

1.142 (a) T
(b) F
(c) T
(d) T
(e) T

1.143 (a) T
(b) T
(c) T
(d) T
(e) T

1.144 (a) T
(b) T
(c) T
(d) T
(e) T

1.145 (a) T
(b) T
(c) T
(d) T
(e) T

1.146 (a) F
(b) T
(c) T
(d) F
(e) T

1.147 (a) T
(b) T
(c) T
(d) T
(e) T

1.148 (a) F
(b) F
(c) T
(d) T
(e) T

1.149 (a) T
(b) T
(c) T
(d) T
(e) F

1.150 (a) T
(b) T
(c) T
(d) F
(e) T

1.151 (a) F
(b) T
(c) T
(d) T
(e) T

1.152 (a) F
(b) F
(c) F
(d) F
(e) F

1.153	(a) T	**1.161**	(a) T	**1.169**	(a) F	**1.177**	(a) F
	(b) T		(b) T		(b) F		(b) F
	(c) T		(c) T		(c) F		(c) F
	(d) F		(d) T		(d) T		(d) T
	(e) T		(e) T		(e) T		(e) T
1.154	(a) T	**1.162**	(a) T	**1.170**	(a) T	**1.178**	(a) T
	(b) T		(b) T		(b) T		(b) T
	(c) T		(c) T		(c) T		(c) T
	(d) T		(d) T		(d) T		(d) T
	(e) F		(e) T		(e) T		(e) T
1.155	(a) T	**1.163**	(a) T	**1.171**	(a) T	**1.179**	(a) F
	(b) F		(b) T		(b) T		(b) T
	(c) T		(c) T		(c) T		(c) T
	(d) T		(d) T		(d) F		(d) T
	(e) T		(e) F		(e) T		(e) T
1.156	(a) T	**1.164**	(a) F	**1.172**	(a) T	**1.180**	(a) T
	(b) T		(b) T		(b) F		(b) T
	(c) T		(c) T		(c) F		(c) T
	(d) T		(d) T		(d) T		(d) F
	(e) T		(e) T		(e) F		(e) T
1.57	(a) F	**1.165**	(a) T	**1.173**	(a) T	**1.181**	(a) T
	(b) T		(b) T		(b) T		(b) T
	(c) T		(c) T		(c) T		(c) T
	(d) T		(d) T		(d) T		(d) T
	(e) T		(e) T		(e) F		(e) T
1.158	(a) T	**1.166**	(a) F	**1.174**	(a) T	**1.182**	(a) F
	(b) T		(b) T		(b) T		(b) F
	(c) T		(c) T		(c) T		(c) T
	(d) T		(d) F		(d) F		(d) F
	(e) T		(e) F		(e) F		(e) T
1.159	(a) T	**1.167**	(a) F	**1.175**	(a) T	**1.183**	(a) F
	(b) T		(b) T		(b) T		(b) F
	(c) T		(c) T		(c) F		(c) F
	(d) T		(d) T		(d) T		(d) T
	(e) T		(e) T		(e) T		(e) T
1.160	(a) F	**1.168**	(a) T	**1.176**	(a) F	**1.184**	(a) T
	(b) T		(b) T		(b) F		(b) F
	(c) T		(c) T		(c) T		(c) T
	(d) T		(d) T		(d) T		(d) F
	(e) F		(e) T		(e) T		(e) F

1.185	(a) F	**1.191**	(a) T	**1.197**	(a) T	**1.203**	(a) T
	(b) F		(b) T		(b) T		(b) T
	(c) F		(c) T		(c) T		(c) T
	(d) T		(d) T		(d) T		(d) T
	(e) T		(e) T		(e) T		(e) T
1.186	(a) F	**1.192**	(a) T	**1.198**	(a) F	**1.204**	(a) T
	(b) F		(b) F		(b) F		(b) T
	(c) F		(c) F		(c) T		(c) T
	(d) T		(d) F		(d) T		(d) F
	(e) F		(e) F		(e) T		(e) F
1.187	(a) F	**1.193**	(a) T	**1.199**	(a) F	**1.205**	(a) T
	(b) F		(b) T		(b) F		(b) T
	(c) F		(c) T		(c) T		(c) T
	(d) T		(d) T		(d) F		(d) T
	(e) F		(e) F		(e) F		(e) F
1.188	(a) T	**1.194**	(a) F	**1.200**	(a) T	**1.206**	(a) F
	(b) T		(b) T		(b) F		(b) F
	(c) T		(c) T		(c) F		(c) T
	(d) T		(d) T		(d) T		(d) T
	(e) T		(e) T		(e) T		(e) T
1.189	(a) F	**1.195**	(a) T	**1.201**	(a) T	**1.207**	(a) T
	(b) F		(b) T		(b) T		(b) F
	(c) T		(c) T		(c) T		(c) T
	(d) T		(d) T		(d) T		(d) T
	(e) T		(e) F		(e) T		(e) T
1.190	(a) T	**1.196**	(a) T	**1.202**	(a) T	**1.208**	(a) T
	(b) F		(b) T		(b) F		(b) T
	(c) F		(c) T		(c) F		(c) T
	(d) T		(d) T		(d) F		(d) F
	(e) F		(e) T		(e) T		(e) T

Cell and Molecular Biology Genetic Disorders and Immunology
Answers

2.1 (a) T	**2.7** (a) T	**2.13** (a) T	**2.19** (a) T
(b) T	(b) T	(b) T	(b) T
(c) T	(c) T	(c) T	(c) T
(d) T	(d) T	(d) T	(d) F
(e) T	(e) T	(e) T	(e) F
2.2 (a) T	**2.8** (a) F	**2.14** (a) F	**2.20** (a) F
(b) T	(b) F	(b) T	(b) T
(c) T	(c) F	(c) T	(c) F
(d) T	(d) F	(d) T	(d) F
(e) F	(e) T	(e) F	(e) T
2.3 (a) T	**2.9** (a) T	**2.15** (a) T	**2.21** (a) T
(b) T	(b) T	(b) T	(b) T
(c) T	(c) T	(c) T	(c) T
(d) T	(d) F	(d) T	(d) F
(e) F	(e) F	(e) F	(e) T
2.4 (a) T	**2.10** (a) T	**2.16** (a) T	**2.22** (a) T
(b) T	(b) T	(b) T	(b) T
(c) T	(c) T	(c) T	(c) T
(d) F	(d) T	(d) T	(d) T
(e) F	(e) T	(e) T	(e) T
2.5 (a) F	**2.11** (a) T	**2.17** (a) T	**2.23** (a) T
(b) T	(b) T	(b) T	(b) T
(c) T	(c) T	(c) T	(c) T
(d) T	(d) T	(d) F	(d) T
(e) T	(e) T	(e) F	(e) T
2.6 (a) T	**2.12** (a) F	**2.18** (a) T	**2.24** (a) F
(b) T	(b) F	(b) T	(b) F
(c) T	(c) F	(c) T	(c) T
(d) T	(d) T	(d) T	(d) T
(e) T	(e) T	(e) T	(e) F

2.25			2.33			2.41			2.49		
	(a)	T		(a)	T		(a)	F		(a)	T
	(b)	T		(b)	F		(b)	T		(b)	F
	(c)	T		(c)	T		(c)	T		(c)	T
	(d)	F		(d)	T		(d)	T		(d)	T
	(e)	T		(e)	T		(e)	T		(e)	T
2.26	(a)	T	2.34	(a)	T	2.42	(a)	F	2.50	(a)	T
	(b)	T		(b)	F		(b)	F		(b)	T
	(c)	F		(c)	F		(c)	F		(c)	T
	(d)	T		(d)	T		(d)	F		(d)	T
	(e)	T		(e)	F		(e)	F		(e)	T
2.27	(a)	F	2.35	(a)	T	2.43	(a)	F	2.51	(a)	F
	(b)	F		(b)	T		(b)	F		(b)	T
	(c)	T		(c)	F		(c)	F		(c)	T
	(d)	T		(d)	T		(d)	F		(d)	T
	(e)	T		(e)	T		(e)	F		(e)	T
2.28	(a)	T	2.36	(a)	F	2.44	(a)	T	2.52	(a)	T
	(b)	T		(b)	F		(b)	T		(b)	T
	(c)	T		(c)	F		(c)	T		(c)	F
	(d)	T		(d)	F		(d)	T		(d)	F
	(e)	T		(e)	T		(e)	T		(e)	F
2.29	(a)	F	2.37	(a)	T	2.45	(a)	T	2.53	(a)	T
	(b)	T		(b)	T		(b)	F		(b)	T
	(c)	T		(c)	T		(c)	F		(c)	F
	(d)	F		(d)	T		(d)	F		(d)	F
	(e)	F		(e)	T		(e)	F		(e)	T
2.30	(a)	T	2.38	(a)	T	2.46	(a)	T	2.54	(a)	F
	(b)	F		(b)	T		(b)	T		(b)	T
	(c)	T		(c)	F		(c)	F		(c)	T
	(d)	T		(d)	T		(d)	T		(d)	T
	(e)	T		(e)	T		(e)	T		(e)	T
2.31	(a)	T	2.39	(a)	T	2.47	(a)	F	2.55	(a)	T
	(b)	F		(b)	T		(b)	F		(b)	T
	(c)	T		(c)	T		(c)	F		(c)	T
	(d)	F		(d)	T		(d)	T		(d)	F
	(e)	T		(e)	T		(e)	T		(e)	F
2.32	(a)	T	2.40	(a)	T	2.48	(a)	F	2.56	(a)	T
	(b)	T		(b)	T		(b)	T		(b)	T
	(c)	T		(c)	T		(c)	T		(c)	T
	(d)	F		(d)	T		(d)	T		(d)	T
	(e)	T		(e)	F		(e)	T		(e)	T

2.57	(a) T	**2.65**	(a) T	**2.73**	(a) T	**2.81**	(a) T
	(b) T		(b) F		(b) T		(b) T
	(c) T		(c) T		(c) T		(c) T
	(d) T		(d) T		(d) T		(d) F
	(e) T		(e) F		(e) F		(e) T

2.58	(a) T	**2.66**	(a) T	**2.74**	(a) F	**2.82**	(a) T
	(b) T		(b) T		(b) T		(b) F
	(c) T		(c) T		(c) T		(c) F
	(d) T		(d) T		(d) T		(d) F
	(e) T		(e) T		(e) T		(e) T

2.59	(a) T	**2.67**	(a) T	**2.75**	(a) T	**2.83**	(a) F
	(b) T		(b) T		(b) F		(b) T
	(c) T		(c) T		(c) F		(c) T
	(d) T		(d) T		(d) T		(d) T
	(e) T		(e) T		(e) T		(e) F

2.60	(a) F	**2.68**	(a) F	**2.76**	(a) F	**2.84**	(a) F
	(b) T		(b) T		(b) T		(b) F
	(c) T		(c) T		(c) T		(c) T
	(d) F		(d) T		(d) T		(d) T
	(e) T		(e) T		(e) T		(e) T

2.61	(a) T	**2.69**	(a) T	**2.77**	(a) F	**2.85**	(a) F
	(b) T		(b) T		(b) T		(b) T
	(c) T		(c) T		(c) T		(c) T
	(d) T		(d) T		(d) T		(d) T
	(e) T		(e) T		(e) T		(e) T

2.62	(a) T	**2.70**	(a) T	**2.78**	(a) F	**2.86**	(a) F
	(b) T		(b) T		(b) T		(b) T
	(c) T		(c) T		(c) F		(c) T
	(d) T		(d) F		(d) T		(d) T
	(e) T		(e) T		(e) T		(e) T

2.63	(a) T	**2.71**	(a) T	**2.79**	(a) T	**2.87**	(a) T
	(b) T		(b) T		(b) T		(b) T
	(c) T		(c) F		(c) T		(c) T
	(d) T		(d) T		(d) F		(d) T
	(e) T		(e) F		(e) T		(e) F

2.64	(a) F	**2.72**	(a) T	**2.80**	(a) F	**2.88**	(a) F
	(b) F		(b) T		(b) T		(b) F
	(c) T		(c) F		(c) T		(c) T
	(d) T		(d) T		(d) F		(d) T
	(e) T		(e) T		(e) T		(e) T

2.89	(a) T	2.97	(a) F	2.105	(a) T	2.113	(a) T
	(b) T		(b) F		(b) T		(b) T
	(c) T		(c) T		(c) T		(c) T
	(d) T		(d) T		(d) T		(d) T
	(e) F		(e) T		(e) T		(e) T

2.90	(a) T	2.98	(a) F	2.106	(a) T	2.114	(a) F
	(b) T		(b) T		(b) F		(b) T
	(c) T		(c) F		(c) T		(c) T
	(d) T		(d) T		(d) T		(d) T
	(e) T		(e) T		(e) T		(e) T

2.91	(a) T	2.99	(a) F	2.107	(a) F	2.115	(a) T
	(b) T		(b) T		(b) F		(b) F
	(c) T		(c) T		(c) T		(c) F
	(d) T		(d) T		(d) T		(d) F
	(e) F		(e) T		(e) F		(e) F

2.92	(a) F	2.100	(a) T	2.108	(a) T	2.116	(a) F
	(b) F		(b) T		(b) F		(b) T
	(c) T		(c) T		(c) T		(c) F
	(d) F		(d) T		(d) T		(d) T
	(e) T		(e) T		(e) T		(e) F

2.93	(a) F	2.101	(a) T	2.109	(a) F	2.117	(a) T
	(b) F		(b) F		(b) F		(b) T
	(c) F		(c) T		(c) T		(c) T
	(d) T		(d) T		(d) T		(d) F
	(e) F		(e) T		(e) T		(e) T

2.94	(a) F	2.102	(a) T	2.110	(a) F	2.118	(a) T
	(b) F		(b) T		(b) T		(b) T
	(c) T		(c) T		(c) T		(c) T
	(d) T		(d) T		(d) T		(d) F
	(e) T		(e) T		(e) T		(e) F

2.95	(a) T	2.103	(a) T	2.111	(a) F	2.119	(a) F
	(b) T		(b) T		(b) T		(b) F
	(c) T		(c) T		(c) T		(c) T
	(d) T		(d) F		(d) T		(d) T
	(e) T		(e) F		(e) T		(e) T

2.96	(a) F	2.104	(a) T	2.112	(a) T	2.120	(a) F
	(b) T		(b) F		(b) T		(b) T
	(c) T		(c) T		(c) T		(c) T
	(d) F		(d) T		(d) T		(d) T
	(e) T		(e) T		(e) T		(e) T

2.121	(a) F	**2.129**	(a) T	**2.137**	(a) F	**2.145**	(a) F
	(b) F		(b) T		(b) F		(b) F
	(c) T		(c) T		(c) T		(c) F
	(d) T		(d) T		(d) T		(d) F
	(e) T		(e) T		(e) T		(e) T
2.122	(a) T	**2.130**	(a) T	**2.138**	(a) T	**2.146**	(a) T
	(b) F		(b) T		(b) T		(b) T
	(c) T		(c) T		(c) T		(c) T
	(d) T		(d) T		(d) T		(d) F
	(e) T		(e) T		(e) T		(e) F
2.123	(a) T	**2.131**	(a) T	**2.139**	(a) T	**2.147**	(a) F
	(b) F		(b) T		(b) T		(b) F
	(c) T		(c) T		(c) T		(c) T
	(d) T		(d) F		(d) F		(d) T
	(e) T		(e) F		(e) F		(e) T
2.124	(a) T	**2.132**	(a) T	**2.140**	(a) F	**2.148**	(a) T
	(b) F		(b) T		(b) T		(b) T
	(c) F		(c) F		(c) T		(c) T
	(d) T		(d) F		(d) T		(d) T
	(e) T		(e) T		(e) F		(e) T
2.125	(a) T	**2.133**	(a) T	**2.141**	(a) T	**2.149**	(a) T
	(b) T		(b) T		(b) T		(b) T
	(c) T		(c) T		(c) T		(c) T
	(d) T		(d) T		(d) T		(d) T
	(e) T		(e) T		(e) F		(e) F
2.126	(a) T	**2.134**	(a) F	**2.142**	(a) F		
	(b) T		(b) T		(b) F		
	(c) T		(c) F		(c) F		
	(d) T		(d) T		(d) F		
	(e) T		(e) T		(e) T		
2.127	(a) T	**2.135**	(a) T	**2.143**	(a) T		
	(b) T		(b) T		(b) T		
	(c) T		(c) T		(c) T		
	(d) F		(d) T		(d) F		
	(e) T		(e) T		(e) F		
2.128	(a) T	**2.136**	(a) T	**2.144**	(a) T		
	(b) T		(b) T		(b) F		
	(c) T		(c) T		(c) F		
	(d) T		(d) T		(d) T		
	(e) T		(e) T		(e) T		

Nutrition
Answers

3.1 (a) T	**3.8** (a) F	**3.15** (a) T	**3.22** (a) T
(b) T	(b) F	(b) F	(b) F
(c) T	(c) T	(c) F	(c) F
(d) T	(d) T	(d) F	(d) T
(e) T	(e) T	(e) F	(e) F
3.2 (a) T	**3.9** (a) F	**3.16** (a) F	**3.23** (a) F
(b) T	(b) T	(b) F	(b) T
(c) T	(c) T	(c) T	(c) T
(d) T	(d) T	(d) T	(d) T
(e) F	(e) F	(e) F	(e) F
3.3 (a) F	**3.10** (a) F	**3.17** (a) T	**3.24** (a) T
(b) T	(b) F	(b) T	(b) T
(c) T	(c) T	(c) T	(c) T
(d) T	(d) T	(d) T	(d) T
(e) T	(e) F	(e) F	(e) T
3.4 (a) T	**3.11** (a) T	**3.18** (a) F	**3.25** (a) T
(b) T	(b) F	(b) F	(b) T
(c) F	(c) T	(c) T	(c) T
(d) T	(d) T	(d) T	(d) T
(e) F	(e) F	(e) F	(e) T
3.5 (a) T	**3.12** (a) F	**3.19** (a) F	**3.26** (a) T
(b) T	(b) T	(b) T	(b) T
(c) T	(c) T	(c) T	(c) T
(d) T	(d) T	(d) T	(d) T
(e) F	(e) T	(e) T	(e) F
3.6 (a) T	**3.13** (a) T	**3.20** (a) F	**3.27** (a) T
(b) F	(b) T	(b) F	(b) T
(c) T	(c) T	(c) F	(c) T
(d) F	(d) T	(d) T	(d) F
(e) F	(e) T	(e) F	(e) T
3.7 (a) F	**3.14** (a) T	**3.21** (a) F	**3.28** (a) F
(b) T	(b) T	(b) T	(b) T
(c) F	(c) T	(c) T	(c) T
(d) T	(d) T	(d) T	(d) T
(e) T	(e) T	(e) F	(e) F

3.29 (a) F	**3.37** (a) F	**3.45** (a) F	**3.53** (a) T
(b) F	(b) T	(b) T	(b) T
(c) T	(c) F	(c) T	(c) T
(d) T	(d) T	(d) F	(d) T
(e) F	(e) T	(e) T	(e) T
3.30 (a) F	**3.38** (a) T	**3.46** (a) T	**3.54** (a) T
(b) F	(b) T	(b) T	(b) F
(c) T	(c) T	(c) T	(c) T
(d) F	(d) T	(d) T	(d) T
(e) F	(e) T	(e) T	(e) F
3.31 (a) T	**3.39** (a) T	**3.47** (a) T	**3.55** (a) F
(b) T	(b) T	(b) F	(b) T
(c) T	(c) T	(c) T	(c) T
(d) T	(d) T	(d) T	(d) T
(e) T	(e) T	(e) T	(e) T
3.32 (a) T	**3.40** (a) T	**3.48** (a) F	**3.56** (a) F
(b) F	(b) F	(b) T	(b) T
(c) T	(c) F	(c) T	(c) F
(d) F	(d) T	(d) T	(d) T
(e) T	(e) T	(e) T	(e) T
3.33 (a) T	**3.41** (a) T	**3.49** (a) T	**3.57** (a) T
(b) T	(b) T	(b) T	(b) T
(c) T	(c) T	(c) T	(c) T
(d) F	(d) T	(d) T	(d) T
(e) T	(e) T	(e) T	(e) T
3.34 (a) T	**3.42** (a) T	**3.50** (a) F	**3.58** (a) T
(b) T	(b) T	(b) F	(b) F
(c) T	(c) T	(c) T	(c) T
(d) F	(d) T	(d) T	(d) F
(e) T	(e) T	(e) T	(e) F
3.35 (a) T	**3.43** (a) T	**3.51** (a) F	**3.59** (a) T
(b) T	(b) T	(b) T	(b) T
(c) T	(c) T	(c) T	(c) F
(d) T	(d) T	(d) T	(d) T
(e) T	(e) T	(e) T	(e) T
3.36 (a) T	**3.44** (a) F	**3.52** (a) T	**3.60** (a) F
(b) F	(b) T	(b) T	(b) F
(c) T	(c) T	(c) T	(c) T
(d) F	(d) T	(d) T	(d) T
(e) T	(e) F	(e) F	(e) T

3.61 (a) T
(b) T
(c) F
(d) T
(e) T

3.62 (a) T
(b) T
(c) T
(d) T
(e) F

3.63 (a) T
(b) T
(c) T
(d) T
(e) T

3.64 (a) T
(b) T
(c) T
(d) T
(e) T

3.65 (a) T
(b) F
(c) T
(d) F
(e) T

3.66 (a) T
(b) T
(c) T
(d) T
(e) T

3.67 (a) F
(b) T
(c) T
(d) T
(e) T

3.68 (a) T
(b) T
(c) T
(d) T
(e) F

3.69 (a) T
(b) F
(c) T
(d) T
(e) T

3.70 (a) F
(b) T
(c) T
(d) F
(e) T

3.71 (a) T
(b) T
(c) T
(d) T
(e) T

3.72 (a) T
(b) T
(c) T
(d) F
(e) F

3.73 (a) T
(b) T
(c) T
(d) T
(e) T

3.74 (a) T
(b) T
(c) T
(d) T
(e) T

3.75 (a) T
(b) T
(c) T
(d) T
(e) T

Gastroenterology
Answers

4.1 (a) F		**4.8** (a) T		**4.15** (a) F		**4.22** (a) T	
(b) T		(b) T		(b) T		(b) T	
(c) T		(c) T		(c) T		(c) T	
(d) T		(d) T		(d) T		(d) T	
(e) F		(e) T		(e) T		(e) T	
4.2 (a) T		**4.9** (a) F		**4.16** (a) F		**4.23** (a) T	
(b) T		(b) T		(b) T		(b) T	
(c) T		(c) T		(c) T		(c) T	
(d) T		(d) T		(d) T		(d) T	
(e) T		(e) T		(e) T		(e) F	
4.3 (a) F		**4.10** (a) F		**4.17** (a) F		**4.24** (a) F	
(b) T		(b) T		(b) F		(b) T	
(c) T		(c) T		(c) T		(c) F	
(d) T		(d) F		(d) T		(d) T	
(e) F		(e) F		(e) T		(e) T	
4.4 (a) F		**4.11** (a) F		**4.18** (a) T		**4.25** (a) T	
(b) T		(b) T		(b) F		(b) F	
(c) F		(c) T		(c) F		(c) F	
(d) T		(d) T		(d) T		(d) T	
(e) T		(e) T		(e) T		(e) T	
4.5 (a) T		**4.12** (a) F		**4.19** (a) F		**4.26** (a) T	
(b) F		(b) F		(b) F		(b) T	
(c) T		(c) F		(c) T		(c) F	
(d) T		(d) T		(d) F		(d) T	
(e) T		(e) T		(e) T		(e) T	
4.6 (a) T		**4.13** (a) T		**4.20** (a) T		**4.27** (a) F	
(b) F		(b) T		(b) T		(b) F	
(c) F		(c) T		(c) T		(c) T	
(d) T		(d) T		(d) T		(d) T	
(e) T		(e) T		(e) F		(e) F	
4.7 (a) T		**4.14** (a) T		**4.21** (a) T		**4.28** (a) F	
(b) F		(b) T		(b) T		(b) F	
(c) F		(c) T		(c) T		(c) T	
(d) T		(d) F		(d) T		(d) T	
(e) T		(e) T		(e) F		(e) T	

4.29 (a) F
(b) F
(c) T
(d) T
(e) T

4.30 (a) T
(b) F
(c) F
(d) T
(e) T

4.31 (a) F
(b) F
(c) T
(d) T
(e) T

4.32 (a) T
(b) T
(c) T
(d) T
(e) F

4.33 (a) F
(b) F
(c) T
(d) T
(e) F

4.34 (a) T
(b) T
(c) F
(d) F
(e) F

4.35 (a) T
(b) T
(c) T
(d) T
(e) F

4.36 (a) T
(b) F
(c) T
(d) T
(e) F

4.37 (a) T
(b) T
(c) T
(d) T
(e) T

4.38 (a) F
(b) F
(c) T
(d) T
(e) T

4.39 (a) T
(b) F
(c) T
(d) T
(e) F

4.40 (a) T
(b) F
(c) T
(d) T
(e) F

4.41 (a) F
(b) F
(c) F
(d) F
(e) F

4.42 (a) T
(b) T
(c) F
(d) T
(e) F

4.43 (a) F
(b) T
(c) F
(d) T
(e) T

4.44 (a) T
(b) F
(c) T
(d) T
(e) F

4.45 (a) T
(b) T
(c) T
(d) T
(e) T

4.46 (a) T
(b) F
(c) T
(d) T
(e) T

4.47 (a) F
(b) F
(c) T
(d) F
(e) F

4.48 (a) T
(b) T
(c) T
(d) T
(e) T

4.49 (a) T
(b) T
(c) T
(d) T
(e) T

4.50 (a) T
(b) T
(c) T
(d) T
(e) T

4.51 (a) F
(b) F
(c) T
(d) T
(e) T

4.52 (a) F
(b) T
(c) T
(d) F
(e) T

4.53 (a) F
(b) T
(c) T
(d) F
(e) T

4.54 (a) F
(b) T
(c) T
(d) F
(e) T

4.55 (a) T
(b) T
(c) T
(d) T
(e) T

4.56 (a) T
(b) T
(c) T
(d) F
(e) T

4.57	(a) T	**4.64**	(a) T	**4.71**	(a) T	**4.78**	(a) T
	(b) T		(b) F		(b) F		(b) T
	(c) T		(c) T		(c) F		(c) T
	(d) F		(d) T		(d) F		(d) T
	(e) T		(e) F		(e) F		(e) T
4.58	(a) T	**4.65**	(a) T	**4.72**	(a) T	**4.79**	(a) F
	(b) F		(b) F		(b) F		(b) F
	(c) T		(c) T		(c) T		(c) T
	(d) T		(d) F		(d) T		(d) F
	(e) T		(e) T		(e) T		(e) T
4.59	(a) T	**4.66**	(a) F	**4.73**	(a) F	**4.80**	(a) T
	(b) T		(b) T		(b) T		(b) F
	(c) T		(c) T		(c) T		(c) T
	(d) F		(d) T		(d) T		(d) T
	(e) T		(e) T		(e) T		(e) F
4.60	(a) F	**4.67**	(a) T	**4.74**	(a) T	**4.81**	(a) T
	(b) T		(b) T		(b) T		(b) T
	(c) T		(c) T		(c) F		(c) T
	(d) T		(d) T		(d) F		(d) T
	(e) T		(e) T		(e) T		(e) T
4.61	(a) T	**4.68**	(a) T	**4.75**	(a) T	**4.82**	(a) F
	(b) T		(b) T		(b) T		(b) F
	(c) T		(c) T		(c) T		(c) F
	(d) T		(d) T		(d) T		(d) T
	(e) T		(e) T		(e) F		(e) F
4.62	(a) T	**4.69**	(a) T	**4.76**	(a) T	**4.83**	(a) T
	(b) T		(b) T		(b) T		(b) T
	(c) F		(c) T		(c) F		(c) T
	(d) F		(d) T		(d) T		(d) T
	(e) F		(e) T		(e) T		(e) T
4.63	(a) F	**4.70**	(a) T	**4.77**	(a) T	**4.84**	(a) T
	(b) F		(b) T		(b) T		(b) T
	(c) F		(c) T		(c) T		(c) T
	(d) F		(d) T		(d) F		(d) T
	(e) T		(e) T		(e) F		(e) F

4.85 (a) T
(b) T
(c) T
(d) T
(e) T

4.86 (a) F
(b) T
(c) T
(d) F
(e) T

4.87 (a) T
(b) T
(c) T
(d) T
(e) T

4.88 (a) T
(b) T
(c) T
(d) T
(e) T

4.89 (a) T
(b) T
(c) T
(d) T
(e) F

4.90 (a) F
(b) F
(c) T
(d) F
(e) T

4.91 (a) F
(b) T
(c) T
(d) T
(e) F

4.92 (a) F
(b) T
(c) F
(d) F
(e) F

4.93 (a) F
(b) F
(c) F
(d) F
(e) F

4.94 (a) F
(b) F
(c) T
(d) F
(e) F

4.95 (a) T
(b) F
(c) F
(d) F
(e) T

4.96 (a) F
(b) T
(c) T
(d) T
(e) F

Liver, Biliary Tract and Pancreatic Diseases
Answers

5.1 (a) F
(b) F
(c) F
(d) T
(e) F

5.2 (a) T
(b) T
(c) T
(d) T
(e) F

5.3 (a) T
(b) T
(c) T
(d) T
(e) T

5.4 (a) T
(b) T
(c) F
(d) T
(e) F

5.5 (a) F
(b) T
(c) F
(d) T
(e) T

5.6 (a) T
(b) T
(c) T
(d) T
(e) T

5.7 (a) F
(b) F
(c) T
(d) T
(e) T

5.8 (a) T
(b) T
(c) T
(d) F
(e) F

5.9 (a) T
(b) T
(c) T
(d) T
(e) F

5.10 (a) T
(b) T
(c) T
(d) T
(e) F

5.11 (a) F
(b) F
(c) T
(d) T
(e) T

5.12 (a) F
(b) T
(c) T
(d) F
(e) T

5.13 (a) T
(b) T
(c) T
(d) T
(e) T

5.14 (a) T
(b) T
(c) T
(d) F
(e) T

5.15 (a) F
(b) T
(c) T
(d) T
(e) T

5.16 (a) T
(b) T
(c) T
(d) T
(e) F

5.17 (a) T
(b) T
(c) T
(d) T
(e) T

5.18 (a) F
(b) T
(c) T
(d) T
(e) T

5.19 (a) F
(b) T
(c) T
(d) T
(e) T

5.20 (a) F
(b) T
(c) T
(d) T
(e) T

5.21 (a) T
(b) T
(c) T
(d) T
(e) F

5.22 (a) T
(b) T
(c) T
(d) T
(e) T

5.23 (a) T
(b) T
(c) T
(d) T
(e) T

5.24 (a) T
(b) T
(c) F
(d) F
(e) T

5.25	(a) F	5.33	(a) F	5.41	(a) F	5.49	(a) T
	(b) T		(b) T		(b) F		(b) T
	(c) T		(c) T		(c) T		(c) T
	(d) F		(d) F		(d) T		(d) F
	(e) F		(e) T		(e) T		(e) F

5.26	(a) T	5.34	(a) T	5.42	(a) F	5.50	(a) T
	(b) T		(b) T		(b) T		(b) T
	(c) T		(c) T		(c) T		(c) T
	(d) T		(d) T		(d) T		(d) T
	(e) T		(e) T		(e) F		(e) T

5.27	(a) F	5.35	(a) T	5.43	(a) T	5.51	(a) T
	(b) T		(b) T		(b) T		(b) T
	(c) F		(c) T		(c) T		(c) T
	(d) T		(d) T		(d) T		(d) T
	(e) F		(e) T		(e) T		(e) T

5.28	(a) F	5.36	(a) T	5.44	(a) T	5.52	(a) T
	(b) T		(b) T		(b) T		(b) T
	(c) T		(c) T		(c) T		(c) T
	(d) T		(d) T		(d) T		(d) F
	(e) F		(e) T		(e) T		(e) F

5.29	(a) T	5.37	(a) T	5.45	(a) T	5.53	(a) T
	(b) T		(b) T		(b) T		(b) F
	(c) T		(c) F		(c) T		(c) T
	(d) T		(d) F		(d) T		(d) F
	(e) T		(e) T		(e) T		(e) F

5.30	(a) F	5.38	(a) F	5.46	(a) T	5.54	(a) T
	(b) F		(b) F		(b) T		(b) F
	(c) T		(c) F		(c) T		(c) F
	(d) T		(d) F		(d) T		(d) F
	(e) T		(e) T		(e) T		(e) F

5.31	(a) T	5.39	(a) F	5.47	(a) T	5.55	(a) T
	(b) T		(b) T		(b) T		(b) F
	(c) T		(c) F		(c) T		(c) T
	(d) T		(d) F		(d) F		(d) T
	(e) T		(e) T		(e) F		(e) T

5.32	(a) T	5.40	(a) T	5.48	(a) T	5.56	(a) T
	(b) T		(b) T		(b) T		(b) T
	(c) T		(c) T		(c) F		(c) T
	(d) T		(d) T		(d) T		(d) F
	(e) T		(e) T		(e) T		(e) F

5.57	(a) T	**5.65**	(a) T	**5.73**	(a) T	**5.81**	(a) T
	(b) F		(b) T		(b) T		(b) T
	(c) F		(c) T		(c) T		(c) T
	(d) F		(d) T		(d) T		(d) T
	(e) T		(e) F		(e) T		(e) T
5.58	(a) T	**5.66**	(a) T	**5.74**	(a) T	**5.82**	(a) T
	(b) T		(b) T		(b) T		(b) T
	(c) T		(c) F		(c) T		(c) T
	(d) T		(d) F		(d) T		(d) T
	(e) T		(e) F		(e) T		(e) T
5.59	(a) T	**5.67**	(a) T	**5.75**	(a) T	**5.83**	(a) T
	(b) T		(b) T		(b) T		(b) T
	(c) T		(c) T		(c) T		(c) F
	(d) T		(d) T		(d) T		(d) T
	(e) F		(e) T		(e) T		(e) F
5.60	(a) F	**5.68**	(a) F	**5.76**	(a) T	**5.84**	(a) F
	(b) T		(b) T		(b) T		(b) T
	(c) T		(c) T		(c) T		(c) T
	(d) T		(d) T		(d) T		(d) T
	(e) F		(e) F		(e) T		(e) T
5.61	(a) F	**5.69**	(a) T	**5.77**	(a) F	**5.85**	(a) T
	(b) T		(b) F		(b) T		(b) T
	(c) T		(c) T		(c) T		(c) T
	(d) T		(d) T		(d) T		(d) T
	(e) F		(e) F		(e) F		(e) T
5.62	(a) F	**5.70**	(a) T	**5.78**	(a) F	**5.86**	(a) T
	(b) T		(b) T		(b) F		(b) T
	(c) T		(c) T		(c) T		(c) T
	(d) T		(d) F		(d) T		(d) T
	(e) F		(e) T		(e) T		(e) F
5.63	(a) F	**5.71**	(a) T	**5.79**	(a) T	**5.87**	(a) F
	(b) T		(b) T		(b) T		(b) T
	(c) T		(c) F		(c) T		(c) T
	(d) T		(d) T		(d) T		(d) T
	(e) F		(e) T		(e) T		(e) F
5.64	(a) F	**5.72**	(a) T	**5.80**	(a) T	**5.88**	(a) F
	(b) T		(b) T		(b) T		(b) T
	(c) T		(c) F		(c) T		(c) T
	(d) F		(d) F		(d) T		(d) F
	(e) F		(e) T		(e) T		(e) T

5.89 (a) T	**5.97** (a) T	**5.105** (a) F	**5.113** (a) T
(b) T	(b) T	(b) T	(b) T
(c) F	(c) T	(c) F	(c) T
(d) F	(d) T	(d) T	(d) T
(e) F	(e) T	(e) T	(e) T
5.90 (a) T	**5.98** (a) T	**5.106** (a) F	**5.114** (a) F
(b) F	(b) T	(b) T	(b) T
(c) T	(c) T	(c) T	(c) T
(d) F	(d) T	(d) T	(d) T
(e) T	(e) T	(e) T	(e) T
5.91 (a) T	**5.99** (a) T	**5.107** (a) F	**5.115** (a) F
(b) T	(b) T	(b) F	(b) F
(c) T	(c) T	(c) T	(c) T
(d) T	(d) T	(d) T	(d) T
(e) T	(e) F	(e) T	(e) F
5.92 (a) T	**5.100** (a) T	**5.108** (a) F	**5.116** (a) T
(b) T	(b) T	(b) T	(b) T
(c) T	(c) T	(c) F	(c) T
(d) T	(d) T	(d) T	(d) T
(e) F	(e) T	(e) F	(e) F
5.93 (a) T	**5.101** (a) T	**5.109** (a) T	**5.117** (a) F
(b) T	(b) T	(b) T	(b) T
(c) T	(c) T	(c) T	(c) T
(d) T	(d) T	(d) T	(d) T
(e) T	(e) T	(e) T	(e) T
5.94 (a) F	**5.102** (a) F	**5.110** (a) T	**5.118** (a) T
(b) T	(b) T	(b) T	(b) T
(c) T	(c) T	(c) F	(c) F
(d) T	(d) T	(d) T	(d) T
(e) F	(e) F	(e) T	(e) T
5.95 (a) T	**5.103** (a) F	**5.111** (a) T	**5.119** (a) T
(b) T	(b) T	(b) T	(b) T
(c) T	(c) T	(c) T	(c) T
(d) T	(d) T	(d) T	(d) T
(e) T	(e) T	(e) T	(e) T
5.96 (a) T	**5.104** (a) F	**5.112** (a) T	**5.120** (a) F
(b) F	(b) F	(b) T	(b) T
(c) T	(c) T	(c) T	(c) T
(d) T	(d) T	(d) T	(d) T
(e) T	(e) T	(e) T	(e) F

5.121 (a) F
(b) T
(c) T
(d) F
(e) F

5.129 (a) T
(b) F
(c) T
(d) T
(e) T

5.137 (a) T
(b) T
(c) T
(d) T
(e) T

5.145 (a) T
(b) T
(c) T
(d) T
(e) T

5.122 (a) T
(b) T
(c) T
(d) T
(e) T

5.130 (a) F
(b) F
(c) F
(d) T
(e) T

5.138 (a) F
(b) T
(c) T
(d) F
(e) F

5.146 (a) F
(b) F
(c) T
(d) T
(e) T

5.123 (a) T
(b) F
(c) T
(d) F
(e) T

5.131 (a) T
(b) T
(c) T
(d) F
(e) T

5.139 (a) T
(b) T
(c) T
(d) T
(e) T

5.147 (a) T
(b) T
(c) T
(d) F
(e) F

5.124 (a) F
(b) T
(c) T
(d) T
(e) T

5.132 (a) F
(b) T
(c) T
(d) T
(e) T

5.140 (a) T
(b) T
(c) T
(d) T
(e) F

5.148 (a) T
(b) T
(c) T
(d) T
(e) T

5.125 (a) T
(b) T
(c) F
(d) T
(e) F

5.133 (a) T
(b) T
(c) T
(d) T
(e) T

5.141 (a) T
(b) T
(c) T
(d) T
(e) T

5.149 (a) T
(b) T
(c) T
(d) T
(e) T

5.126 (a) F
(b) T
(c) T
(d) T
(e) T

5.134 (a) T
(b) T
(c) T
(d) T
(e) T

5.142 (a) T
(b) F
(c) T
(d) T
(e) T

5.150 (a) T
(b) T
(c) T
(d) T
(e) T

5.127 (a) T
(b) T
(c) T
(d) T
(e) T

5.135 (a) T
(b) T
(c) T
(d) T
(e) T

5.143 (a) T
(b) T
(c) T
(d) T
(e) T

5.151 (a) F
(b) T
(c) T
(d) T
(e) T

5.128 (a) T
(b) T
(c) T
(d) T
(e) T

5.136 (a) T
(b) T
(c) T
(d) F
(e) T

5.144 (a) T
(b) T
(c) T
(d) T
(e) T

5.152 (a) F
(b) T
(c) T
(d) T
(e) T

5.153 (a) T
(b) T
(c) T
(d) F
(e) F

5.154 (a) T
(b) T
(c) T
(d) T
(e) T

5.155 (a) T
(b) T
(c) T
(d) F
(e) F

5.156 (a) F
(b) F
(c) F
(d) F
(e) T

5.157 (a) F
(b) F
(c) F
(d) F
(e) T

5.158 (a) T
(b) F
(c) F
(d) T
(e) F

Haematological Disease
Answers

6.1 (a) F	**6.8** (a) F	**6.15** (a) T	**6.22** (a) F
(b) F	(b) T	(b) T	(b) F
(c) T	(c) F	(c) T	(c) T
(d) T	(d) F	(d) T	(d) T
(e) T	(e) F	(e) T	(e) T
6.2 (a) F	**6.9** (a) F	**6.16** (a) F	**6.23** (a) T
(b) T	(b) T	(b) F	(b) T
(c) T	(c) T	(c) T	(c) F
(d) T	(d) T	(d) T	(d) T
(e) F	(e) T	(e) F	(e) T
6.3 (a) F	**6.10** (a) F	**6.17** (a) T	**6.24** (a) T
(b) T	(b) T	(b) T	(b) T
(c) T	(c) F	(c) T	(c) T
(d) F	(d) F	(d) F	(d) T
(e) F	(e) F	(e) T	(e) T
6.4 (a) T	**6.11** (a) F	**6.18** (a) T	**6.25** (a) F
(b) F	(b) F	(b) T	(b) T
(c) F	(c) F	(c) T	(c) T
(d) T	(d) T	(d) F	(d) T
(e) F	(e) T	(e) F	(e) T
6.5 (a) F	**6.12** (a) T	**6.19** (a) F	**6.26** (a) T
(b) F	(b) T	(b) F	(b) F
(c) T	(c) T	(c) F	(c) T
(d) F	(d) T	(d) F	(d) T
(e) T	(e) T	(e) F	(e) T
6.6 (a) T	**6.13** (a) F	**6.20** (a) T	**6.27** (a) T
(b) T	(b) F	(b) T	(b) T
(c) F	(c) F	(c) T	(c) T
(d) T	(d) T	(d) F	(d) F
(e) T	(e) T	(e) F	(e) T
6.7 (a) F	**6.14** (a) F	**6.21** (a) T	**6.28** (a) F
(b) T	(b) F	(b) T	(b) T
(c) T	(c) T	(c) T	(c) T
(d) F	(d) T	(d) T	(d) T
(e) T	(e) T	(e) T	(e) T

6.29 (a) T	**6.37** (a) T	**6.45** (a) T	**6.53** (a) T
(b) T	(b) T	(b) T	(b) T
(c) T	(c) T	(c) T	(c) T
(d) T	(d) T	(d) T	(d) T
(e) T	(e) F	(e) T	(e) T
6.30 (a) F	**6.38** (a) T	**6.46** (a) T	**6.54** (a) T
(b) F	(b) F	(b) T	(b) T
(c) F	(c) T	(c) T	(c) T
(d) T	(d) T	(d) T	(d) T
(e) F	(e) T	(e) T	(e) F
6.31 (a) T	**6.39** (a) F	**6.47** (a) T	**6.55** (a) T
(b) F	(b) T	(b) T	(b) T
(c) T	(c) F	(c) T	(c) T
(d) T	(d) T	(d) T	(d) T
(e) F	(e) T	(e) T	(e) F
6.32 (a) T	**6.40** (a) F	**6.48** (a) T	**6.56** (a) F
(b) F	(b) F	(b) T	(b) F
(c) T	(c) F	(c) F	(c) F
(d) T	(d) T	(d) T	(d) T
(e) T	(e) T	(e) F	(e) F
6.33 (a) T	**6.41** (a) F	**6.49** (a) T	**6.57** (a) T
(b) T	(b) F	(b) T	(b) F
(c) T	(c) T	(c) T	(c) T
(d) T	(d) T	(d) F	(d) F
(e) T	(e) T	(e) T	(e) F
6.34 (a) T	**6.42** (a) F	**6.50** (a) F	**6.58** (a) T
(b) T	(b) F	(b) F	(b) T
(c) T	(c) T	(c) T	(c) T
(d) T	(d) T	(d) F	(d) T
(e) F	(e) F	(e) F	(e) T
6.35 (a) T	**6.43** (a) T	**6.51** (a) T	**6.59** (a) T
(b) T	(b) F	(b) T	(b) T
(c) T	(c) T	(c) T	(c) T
(d) T	(d) F	(d) T	(d) T
(e) T	(e) F	(e) T	(e) T
6.36 (a) T	**6.44** (a) T	**6.52** (a) F	**6.60** (a) T
(b) T	(b) T	(b) F	(b) T
(c) T	(c) T	(c) T	(c) F
(d) F	(d) T	(d) T	(d) F
(e) F	(e) T	(e) T	(e) T

6.61 (a) T
(b) T
(c) T
(d) T
(e) T

6.62 (a) F
(b) F
(c) F
(d) T
(e) T

6.63 (a) T
(b) T
(c) F
(d) T
(e) F

6.64 (a) F
(b) T
(c) F
(d) T
(e) F

6.65 (a) F
(b) F
(c) T
(d) T
(e) T

6.66 (a) F
(b) T
(c) T
(d) T
(e) T

6.67 (a) T
(b) T
(c) T
(d) T
(e) F

6.68 (a) T
(b) F
(c) F
(d) T
(e) T

6.69 (a) T
(b) F
(c) T
(d) T
(e) T

6.70 (a) T
(b) T
(c) T
(d) T
(e) T

6.71 (a) F
(b) F
(c) F
(d) T
(e) T

6.72 (a) F
(b) F
(c) T
(d) T
(e) F

6.73 (a) T
(b) F
(c) T
(d) T
(e) F

6.74 (a) T
(b) T
(c) F
(d) F
(e) T

6.75 (a) T
(b) T
(c) T
(d) T
(e) F

6.76 (a) F
(b) F
(c) T
(d) T
(e) T

6.77 (a) T
(b) F
(c) F
(d) F
(e) T

6.78 (a) F
(b) T
(c) T
(d) F
(e) T

6.79 (a) F
(b) T
(c) T
(d) T
(e) F

6.80 (a) T
(b) T
(c) T
(d) T
(e) F

6.81 (a) T
(b) F
(c) F
(d) T
(e) F

6.82 (a) T
(b) F
(c) T
(d) F
(e) F

6.83 (a) T
(b) F
(c) T
(d) T
(e) T

6.84 (a) T
(b) T
(c) T
(d) T
(e) T

6.85 (a) T
(b) F
(c) T
(d) T
(e) T

6.86 (a) T
(b) T
(c) F
(d) F
(e) F

6.87 (a) T
(b) T
(c) F
(d) F
(e) F

6.88 (a) T
(b) T
(c) T
(d) T
(e) T

6.89 (a) T
(b) T
(c) T
(d) T
(e) T

6.90 (a) T
(b) T
(c) T
(d) F
(e) F

6.91 (a) F
(b) F
(c) T
(d) T
(e) T

6.92 (a) T
(b) T
(c) F
(d) F
(e) T

6.93	(a) T	**6.101**	(a) T	**6.109**	(a) T	**6.117**	(a) T
	(b) T		(b) T		(b) T		(b) F
	(c) T		(c) T		(c) T		(c) T
	(d) T		(d) T		(d) T		(d) T
	(e) T		(e) T		(e) T		(e) T
6.94	(a) T	**6.102**	(a) T	**6.110**	(a) T	**6.118**	(a) T
	(b) T		(b) F		(b) T		(b) T
	(c) T		(c) F		(c) T		(c) T
	(d) T		(d) F		(d) T		(d) T
	(e) T		(e) T		(e) T		(e) F
6.95	(a) T	**6.103**	(a) T	**6.111**	(a) T	**6.119**	(a) F
	(b) F		(b) T		(b) T		(b) T
	(c) T		(c) T		(c) F		(c) F
	(d) T		(d) T		(d) T		(d) F
	(e) T		(e) T		(e) F		(e) T
6.96	(a) F	**6.104**	(a) F	**6.112**	(a) T	**6.120**	(a) F
	(b) F		(b) F		(b) T		(b) T
	(c) F		(c) F		(c) F		(c) T
	(d) T		(d) F		(d) T		(d) T
	(e) T		(e) T		(e) F		(e) F
6.97	(a) F	**6.105**	(a) T	**6.113**	(a) F	**6.121**	(a) T
	(b) T		(b) T		(b) F		(b) F
	(c) T		(c) T		(c) F		(c) T
	(d) F		(d) T		(d) T		(d) F
	(e) T		(e) T		(e) T		(e) T
6.98	(a) T	**6.106**	(a) T	**6.114**	(a) T	**6.122**	(a) T
	(b) T		(b) T		(b) T		(b) F
	(c) T		(c) F		(c) T		(c) T
	(d) T		(d) F		(d) T		(d) F
	(e) F		(e) F		(e) T		(e) T
6.99	(a) T	**6.107**	(a) T	**6.115**	(a) F	**6.123**	(a) T
	(b) T		(b) F		(b) T		(b) T
	(c) T		(c) F		(c) T		(c) F
	(d) T		(d) F		(d) T		(d) F
	(e) T		(e) F		(e) T		(e) T
6.100	(a) T	**6.108**	(a) F	**6.116**	(a) T	**6.124**	(a) T
	(b) T		(b) T		(b) T		(b) T
	(c) T		(c) T		(c) T		(c) F
	(d) T		(d) T		(d) T		(d) F
	(e) T		(e) F		(e) T		(e) F

6.125 (a) T
    (b) T
    (c) T
    (d) F
    (e) T

6.126 (a) F
    (b) T
    (c) T
    (d) T
    (e) T

Medical Oncology
Answers

7.1 (a) T
    (b) T
    (c) T
    (d) T
    (e) T

7.2 (a) F
    (b) F
    (c) T
    (d) T
    (e) T

7.3 (a) F
    (b) F
    (c) T
    (d) T
    (e) T

7.4 (a) T
    (b) T
    (c) T
    (d) T
    (e) T

7.5 (a) T
    (b) F
    (c) T
    (d) T
    (e) F

7.6 (a) T
    (b) T
    (c) T
    (d) T
    (e) T

7.7 (a) F
    (b) T
    (c) T
    (d) T
    (e) F

7.8 (a) T
    (b) T
    (c) T
    (d) T
    (e) F

7.9 (a) T
    (b) T
    (c) T
    (d) T
    (e) T

7.10 (a) T
    (b) T
    (c) T
    (d) T
    (e) T

7.11 (a) T
    (b) T
    (c) T
    (d) T
    (e) T

7.12 (a) F
    (b) T
    (c) T
    (d) T
    (e) T

7.13 (a) T
    (b) T
    (c) T
    (d) T
    (e) T

7.14 (a) T
    (b) T
    (c) T
    (d) T
    (e) T

7.15 (a) T
    (b) T
    (c) T
    (d) T
    (e) F

7.16 (a) F
    (b) F
    (c) F
    (d) F
    (e) F

7.17 (a) F
    (b) T
    (c) T
    (d) T
    (e) T

7.18 (a) T
    (b) T
    (c) T
    (d) F
    (e) T

7.19 (a) T
    (b) T
    (c) T
    (d) F
    (e) T

7.20 (a) T
    (b) T
    (c) T
    (d) T
    (e) T

7.21 (a) F
    (b) T
    (c) T
    (d) T
    (e) F

7.22 (a) T
    (b) T
    (c) F
    (d) T
    (e) T

7.23 (a) T
    (b) T
    (c) T
    (d) T
    (e) F

7.24 (a) F
    (b) F
    (c) T
    (d) F
    (e) F

7.25 (a) T
    (b) T
    (c) T
    (d) T
    (e) T

7.26 (a) F
    (b) T
    (c) T
    (d) T
    (e) F

7.27 (a) F
    (b) T
    (c) F
    (d) F
    (e) T

7.28 (a) F
    (b) T
    (c) T
    (d) T
    (e) T

7.29			7.36			7.43			7.50		
	(a)	F		(a)	T		(a)	F		(a)	F
	(b)	F		(b)	T		(b)	F		(b)	T
	(c)	T		(c)	T		(c)	F		(c)	T
	(d)	T		(d)	T		(d)	T		(d)	T
	(e)	T		(e)	T		(e)	T		(e)	T
7.30	(a)	T	7.37	(a)	T	7.44	(a)	T	7.51	(a)	T
	(b)	T		(b)	T		(b)	T		(b)	T
	(c)	F		(c)	F		(c)	T		(c)	F
	(d)	T		(d)	F		(d)	T		(d)	T
	(e)	T		(e)	T		(e)	T		(e)	T
7.31	(a)	T	7.38	(a)	F	7.45	(a)	F	7.52	(a)	F
	(b)	F		(b)	T		(b)	T		(b)	T
	(c)	F		(c)	T		(c)	T		(c)	F
	(d)	T		(d)	F		(d)	T		(d)	T
	(e)	T		(e)	F		(e)	T		(e)	T
7.32	(a)	T	7.39	(a)	F	7.46	(a)	T	7.53	(a)	T
	(b)	T		(b)	F		(b)	T		(b)	T
	(c)	F		(c)	F		(c)	T		(c)	T
	(d)	T		(d)	T		(d)	T		(d)	T
	(e)	T		(e)	T		(e)	T		(e)	F
7.33	(a)	T	7.40	(a)	F	7.47	(a)	F	7.54	(a)	T
	(b)	T		(b)	F		(b)	F		(b)	T
	(c)	T		(c)	T		(c)	T		(c)	T
	(d)	T		(d)	F		(d)	F		(d)	T
	(e)	T		(e)	T		(e)	F		(e)	F
7.34	(a)	T	7.41	(a)	F	7.48	(a)	T			
	(b)	T		(b)	F		(b)	T			
	(c)	T		(c)	T		(c)	T			
	(d)	T		(d)	T		(d)	T			
	(e)	T		(e)	T		(e)	T			
7.35	(a)	T	7.42	(a)	T	7.49	(a)	T			
	(b)	T		(b)	T		(b)	F			
	(c)	T		(c)	F		(c)	T			
	(d)	T		(d)	T		(d)	T			
	(e)	T		(e)	T		(e)	F			

Rheumatology and Bone Disease
Answers

8.1	(a) F	**8.7**	(a) T	**8.13**	(a) F	**8.19**	(a) F
	(b) F		(b) T		(b) F		(b) T
	(c) F		(c) T		(c) F		(c) T
	(d) T		(d) T		(d) F		(d) T
	(e) T		(e) T		(e) F		(e) T
8.2	(a) T	**8.8**	(a) T	**8.14**	(a) T	**8.20**	(a) F
	(b) T		(b) T		(b) F		(b) F
	(c) T		(c) T		(c) T		(c) T
	(d) T		(d) F		(d) T		(d) T
	(e) T		(e) F		(e) T		(e) T
8.3	(a) T	**8.9**	(a) T	**8.15**	(a) F	**8.21**	(a) T
	(b) T		(b) T		(b) F		(b) T
	(c) T		(c) T		(c) T		(c) T
	(d) F		(d) T		(d) F		(d) T
	(e) T		(e) T		(e) T		(e) T
8.4	(a) T	**8.10**	(a) T	**8.16**	(a) T	**8.22**	(a) F
	(b) T		(b) F		(b) T		(b) T
	(c) T		(c) T		(c) T		(c) T
	(d) F		(d) T		(d) T		(d) T
	(e) F		(e) T		(e) T		(e) T
8.5	(a) F	**8.11**	(a) T	**8.17**	(a) T	**8.23**	(a) F
	(b) T		(b) T		(b) T		(b) F
	(c) F		(c) T		(c) T		(c) F
	(d) F		(d) T		(d) T		(d) T
	(e) T		(e) T		(e) F		(e) F
8.6	(a) F	**8.12**	(a) F	**8.18**	(a) F	**8.24**	(a) F
	(b) T		(b) T		(b) F		(b) T
	(c) T		(c) T		(c) F		(c) T
	(d) T		(d) T		(d) F		(d) T
	(e) F		(e) F		(e) F		(e) F

8.25 (a) F
(b) T
(c) F
(d) T
(e) T

8.26 (a) T
(b) T
(c) F
(d) F
(e) F

8.27 (a) T
(b) T
(c) T
(d) T
(e) T

8.28 (a) T
(b) T
(c) T
(d) T
(e) T

8.29 (a) F
(b) F
(c) T
(d) F
(e) T

8.30 (a) T
(b) T
(c) T
(d) T
(e) F

8.31 (a) T
(b) F
(c) T
(d) F
(e) F

8.32 (a) F
(b) T
(c) T
(d) T
(e) F

8.33 (a) T
(b) T
(c) F
(d) F
(e) T

8.34 (a) F
(b) T
(c) T
(d) T
(e) F

8.35 (a) T
(b) T
(c) T
(d) T
(e) T

8.36 (a) F
(b) T
(c) T
(d) T
(e) T

8.37 (a) T
(b) T
(c) F
(d) F
(e) F

8.38 (a) F
(b) T
(c) T
(d) T
(e) F

8.39 (a) T
(b) T
(c) T
(d) F
(e) F

8.40 (a) T
(b) T
(c) T
(d) T
(e) T

8.41 (a) T
(b) T
(c) T
(d) T
(e) T

8.42 (a) F
(b) F
(c) F
(d) F
(e) F

8.43 (a) F
(b) F
(c) F
(d) T
(e) T

8.44 (a) T
(b) F
(c) T
(d) F
(e) T

8.45 (a) F
(b) T
(c) T
(d) T
(e) F

8.46 (a) T
(b) T
(c) T
(d) T
(e) T

8.47 (a) T
(b) T
(c) T
(d) T
(e) T

8.48 (a) T
(b) T
(c) T
(d) T
(e) F

8.49 (a) F
(b) T
(c) T
(d) T
(e) F

8.50 (a) F
(b) T
(c) T
(d) T
(e) T

8.51 (a) F
(b) T
(c) T
(d) T
(e) T

8.52 (a) T
(b) T
(c) F
(d) F
(e) T

8.53 (a) T
(b) T
(c) T
(d) T
(e) T

8.54 (a) T
(b) T
(c) T
(d) F
(e) F

8.55 (a) T
(b) T
(c) T
(d) F
(e) F

8.56 (a) F
(b) F
(c) F
(d) F
(e) F

8.57	(a) T	8.65	(a) F	8.73	(a) T	8.81	(a) T
	(b) T		(b) T		(b) T		(b) T
	(c) T		(c) T		(c) T		(c) F
	(d) F		(d) T		(d) F		(d) T
	(e) F		(e) T		(e) F		(e) F
8.58	(a) F	8.66	(a) T	8.74	(a) F	8.82	(a) T
	(b) F		(b) T		(b) T		(b) T
	(c) T		(c) T		(c) T		(c) F
	(d) T		(d) T		(d) T		(d) F
	(e) T		(e) T		(e) F		(e) T
8.59	(a) T	8.67	(a) T	8.75	(a) T	8.83	(a) T
	(b) F		(b) T		(b) T		(b) T
	(c) T		(c) T		(c) F		(c) T
	(d) T		(d) T		(d) F		(d) T
	(e) T		(e) F		(e) F		(e) T
8.60	(a) T	8.68	(a) T	8.76	(a) T	8.84	(a) T
	(b) T		(b) F		(b) F		(b) T
	(c) T		(c) T		(c) T		(c) T
	(d) T		(d) T		(d) F		(d) T
	(e) T		(e) T		(e) T		(e) T
8.61	(a) T	8.69	(a) F	8.77	(a) F	8.85	(a) T
	(b) T		(b) T		(b) T		(b) T
	(c) T		(c) F		(c) F		(c) T
	(d) T		(d) F		(d) T		(d) F
	(e) T		(e) T		(e) T		(e) F
8.62	(a) F	8.70	(a) T	8.78	(a) T	8.86	(a) T
	(b) T		(b) T		(b) T		(b) T
	(c) F		(c) T		(c) F		(c) T
	(d) F		(d) T		(d) F		(d) T
	(e) T		(e) T		(e) F		(e) T
8.63	(a) F	8.71	(a) F	8.79	(a) T	8.87	(a) F
	(b) T		(b) T		(b) F		(b) F
	(c) T		(c) F		(c) T		(c) T
	(d) T		(d) F		(d) T		(d) T
	(e) T		(e) T		(e) F		(e) T
8.64	(a) T	8.72	(a) T	8.80	(a) T	8.88	(a) T
	(b) T		(b) T		(b) T		(b) F
	(c) T		(c) T		(c) F		(c) F
	(d) F		(d) T		(d) T		(d) F
	(e) T		(e) T		(e) T		(e) T

8.89 (a) F
(b) T
(c) T
(d) T
(e) F

8.90 (a) T
(b) T
(c) T
(d) T
(e) T

8.91 (a) F
(b) T
(c) T
(d) T
(e) F

8.92 (a) T
(b) T
(c) T
(d) F
(e) F

8.93 (a) T
(b) T
(c) T
(d) T
(e) F

8.94 (a) T
(b) T
(c) T
(d) T
(e) T

8.95 (a) T
(b) T
(c) T
(d) T
(e) F

8.96 (a) T
(b) T
(c) F
(d) T
(e) T

8.97 (a) T
(b) T
(c) T
(d) F
(e) T

8.98 (a) F
(b) T
(c) T
(d) T
(e) F

8.99 (a) T
(b) T
(c) T
(d) T
(e) F

8.100 (a) T
(b) T
(c) T
(d) T
(e) T

8.101 (a) T
(b) T
(c) T
(d) T
(e) F

8.102 (a) F
(b) T
(c) F
(d) T
(e) T

8.103 (a) F
(b) T
(c) F
(d) T
(e) T

8.104 (a) F
(b) T
(c) T
(d) T
(e) F

8.105 (a) F
(b) T
(c) F
(d) F
(e) T

8.106 (a) F
(b) T
(c) T
(d) F
(e) F

8.107 (a) T
(b) T
(c) T
(d) T
(e) T

8.108 (a) F
(b) F
(c) T
(d) T
(e) F

8.109 (a) F
(b) T
(c) T
(d) T
(e) F

8.110 (a) T
(b) T
(c) T
(d) F
(e) F

8.111 (a) F
(b) T
(c) F
(d) T
(e) F

8.112 (a) F
(b) F
(c) F
(d) F
(e) T

8.113 (a) T
(b) T
(c) T
(d) F
(e) F

Renal Disease
Answers

9.1 (a) F
(b) T
(c) T
(d) F
(e) T

9.2 (a) T
(b) T
(c) T
(d) T
(e) T

9.3 (a) F
(b) F
(c) F
(d) F
(e) F

9.4 (a) T
(b) F
(c) T
(d) T
(e) F

9.5 (a) F
(b) F
(c) T
(d) T
(e) T

9.6 (a) T
(b) F
(c) F
(d) F
(e) F

9.7 (a) T
(b) T
(c) T
(d) T
(e) F

9.8 (a) T
(b) T
(c) T
(d) T
(e) T

9.9 (a) F
(b) F
(c) T
(d) T
(e) T

9.10 (a) F
(b) T
(c) T
(d) T
(e) F

9.11 (a) F
(b) F
(c) F
(d) T
(e) T

9.12 (a) T
(b) T
(c) T
(d) T
(e) F

9.13 (a) T
(b) F
(c) T
(d) T
(e) T

9.14 (a) T
(b) T
(c) T
(d) T
(e) T

9.15 (a) T
(b) T
(c) T
(d) T
(e) T

9.16 (a) F
(b) T
(c) T
(d) F
(e) F

9.17 (a) T
(b) T
(c) T
(d) T
(e) T

9.18 (a) F
(b) F
(c) T
(d) T
(e) T

9.19 (a) F
(b) F
(c) T
(d) T
(e) F

9.20 (a) T
(b) T
(c) F
(d) F
(e) F

9.21 (a) F
(b) T
(c) T
(d) T
(e) T

9.22 (a) F
(b) T
(c) T
(d) F
(e) F

9.23 (a) T
(b) T
(c) T
(d) T
(e) T

9.24 (a) F
(b) F
(c) F
(d) T
(e) F

9.25 (a) T
(b) F
(c) F
(d) T
(e) T

9.26 (a) T
(b) T
(c) T
(d) T
(e) T

9.27 (a) T
(b) T
(c) T
(d) F
(e) F

9.28 (a) T
(b) T
(c) F
(d) F
(e) T

9.29 (a) T
(b) T
(c) T
(d) T
(e) T

9.30 (a) T
(b) F
(c) T
(d) F
(e) T

9.31 (a) F
(b) T
(c) F
(d) T
(e) T

9.32 (a) T
(b) F
(c) F
(d) F
(e) T

9.33 (a) T
(b) T
(c) T
(d) T
(e) T

9.34 (a) F
(b) F
(c) T
(d) T
(e) T

9.35 (a) T
(b) F
(c) T
(d) F
(e) T

9.36 (a) T
(b) T
(c) F
(d) T
(e) F

9.37 (a) F
(b) T
(c) T
(d) T
(e) T

9.38 (a) T
(b) T
(c) T
(d) T
(e) T

9.39 (a) T
(b) T
(c) T
(d) F
(e) F

9.40 (a) T
(b) T
(c) T
(d) T
(e) T

9.41 (a) F
(b) F
(c) T
(d) F
(e) T

9.42 (a) F
(b) F
(c) F
(d) F
(e) F

9.43 (a) F
(b) T
(c) T
(d) T
(e) T

9.44 (a) F
(b) F
(c) F
(d) F
(e) T

9.45 (a) T
(b) T
(c) T
(d) T
(e) T

9.46 (a) T
(b) F
(c) T
(d) F
(e) F

9.47 (a) F
(b) T
(c) T
(d) T
(e) F

9.48 (a) F
(b) T
(c) T
(d) T
(e) T

9.49 (a) T
(b) T
(c) T
(d) T
(e) T

9.50 (a) F
(b) T
(c) F
(d) T
(e) F

9.51 (a) T
(b) T
(c) F
(d) T
(e) T

9.52 (a) T
(b) F
(c) T
(d) F
(e) T

9.53 (a) T
(b) T
(c) T
(d) T
(e) T

9.54 (a) T
(b) T
(c) F
(d) T
(e) F

9.55 (a) T
(b) T
(c) T
(d) F
(e) F

9.56 (a) T
(b) T
(c) F
(d) T
(e) T

9.57 (a) T
(b) T
(c) F
(d) T
(e) F

9.58 (a) T
(b) F
(c) T
(d) T
(e) T

9.59 (a) F
(b) T
(c) T
(d) F
(e) F

9.60 (a) T
(b) T
(c) T
(d) T
(e) T

9.61 (a) T
    (b) T
    (c) T
    (d) T
    (e) T

9.62 (a) T
    (b) T
    (c) T
    (d) T
    (e) T

9.63 (a) T
    (b) T
    (c) T
    (d) T
    (e) F

9.64 (a) F
    (b) T
    (c) T
    (d) T
    (e) T

9.65 (a) F
    (b) T
    (c) T
    (d) F
    (e) T

9.66 (a) F
    (b) T
    (c) T
    (d) T
    (e) F

9.67 (a) F
    (b) T
    (c) T
    (d) F
    (e) T

9.68 (a) F
    (b) T
    (c) T
    (d) F
    (e) T

Water, Electrolytes and Acid-Base Homeostasis
Answers

10.1 (a) T		**10.7** (a) T		**10.13** (a) F		**10.19** (a) F	
(b) F		(b) F		(b) F		(b) T	
(c) F		(c) F		(c) F		(c) T	
(d) T		(d) T		(d) F		(d) F	
(e) T		(e) T		(e) F		(e) F	
10.2 (a) T		**10.8** (a) T		**10.14** (a) T		**10.20** (a) F	
(b) F		(b) T		(b) T		(b) T	
(c) T		(c) F		(c) T		(c) T	
(d) F		(d) T		(d) T		(d) T	
(e) F		(e) F		(e) T		(e) T	
10.3 (a) T		**10.9** (a) F		**10.15** (a) F		**10.21** (a) F	
(b) F		(b) F		(b) F		(b) T	
(c) T		(c) F		(c) T		(c) T	
(d) F		(d) F		(d) F		(d) T	
(e) T		(e) F		(e) T		(e) T	
10.4 (a) T		**10.10** (a) F		**10.16** (a) F		**10.22** (a) T	
(b) T		(b) T		(b) F		(b) T	
(c) T		(c) T		(c) F		(c) T	
(d) T		(d) T		(d) T		(d) T	
(e) T		(e) F		(e) T		(e) F	
10.5 (a) T		**10.11** (a) F		**10.17** (a) T		**10.23** (a) T	
(b) T		(b) T		(b) T		(b) T	
(c) T		(c) T		(c) T		(c) T	
(d) T		(d) T		(d) F		(d) T	
(e) F		(e) T		(e) T		(e) T	
10.6 (a) F		**10.12** (a) T		**10.18** (a) T		**10.24** (a) T	
(b) F		(b) T		(b) T		(b) F	
(c) F		(c) T		(c) T		(c) F	
(d) T		(d) F		(d) F		(d) T	
(e) T		(e) F		(e) T		(e) T	

10.25 (a) T
(b) T
(c) F
(d) F
(e) T

10.26 (a) T
(b) T
(c) T
(d) T
(e) F

10.27 (a) F
(b) T
(c) T
(d) T
(e) T

10.28 (a) T
(b) T
(c) T
(d) T
(e) T

10.29 (a) T
(b) F
(c) T
(d) F
(e) F

10.30 (a) T
(b) T
(c) T
(d) T
(e) T

10.31 (a) F
(b) T
(c) F
(d) T
(e) T

10.32 (a) F
(b) T
(c) F
(d) F
(e) T

10.33 (a) T
(b) T
(c) F
(d) T
(e) T

10.34 (a) T
(b) T
(c) T
(d) T
(e) T

10.35 (a) T
(b) T
(c) T
(d) F
(e) T

10.36 (a) T
(b) T
(c) T
(d) T
(e) F

10.37 (a) T
(b) F
(c) T
(d) T
(e) F

10.38 (a) T
(b) F
(c) T
(d) T
(e) T

10.39 (a) T
(b) T
(c) F
(d) T
(e) T

10.40 (a) T
(b) T
(c) F
(d) T
(e) F

10.41 (a) T
(b) F
(c) T
(d) T
(e) T

10.42 (a) T
(b) T
(c) T
(d) T
(e) T

10.43 (a) T
(b) F
(c) T
(d) F
(e) F

10.44 (a) F
(b) F
(c) T
(d) F
(e) F

10.45 (a) T
(b) T
(c) T
(d) T
(e) T

10.46 (a) T
(b) T
(c) T
(d) T
(e) T

10.47 (a) F
(b) F
(c) F
(d) F
(e) F

10.48 (a) T
(b) F
(c) T
(d) T
(e) T

10.49 (a) T
(b) F
(c) F
(d) T
(e) F

Cardiovascular Disease
Answers

11.1 (a) T
(b) F
(c) F
(d) F
(e) T

11.2 (a) F
(b) F
(c) T
(d) F
(e) F

11.3 (a) F
(b) F
(c) F
(d) T
(e) F

11.4 (a) T
(b) T
(c) F
(d) F
(e) T

11.5 (a) T
(b) T
(c) F
(d) F
(e) T

11.6 (a) F
(b) T
(c) T
(d) T
(e) F

11.7 (a) F
(b) T
(c) F
(d) T
(e) T

11.8 (a) T
(b) F
(c) T
(d) F
(e) F

11.9 (a) F
(b) T
(c) T
(d) F
(e) F

11.10 (a) T
(b) F
(c) F
(d) T
(e) F

11.11 (a) T
(b) T
(c) T
(d) F
(e) T

11.12 (a) T
(b) T
(c) T
(d) T
(e) T

11.13 (a) T
(b) T
(c) T
(d) T
(e) F

11.14 (a) T
(b) T
(c) T
(d) T
(e) T

11.15 (a) T
(b) T
(c) T
(d) T
(e) T

11.16 (a) T
(b) T
(c) T
(d) T
(e) F

11.17 (a) T
(b) T
(c) T
(d) T
(e) T

11.18 (a) T
(b) T
(c) T
(d) T
(e) F

11.19 (a) F
(b) T
(c) F
(d) T
(e) F

11.20 (a) T
(b) T
(c) T
(d) T
(e) T

11.21 (a) T
(b) T
(c) F
(d) F
(e) T

11.22 (a) F
(b) F
(c) T
(d) T
(e) F

11.23 (a) T
(b) T
(c) T
(d) F
(e) T

11.24 (a) T
(b) F
(c) F
(d) T
(e) F

11.25 (a) F
(b) T
(c) T
(d) T
(e) T

11.26 (a) T
(b) T
(c) F
(d) T
(e) T

11.27 (a) F
(b) T
(c) T
(d) T
(e) T

11.28 (a) T
(b) T
(c) T
(d) F
(e) F

11.29 (a) F	**11.36** (a) F	**11.43** (a) T	**11.50** (a) F
(b) T	(b) T	(b) T	(b) F
(c) T	(c) T	(c) T	(c) T
(d) T	(d) T	(d) T	(d) T
(e) F	(e) T	(e) F	(e) T
11.30 (a) T	**11.37** (a) F	**11.44** (a) F	**11.51** (a) T
(b) T	(b) T	(b) T	(b) F
(c) T	(c) T	(c) T	(c) F
(d) T	(d) T	(d) T	(d) F
(e) T	(e) T	(e) T	(e) T
11.31 (a) T	**11.38** (a) F	**11.45** (a) T	**11.52** (a) T
(b) T	(b) T	(b) T	(b) T
(c) F	(c) T	(c) T	(c) F
(d) F	(d) F	(d) T	(d) T
(e) F	(e) F	(e) T	(e) F
11.32 (a) F	**11.39** (a) T	**11.46** (a) T	**11.53** (a) F
(b) F	(b) F	(b) T	(b) T
(c) T	(c) T	(c) T	(c) T
(d) F	(d) T	(d) T	(d) T
(e) F	(e) T	(e) F	(e) T
11.33 (a) T	**11.40** (a) F	**11.47** (a) T	**11.54** (a) T
(b) T	(b) F	(b) F	(b) T
(c) T	(c) T	(c) F	(c) F
(d) T	(d) T	(d) F	(d) T
(e) T	(e) F	(e) T	(e) F
11.34 (a) F	**11.41** (a) T	**11.48** (a) F	**11.55** (a) T
(b) T	(b) F	(b) T	(b) T
(c) F	(c) T	(c) T	(c) T
(d) T	(d) T	(d) T	(d) F
(e) T	(e) F	(e) F	(e) T
11.35 (a) F	**11.42** (a) T	**11.49** (a) F	**11.56** (a) T
(b) F	(b) T	(b) F	(b) T
(c) F	(c) T	(c) T	(c) F
(d) T	(d) T	(d) T	(d) T
(e) T	(e) T	(e) T	(e) T

11.57	(a)	T		**11.64**	(a)	F		**11.71**	(a)	F		**11.78**	(a)	T
	(b)	T			(b)	T			(b)	F			(b)	T
	(c)	T			(c)	T			(c)	F			(c)	T
	(d)	T			(d)	F			(d)	T			(d)	F
	(e)	T			(e)	F			(e)	F			(e)	T
11.58	(a)	T		**11.65**	(a)	T		**11.72**	(a)	F		**11.79**	(a)	F
	(b)	T			(b)	T			(b)	F			(b)	T
	(c)	F			(c)	T			(c)	T			(c)	F
	(d)	T			(d)	T			(d)	T			(d)	T
	(e)	T			(e)	T			(e)	T			(e)	T
11.59	(a)	T		**11.66**	(a)	T		**11.73**	(a)	F		**11.80**	(a)	T
	(b)	T			(b)	T			(b)	T			(b)	T
	(c)	T			(c)	T			(c)	F			(c)	T
	(d)	F			(d)	F			(d)	T			(d)	T
	(e)	F			(e)	T			(e)	T			(e)	F
11.60	(a)	F		**11.67**	(a)	T		**11.74**	(a)	F		**11.81**	(a)	T
	(b)	F			(b)	T			(b)	T			(b)	T
	(c)	T			(c)	T			(c)	T			(c)	T
	(d)	T			(d)	T			(d)	T			(d)	T
	(e)	T			(e)	T			(e)	T			(e)	F
11.61	(a)	T		**11.68**	(a)	T		**11.75**	(a)	T		**11.82**	(a)	F
	(b)	T			(b)	T			(b)	F			(b)	T
	(c)	F			(c)	T			(c)	F			(c)	T
	(d)	T			(d)	T			(d)	T			(d)	T
	(e)	F			(e)	F			(e)	T			(e)	T
11.62	(a)	F		**11.69**	(a)	T		**11.76**	(a)	T		**11.83**	(a)	F
	(b)	F			(b)	F			(b)	F			(b)	T
	(c)	T			(c)	T			(c)	F			(c)	T
	(d)	T			(d)	T			(d)	F			(d)	F
	(e)	T			(e)	T			(e)	F			(e)	F
11.63	(a)	F		**11.70**	(a)	T		**11.77**	(a)	F		**11.84**	(a)	T
	(b)	F			(b)	T			(b)	T			(b)	T
	(c)	T			(c)	T			(c)	F			(c)	T
	(d)	F			(d)	F			(d)	T			(d)	F
	(e)	T			(e)	T			(e)	T			(e)	T

11.85 (a) T
(b) F
(c) T
(d) T
(e) F

11.86 (a) F
(b) T
(c) T
(d) F
(e) F

11.87 (a) T
(b) T
(c) T
(d) T
(e) T

11.88 (a) F
(b) F
(c) F
(d) T
(e) T

11.89 (a) F
(b) T
(c) F
(d) T
(e) T

11.90 (a) T
(b) F
(c) T
(d) T
(e) T

11.91 (a) T
(b) T
(c) F
(d) F
(e) T

11.92 (a) F
(b) F
(c) T
(d) F
(e) F

11.93 (a) T
(b) T
(c) T
(d) T
(e) T

11.94 (a) F
(b) T
(c) T
(d) F
(e) T

11.95 (a) T
(b) T
(c) T
(d) T
(e) T

11.96 (a) F
(b) F
(c) F
(d) F
(e) T

11.97 (a) F
(b) F
(c) F
(d) F
(e) T

11.98 (a) T
(b) F
(c) T
(d) T
(e) F

11.99 (a) T
(b) T
(c) T
(d) T
(e) T

11.100 (a) F
(b) T
(c) T
(d) T
(e) F

11.101 (a) F
(b) T
(c) F
(d) T
(e) T

11.102 (a) T
(b) T
(c) T
(d) T
(e) T

11.103 (a) F
(b) T
(c) T
(d) F
(e) F

11.104 (a) F
(b) T
(c) T
(d) F
(e) T

11.105 (a) T
(b) T
(c) F
(d) F
(e) F

11.106 (a) F
(b) T
(c) T
(d) F
(e) T

11.107 (a) T
(b) T
(c) T
(d) T
(e) T

11.108 (a) T
(b) T
(c) F
(d) T
(e) T

11.109 (a) T
(b) T
(c) F
(d) T
(e) T

11.110 (a) F
(b) F
(c) F
(d) F
(e) T

11.111 (a) F
(b) T
(c) T
(d) F
(e) F

11.112 (a) T
(b) T
(c) T
(d) T
(e) T

11.113	(a) F	11.120	(a) T	11.127	(a) T	11.134	(a) T
	(b) T		(b) T		(b) T		(b) T
	(c) T		(c) T		(c) T		(c) T
	(d) T		(d) T		(d) T		(d) T
	(e) F		(e) T		(e) T		(e) T
11.114	(a) T	11.121	(a) T	11.128	(a) F	11.135	(a) F
	(b) T		(b) T		(b) T		(b) T
	(c) F		(c) F		(c) F		(c) T
	(d) T		(d) T		(d) T		(d) T
	(e) T		(e) F		(e) T		(e) F
11.115	(a) T	11.122	(a) T	11.129	(a) T	11.136	(a) T
	(b) T		(b) T		(b) F		(b) T
	(c) T		(c) T		(c) T		(c) T
	(d) F		(d) T		(d) T		(d) T
	(e) F		(e) T		(e) T		(e) T
11.116	(a) T	11.123	(a) T	11.130	(a) T	11.137	(a) F
	(b) F		(b) T		(b) T		(b) T
	(c) F		(c) F		(c) F		(c) T
	(d) T		(d) T		(d) F		(d) T
	(e) T		(e) T		(e) T		(e) T
11.117	(a) T	11.124	(a) F	11.131	(a) T	11.138	(a) T
	(b) T		(b) F		(b) T		(b) T
	(c) T		(c) T		(c) F		(c) T
	(d) F		(d) T		(d) T		(d) T
	(e) F		(e) T		(e) F		(e) T
11.118	(a) T	11.125	(a) F	11.132	(a) F	11.139	(a) T
	(b) F		(b) T		(b) T		(b) T
	(c) F		(c) T		(c) T		(c) T
	(d) T		(d) T		(d) T		(d) T
	(e) T		(e) F		(e) T		(e) T
11.119	(a) F	11.126	(a) T	11.133	(a) F	11.140	(a) T
	(b) T		(b) T		(b) T		(b) T
	(c) T		(c) F		(c) F		(c) T
	(d) F		(d) T		(d) F		(d) T
	(e) F		(e) F		(e) T		(e) T

11.141	(a)	F	**11.148**	(a)	T	**11.155**	(a)	T	**11.162**	(a)	T

11.141 (a) F
(b) T
(c) T
(d) T
(e) T

11.142 (a) T
(b) T
(c) T
(d) T
(e) T

11.143 (a) T
(b) F
(c) T
(d) F
(e) F

11.144 (a) F
(b) T
(c) F
(d) F
(e) T

11.145 (a) F
(b) F
(c) T
(d) T
(e) F

11.146 (a) F
(b) T
(c) T
(d) T
(e) T

11.147 (a) F
(b) T
(c) T
(d) T
(e) T

11.148 (a) T
(b) F
(c) F
(d) T
(e) T

11.149 (a) T
(b) F
(c) T
(d) F
(e) T

11.150 (a) T
(b) T
(c) T
(d) T
(e) T

11.151 (a) T
(b) F
(c) T
(d) T
(e) T

11.152 (a) T
(b) T
(c) F
(d) T
(e) T

11.153 (a) T
(b) T
(c) T
(d) F
(e) T

11.154 (a) T
(b) T
(c) T
(d) T
(e) T

11.155 (a) T
(b) T
(c) T
(d) T
(e) T

11.156 (a) T
(b) T
(c) T
(d) T
(e) T

11.157 (a) T
(b) T
(c) T
(d) T
(e) T

11.158 (a) T
(b) T
(c) T
(d) T
(e) T

11.159 (a) F
(b) F
(c) T
(d) T
(e) T

11.160 (a) T
(b) F
(c) F
(d) T
(e) F

11.161 (a) T
(b) T
(c) F
(d) T
(e) F

11.162 (a) T
(b) T
(c) T
(d) T
(e) T

11.163 (a) T
(b) T
(c) T
(d) T
(e) T

11.164 (a) F
(b) T
(c) F
(d) T
(e) T

11.165 (a) T
(b) T
(c) T
(d) F
(e) F

11.166 (a) T
(b) T
(c) T
(d) T
(e) T

11.167 (a) T
(b) F
(c) F
(d) T
(e) T

11.168 (a) T
(b) F
(c) T
(d) T
(e) T

11.169	(a)	F	**11.171**	(a)	T	**11.173**	(a)	T
	(b)	T		(b)	F		(b)	T
	(c)	F		(c)	F		(c)	T
	(d)	F		(d)	T		(d)	F
	(e)	F		(e)	F		(e)	T

11.170	(a)	T	**11.172**	(a)	T
	(b)	F		(b)	T
	(c)	T		(c)	T
	(d)	F		(d)	T
	(e)	T		(e)	F

Respiratory Disease
Answers

12.1	(a)	F	12.8	(a)	T	12.15	(a)	T	12.22	(a)	F
	(b)	T		(b)	F		(b)	T		(b)	F
	(c)	T		(c)	T		(c)	T		(c)	F
	(d)	T		(d)	F		(d)	F		(d)	F
	(e)	F		(e)	T		(e)	T		(e)	F

12.2	(a)	T	12.9	(a)	T	12.16	(a)	T	12.23	(a)	F
	(b)	T		(b)	T		(b)	T		(b)	T
	(c)	T		(c)	T		(c)	F		(c)	T
	(d)	T		(d)	T		(d)	T		(d)	T
	(e)	F		(e)	T		(e)	T		(e)	F

12.3	(a)	T	12.10	(a)	T	12.17	(a)	F	12.24	(a)	F
	(b)	T		(b)	T		(b)	T		(b)	T
	(c)	T		(c)	T		(c)	T		(c)	T
	(d)	T		(d)	T		(d)	T		(d)	T
	(e)	T		(e)	T		(e)	T		(e)	T

12.4	(a)	F	12.11	(a)	T	12.18	(a)	F	12.25	(a)	T
	(b)	T		(b)	T		(b)	T		(b)	T
	(c)	T		(c)	T		(c)	T		(c)	T
	(d)	F		(d)	T		(d)	F		(d)	F
	(e)	F		(e)	F		(e)	T		(e)	F

12.5	(a)	T	12.12	(a)	F	12.19	(a)	T	12.26	(a)	T
	(b)	F		(b)	T		(b)	F		(b)	T
	(c)	T		(c)	T		(c)	T		(c)	T
	(d)	F		(d)	F		(d)	T		(d)	T
	(e)	T		(e)	T		(e)	F		(e)	T

12.6	(a)	T	12.13	(a)	T	12.20	(a)	T	12.27	(a)	T
	(b)	T		(b)	F		(b)	F		(b)	T
	(c)	F		(c)	F		(c)	T		(c)	T
	(d)	T		(d)	T		(d)	F		(d)	T
	(e)	T		(e)	F		(e)	T		(e)	T

12.7	(a)	T	12.14	(a)	F	12.21	(a)	T	12.28	(a)	F
	(b)	T		(b)	T		(b)	F		(b)	F
	(c)	T		(c)	T		(c)	F		(c)	T
	(d)	T		(d)	T		(d)	T		(d)	T
	(e)	F		(e)	F		(e)	F		(e)	T

12.29	(a)	T	**12.37**	(a)	T	**12.45**	(a)	F	**12.53**	(a)	T
	(b)	T		(b)	T		(b)	F		(b)	T
	(c)	T		(c)	T		(c)	T		(c)	T
	(d)	T		(d)	T		(d)	T		(d)	T
	(e)	T		(e)	F		(e)	T		(e)	T
12.30	(a)	F	**12.38**	(a)	F	**12.46**	(a)	T	**12.54**	(a)	T
	(b)	T		(b)	T		(b)	T		(b)	T
	(c)	F		(c)	T		(c)	F		(c)	T
	(d)	T		(d)	F		(d)	F		(d)	T
	(e)	T		(e)	F		(e)	T		(e)	T
12.31	(a)	F	**12.39**	(a)	T	**12.47**	(a)	T	**12.55**	(a)	F
	(b)	T		(b)	T		(b)	T		(b)	F
	(c)	T		(c)	F		(c)	T		(c)	T
	(d)	F		(d)	T		(d)	T		(d)	T
	(e)	T		(e)	T		(e)	T		(e)	T
12.32	(a)	F	**12.40**	(a)	T	**12.48**	(a)	T	**12.56**	(a)	T
	(b)	F		(b)	T		(b)	T		(b)	T
	(c)	F		(c)	F		(c)	T		(c)	T
	(d)	T		(d)	F		(d)	T		(d)	T
	(e)	F		(e)	T		(e)	T		(e)	T
12.33	(a)	T	**12.41**	(a)	F	**12.49**	(a)	T	**12.57**	(a)	T
	(b)	T		(b)	F		(b)	T		(b)	T
	(c)	F		(c)	T		(c)	T		(c)	T
	(d)	F		(d)	F		(d)	T		(d)	F
	(e)	F		(e)	F		(e)	F		(e)	F
12.34	(a)	T	**12.42**	(a)	F	**12.50**	(a)	F	**12.58**	(a)	T
	(b)	T		(b)	T		(b)	T		(b)	T
	(c)	T		(c)	F		(c)	F		(c)	T
	(d)	T		(d)	F		(d)	F		(d)	T
	(e)	T		(e)	F		(e)	T		(e)	T
12.35	(a)	T	**12.43**	(a)	F	**12.51**	(a)	F	**12.59**	(a)	F
	(b)	T		(b)	T		(b)	T		(b)	T
	(c)	T		(c)	F		(c)	T		(c)	T
	(d)	F		(d)	T		(d)	T		(d)	T
	(e)	T		(e)	F		(e)	T		(e)	F
12.36	(a)	T	**12.44**	(a)	F	**12.52**	(a)	T	**12.60**	(a)	T
	(b)	T		(b)	T		(b)	T		(b)	T
	(c)	T		(c)	T		(c)	F		(c)	T
	(d)	F		(d)	T		(d)	T		(d)	T
	(e)	T		(e)	T		(e)	F		(e)	T

12.61	(a)	T	**12.69**	(a)	T	**12.77**	(a)	T	**12.85**	(a)	T
	(b)	T		(b)	T		(b)	F		(b)	T
	(c)	T		(c)	F		(c)	F		(c)	T
	(d)	F		(d)	F		(d)	T		(d)	T
	(e)	T		(e)	T		(e)	T		(e)	F

12.62	(a)	T	**12.70**	(a)	T	**12.78**	(a)	T	**12.86**	(a)	T
	(b)	T		(b)	T		(b)	T		(b)	T
	(c)	T		(c)	T		(c)	T		(c)	T
	(d)	T		(d)	T		(d)	T		(d)	T
	(e)	T		(e)	F		(e)	F		(e)	T

12.63	(a)	F	**12.71**	(a)	T	**12.79**	(a)	F	**12.87**	(a)	F
	(b)	T		(b)	F		(b)	T		(b)	F
	(c)	T		(c)	T		(c)	F		(c)	T
	(d)	T		(d)	T		(d)	F		(d)	T
	(e)	T		(e)	F		(e)	T		(e)	T

12.64	(a)	T	**12.72**	(a)	F	**12.80**	(a)	T	**12.88**	(a)	T
	(b)	T		(b)	F		(b)	T		(b)	T
	(c)	T		(c)	T		(c)	T		(c)	T
	(d)	T		(d)	T		(d)	T		(d)	F
	(e)	T		(e)	T		(e)	F		(e)	T

12.65	(a)	F	**12.73**	(a)	F	**12.81**	(a)	T	**12.89**	(a)	T
	(b)	T		(b)	T		(b)	T		(b)	T
	(c)	T		(c)	T		(c)	T		(c)	T
	(d)	F		(d)	T		(d)	T		(d)	T
	(e)	T		(e)	F		(e)	T		(e)	T

12.66	(a)	F	**12.74**	(a)	T	**12.82**	(a)	T	**12.90**	(a)	T
	(b)	F		(b)	T		(b)	T		(b)	T
	(c)	F		(c)	T		(c)	F		(c)	T
	(d)	F		(d)	T		(d)	T		(d)	T
	(e)	F		(e)	T		(e)	F		(e)	F

12.67	(a)	F	**12.75**	(a)	T	**12.83**	(a)	F	**12.91**	(a)	F
	(b)	T		(b)	F		(b)	T		(b)	T
	(c)	F		(c)	T		(c)	C		(c)	T
	(d)	T		(d)	T		(d)	T		(d)	F
	(e)	F		(e)	T		(e)	T		(e)	F

12.68	(a)	T	**12.76**	(a)	F	**12.84**	(a)	F	**12.92**	(a)	T
	(b)	T		(b)	T		(b)	T		(b)	T
	(c)	T		(c)	T		(c)	T		(c)	T
	(d)	T		(d)	F		(d)	T		(d)	T
	(e)	T		(e)	T		(e)	T		(e)	F

12.93	(a) T	12.101	(a) F	12.109	(a) T	12.117	(a) T
	(b) T		(b) F		(b) T		(b) T
	(c) T		(c) T		(c) T		(c) T
	(d) F		(d) T		(d) T		(d) T
	(e) T		(e) T		(e) T		(e) T
12.94	(a) F	12.102	(a) T	12.110	(a) T	12.118	(a) T
	(b) T		(b) T		(b) F		(b) T
	(c) T		(c) T		(c) T		(c) T
	(d) T		(d) T		(d) T		(d) T
	(e) F		(e) T		(e) F		(e) F
12.95	(a) T	12.103	(a) F	12.111	(a) T	12.119	(a) F
	(b) T		(b) T		(b) T		(b) T
	(c) T		(c) T		(c) T		(c) T
	(d) T		(d) T		(d) T		(d) T
	(e) F		(e) T		(e) T		(e) T
12.96	(a) T	12.104	(a) T	12.112	(a) T	12.120	(a) F
	(b) F		(b) T		(b) T		(b) F
	(c) T		(c) F		(c) T		(c) F
	(d) F		(d) T		(d) T		(d) F
	(e) T		(e) T		(e) F		(e) F
12.97	(a) T	12.105	(a) T	12.113	(a) T	12.121	(a) T
	(b) T		(b) T		(b) T		(b) T
	(c) T		(c) T		(c) T		(c) T
	(d) T		(d) T		(d) T		(d) T
	(e) F		(e) T		(e) T		(e) F
12.98	(a) F	12.106	(a) F	12.114	(a) T	12.122	(a) T
	(b) F		(b) T		(b) F		(b) F
	(c) T		(c) F		(c) T		(c) T
	(d) T		(d) F		(d) T		(d) F
	(e) T		(e) T		(e) T		(e) F
12.99	(a) T	12.107	(a) T	12.115	(a) F	12.123	(a) T
	(b) T		(b) T		(b) T		(b) T
	(c) T		(c) F		(c) T		(c) F
	(d) T		(d) T		(d) T		(d) F
	(e) T		(e) T		(e) T		(e) F
12.100	(a) T	12.108	(a) F	12.116	(a) F	12.124	(a) F
	(b) T		(b) T		(b) F		(b) T
	(c) T		(c) F		(c) T		(c) T
	(d) T		(d) T		(d) T		(d) T
	(e) T		(e) T		(e) T		(e) T

12.125	(a)	T		**12.127**	(a)	T
	(b)	T			(b)	T
	(c)	T			(c)	T
	(d)	T			(d)	T
	(e)	T			(e)	T
12.126	(a)	T		**12.128**	(a)	T
	(b)	T			(b)	F
	(c)	T			(c)	T
	(d)	T			(d)	F
	(e)	T			(e)	F

Intensive Care Medicine
Answers

13.1 (a) T	**13.8** (a) F	**13.15** (a) T	**13.22** (a) T
(b) F	(b) T	(b) T	(b) T
(c) T	(c) F	(c) T	(c) T
(d) F	(d) F	(d) F	(d) T
(e) T	(e) T	(e) T	(e) T
13.2 (a) F	**13.9** (a) T	**13.16** (a) T	**13.23** (a) T
(b) F	(b) T	(b) T	(b) F
(c) T	(c) T	(c) T	(c) T
(d) F	(d) T	(d) T	(d) F
(e) F	(e) F	(e) F	(e) F
13.3 (a) T	**13.10** (a) F	**13.17** (a) T	**13.24** (a) T
(b) T	(b) F	(b) T	(b) T
(c) T	(c) T	(c) T	(c) T
(d) F	(d) T	(d) T	(d) F
(e) F	(e) F	(e) T	(e) T
13.4 (a) F	**13.11** (a) F	**13.18** (a) F	**13.25** (a) T
(b) T	(b) T	(b) F	(b) T
(c) T	(c) F	(c) F	(c) T
(d) T	(d) T	(d) F	(d) T
(e) F	(e) T	(e) F	(e) T
13.5 (a) T	**13.12** (a) T	**13.19** (a) T	**13.26** (a) T
(b) T	(b) T	(b) T	(b) T
(c) T	(c) T	(c) T	(c) T
(d) T	(d) T	(d) T	(d) T
(e) T	(e) T	(e) T	(e) F
13.6 (a) T	**13.13** (a) T	**13.20** (a) F	**13.27** (a) F
(b) T	(b) T	(b) F	(b) T
(c) T	(c) F	(c) F	(c) T
(d) T	(d) T	(d) T	(d) F
(e) F	(e) T	(e) T	(e) T
13.7 (a) F	**13.14** (a) T	**13.21** (a) T	**13.28** (a) F
(b) T	(b) T	(b) T	(b) T
(c) T	(c) T	(c) T	(c) T
(d) T	(d) T	(d) T	(d) T
(e) T	(e) T	(e) T	(e) T

13.29 (a) T
(b) T
(c) F
(d) T
(e) T

13.30 (a) T
(b) F
(c) F
(d) F
(e) F

13.31 (a) F
(b) T
(c) F
(d) T
(e) T

13.32 (a) T
(b) T
(c) T
(d) F
(e) F

13.33 (a) F
(b) T
(c) T
(d) T
(e) F

13.34 (a) F
(b) T
(c) T
(d) T
(e) T

13.35 (a) F
(b) T
(c) F
(d) F
(e) F

13.36 (a) T
(b) T
(c) T
(d) T
(e) T

13.37 (a) F
(b) F
(c) T
(d) F
(e) T

13.38 (a) T
(b) T
(c) T
(d) T
(e) T

13.39 (a) F
(b) F
(c) F
(d) F
(e) F

13.40 (a) T
(b) T
(c) T
(d) T
(e) T

13.41 (a) F
(b) T
(c) T
(d) T
(e) F

13.42 (a) T
(b) F
(c) F
(d) T
(e) T

13.43 (a) T
(b) T
(c) F
(d) F
(e) T

13.44 (a) F
(b) T
(c) F
(d) F
(e) F

13.45 (a) F
(b) F
(c) F
(d) F
(e) T

Adverse Drug Reactions and Poisoning

Answers

14.1 (a) T
(b) T
(c) T
(d) T
(e) T

14.2 (a) T
(b) T
(c) T
(d) T
(e) T

14.3 (a) F
(b) T
(c) F
(d) T
(e) T

14.4 (a) T
(b) T
(c) T
(d) F
(e) F

14.5 (a) F
(b) T
(c) T
(d) T
(e) T

14.6 (a) T
(b) F
(c) F
(d) F
(e) F

14.7 (a) T
(b) T
(c) T
(d) T
(e) T

14.8 (a) T
(b) T
(c) T
(d) T
(e) T

14.9 (a) F
(b) F
(c) T
(d) T
(e) T

14.10 (a) T
(b) T
(c) T
(d) F
(e) F

14.11 (a) F
(b) T
(c) T
(d) T
(e) F

14.12 (a) T
(b) T
(c) T
(d) T
(e) T

14.13 (a) F
(b) T
(c) T
(d) T
(e) T

14.14 (a) T
(b) T
(c) F
(d) F
(e) F

14.15 (a) T
(b) F
(c) T
(d) T
(e) F

14.16 (a) T
(b) T
(c) T
(d) T
(e) T

14.17 (a) T
(b) T
(c) T
(d) T
(e) F

14.18 (a) T
(b) T
(c) T
(d) T
(e) T

14.19 (a) F
(b) T
(c) T
(d) T
(e) F

14.20 (a) F
(b) T
(c) T
(d) T
(e) T

14.21 (a) T
(b) T
(c) T
(d) T
(e) T

14.22 (a) T
(b) T
(c) T
(d) T
(e) T

14.23 (a) F
(b) T
(c) F
(d) T
(e) T

14.24 (a) F
(b) T
(c) F
(d) T
(e) F

14.25	(a)	F	**14.33**	(a)	F	**14.41**	(a)	T	**14.49**	(a)	T
	(b)	F		(b)	T		(b)	F		(b)	T
	(c)	T		(c)	T		(c)	T		(c)	T
	(d)	T		(d)	F		(d)	T		(d)	T
	(e)	T		(e)	F		(e)	F		(e)	T

14.25 (a) F (b) F (c) T (d) T (e) T

14.26 (a) F (b) T (c) T (d) T (e) F

14.27 (a) T (b) T (c) T (d) T (e) T

14.28 (a) F (b) T (c) F (d) T (e) F

14.29 (a) T (b) F (c) F (d) F (e) F

14.30 (a) T (b) T (c) T (d) T (e) T

14.31 (a) F (b) T (c) T (d) T (e) T

14.32 (a) T (b) T (c) T (d) T (e) T

14.33 (a) F (b) T (c) T (d) F (e) F

14.34 (a) F (b) F (c) T (d) T (e) T

14.35 (a) T (b) T (c) F (d) T (e) F

14.36 (a) F (b) T (c) T (d) T (e) F

14.37 (a) T (b) T (c) T (d) T (e) T

14.38 (a) T (b) F (c) F (d) T (e) F

14.39 (a) F (b) T (c) T (d) T (e) F

14.40 (a) T (b) F (c) T (d) T (e) T

14.41 (a) T (b) F (c) T (d) T (e) F

14.42 (a) T (b) T (c) T (d) T (e) T

14.43 (a) T (b) T (c) F (d) T (e) T

14.44 (a) F (b) T (c) F (d) T (e) T

14.45 (a) T (b) T (c) T (d) F (e) T

14.46 (a) T (b) F (c) T (d) F (e) F

14.47 (a) T (b) T (c) T (d) T (e) T

14.48 (a) F (b) T (c) T (d) T (e) F

14.49 (a) T (b) T (c) T (d) T (e) T

14.50 (a) T (b) F (c) F (d) F (e) F

14.51 (a) T (b) T (c) T (d) T (e) T

14.52 (a) F (b) T (c) T (d) F (e) T

14.53 (a) T (b) T (c) T (d) T (e) T

14.54 (a) T (b) T (c) T (d) T (e) T

14.55 (a) T (b) T (c) T (d) T (e) T

14.56 (a) F (b) T (c) F (d) T (e) T

Environmental Medicine
Answers

15.1 (a) T
    (b) F
    (c) F
    (d) T
    (e) T

15.4 (a) F
    (b) F
    (c) F
    (d) F
    (e) F

15.7 (a) F
    (b) T
    (c) T
    (d) T
    (e) F

15.10 (a) F
    (b) T
    (c) F
    (d) T
    (e) F

15.2 (a) T
    (b) T
    (c) T
    (d) T
    (e) T

15.5 (a) F
    (b) T
    (c) T
    (d) T
    (e) T

15.8 (a) T
    (b) T
    (c) T
    (d) T
    (e) F

15.11 (a) F
    (b) T
    (c) T
    (d) T
    (e) F

15.3 (a) T
    (b) F
    (c) F
    (d) T
    (e) T

15.6 (a) F
    (b) F
    (c) T
    (d) T
    (e) T

15.9 (a) T
    (b) T
    (c) T
    (d) T
    (e) T

Endocrinology System
Answers

16.1 (a) T	**16.8** (a) T	**16.15** (a) T	**16.22** (a) T
(b) T	(b) F	(b) T	(b) T
(c) T	(c) T	(c) F	(c) T
(d) T	(d) F	(d) F	(d) T
(e) F	(e) F	(e) T	(e) T
16.2 (a) T	**16.9** (a) T	**16.16** (a) F	**16.23** (a) T
(b) T	(b) T	(b) T	(b) F
(c) T	(c) T	(c) T	(c) F
(d) T	(d) T	(d) T	(d) F
(e) T	(e) T	(e) F	(e) F
16.3 (a) T	**16.10** (a) T	**16.17** (a) T	**16.24** (a) F
(b) T	(b) T	(b) T	(b) T
(c) T	(c) T	(c) T	(c) T
(d) T	(d) T	(d) T	(d) F
(e) T	(e) T	(e) T	(e) F
16.4 (a) T	**16.11** (a) T	**16.18** (a) F	**16.25** (a) F
(b) T	(b) T	(b) F	(b) F
(c) F	(c) T	(c) T	(c) T
(d) F	(d) T	(d) T	(d) F
(e) F	(e) T	(e) T	(e) F
16.5 (a) F	**16.12** (a) F	**16.19** (a) T	**16.26** (a) F
(b) T	(b) F	(b) F	(b) F
(c) T	(c) F	(c) T	(c) F
(d) F	(d) F	(d) T	(d) T
(e) T	(e) F	(e) T	(e) T
16.6 (a) T	**16.13** (a) F	**16.20** (a) F	**16.27** (a) F
(b) T	(b) F	(b) F	(b) T
(c) T	(c) F	(c) T	(c) T
(d) T	(d) F	(d) F	(d) T
(e) T	(e) F	(e) T	(e) F
16.7 (a) F	**16.14** (a) T	**16.21** (a) F	**16.28** (a) F
(b) T	(b) T	(b) T	(b) T
(c) F	(c) T	(c) T	(c) T
(d) T	(d) T	(d) T	(d) T
(e) F	(e) T	(e) T	(e) T

16.29 (a) F		**16.37** (a) T		**16.45** (a) T		**16.53** (a) T	
(b) F		(b) T		(b) T		(b) T	
(c) F		(c) T		(c) T		(c) F	
(d) F		(d) T		(d) T		(d) T	
(e) F		(e) T		(e) T		(e) T	
16.30 (a) F		**16.38** (a) F		**16.46** (a) T		**16.54** (a) F	
(b) T		(b) T		(b) T		(b) T	
(c) T		(c) T		(c) T		(c) F	
(d) T		(d) T		(d) T		(d) T	
(e) F		(e) F		(e) T		(e) T	
16.31 (a) F		**16.39** (a) T		**16.47** (a) F		**16.55** (a) F	
(b) F		(b) T		(b) F		(b) F	
(c) F		(c) T		(c) F		(c) T	
(d) F		(d) T		(d) T		(d) T	
(e) F		(e) T		(e) F		(e) T	
16.32 (a) T		**16.40** (a) F		**16.48** (a) T		**16.56** (a) T	
(b) F		(b) T		(b) T		(b) T	
(c) T		(c) T		(c) T		(c) T	
(d) T		(d) T		(d) T		(d) T	
(e) T		(e) T		(e) T		(e) T	
16.33 (a) F		**16.41** (a) F		**16.49** (a) T		**16.57** (a) F	
(b) F		(b) T		(b) T		(b) F	
(c) F		(c) T		(c) F		(c) F	
(d) T		(d) T		(d) T		(d) F	
(e) T		(e) T		(e) F		(e) T	
16.34 (a) F		**16.42** (a) T		**16.50** (a) T		**16.58** (a) F	
(b) T		(b) T		(b) F		(b) T	
(c) F		(c) T		(c) F		(c) T	
(d) F		(d) T		(d) T		(d) T	
(e) T		(e) T		(e) T		(e) F	
16.35 (a) T		**16.43** (a) F		**16.51** (a) F		**16.59** (a) T	
(b) T		(b) T		(b) T		(b) T	
(c) T		(c) T		(c) F		(c) T	
(d) T		(d) F		(d) T		(d) T	
(e) T		(e) T		(e) T		(e) T	
16.36 (a) F		**16.44** (a) F		**16.52** (a) T		**16.60** (a) F	
(b) T		(b) F		(b) T		(b) F	
(c) F		(c) F		(c) F		(c) T	
(d) T		(d) F		(d) T		(d) T	
(e) T		(e) F		(e) T		(e) F	

16.61	(a) T	**16.69**	(a) F	**16.77**	(a) F	**16.85**	(a) T
	(b) T		(b) T		(b) F		(b) T
	(c) T		(c) T		(c) T		(c) T
	(d) T		(d) T		(d) T		(d) T
	(e) T		(e) T		(e) T		(e) T
16.62	(a) T	**16.70**	(a) F	**16.78**	(a) T	**16.86**	(a) T
	(b) T		(b) F		(b) F		(b) T
	(c) T		(c) F		(c) T		(c) F
	(d) T		(d) T		(d) T		(d) F
	(e) F		(e) T		(e) F		(e) T
16.63	(a) T	**16.71**	(a) F	**16.79**	(a) T	**16.87**	(a) F
	(b) F		(b) F		(b) T		(b) F
	(c) F		(c) T		(c) T		(c) T
	(d) T		(d) T		(d) T		(d) T
	(e) T		(e) F		(e) T		(e) T
16.64	(a) T	**16.72**	(a) T	**16.80**	(a) F	**16.88**	(a) F
	(b) F		(b) F		(b) F		(b) F
	(c) T		(c) F		(c) T		(c) F
	(d) F		(d) F		(d) T		(d) T
	(e) F		(e) F		(e) T		(e) T
16.65	(a) T	**16.73**	(a) T	**16.81**	(a) T	**16.89**	(a) F
	(b) T		(b) T		(b) T		(b) F
	(c) T		(c) T		(c) T		(c) T
	(d) T		(d) T		(d) T		(d) T
	(e) T		(e) F		(e) T		(e) T
16.66	(a) F	**16.74**	(a) T	**16.82**	(a) F	**16.90**	(a) F
	(b) F		(b) F		(b) F		(b) F
	(c) T		(c) T		(c) F		(c) T
	(d) T		(d) F		(d) F		(d) F
	(e) T		(e) T		(e) F		(e) F
16.67	(a) T	**16.75**	(a) T	**16.83**	(a) F	**16.91**	(a) T
	(b) F		(b) F		(b) F		(b) T
	(c) T		(c) F		(c) F		(c) T
	(d) T		(d) F		(d) T		(d) T
	(e) T		(e) F		(e) T		(e) T
16.68	(a) T	**16.76**	(a) F	**16.84**	(a) T	**16.92**	(a) F
	(b) T		(b) T		(b) T		(b) F
	(c) T		(c) T		(c) T		(c) T
	(d) T		(d) T		(d) T		(d) T
	(e) T		(e) F		(e) T		(e) F

16.93	(a) F	**16.101**	(a) T	**16.109**	(a) T	**16.117**	(a) T
	(b) F		(b) T		(b) T		(b) T
	(c) T		(c) T		(c) F		(c) F
	(d) T		(d) T		(d) T		(d) F
	(e) T		(e) T		(e) T		(e) F
16.94	(a) F	**16.102**	(a) F	**16.110**	(a) T	**16.118**	(a) F
	(b) F		(b) T		(b) T		(b) F
	(c) T		(c) F		(c) T		(c) F
	(d) F		(d) T		(d) F		(d) T
	(e) F		(e) T		(e) T		(e) F
16.95	(a) T	**16.103**	(a) T	**16.111**	(a) T	**16.119**	(a) F
	(b) F		(b) T		(b) T		(b) T
	(c) F		(c) T		(c) F		(c) T
	(d) T		(d) F		(d) T		(d) T
	(e) T		(e) F		(e) F		(e) T
16.96	(a) T	**16.104**	(a) T	**16.112**	(a) T	**16.120**	(a) T
	(b) F		(b) F		(b) F		(b) T
	(c) F		(c) F		(c) T		(c) T
	(d) T		(d) F		(d) T		(d) T
	(e) T		(e) F		(e) F		(e) T
16.97	(a) F	**16.105**	(a) F	**16.113**	(a) T	**16.121**	(a) T
	(b) F		(b) F		(b) T		(b) F
	(c) T		(c) T		(c) F		(c) F
	(d) T		(d) T		(d) F		(d) F
	(e) T		(e) F		(e) F		(e) F
16.98	(a) T	**16.106**	(a) F	**16.114**	(a) F	**16.122**	(a) F
	(b) T		(b) T		(b) F		(b) T
	(c) F		(c) T		(c) F		(c) F
	(d) T		(d) T		(d) F		(d) F
	(e) F		(e) T		(e) T		(e) T
16.99	(a) T	**16.107**	(a) T	**16.115**	(a) F	**16.123**	(a) T
	(b) F		(b) F		(b) F		(b) F
	(c) T		(c) T		(c) F		(c) F
	(d) T		(d) F		(d) F		(d) F
	(e) T		(e) F		(e) T		(e) F
16.100	(a) T	**16.108**	(a) T	**16.116**	(a) T	**16.124**	(a) T
	(b) T		(b) T		(b) T		(b) T
	(c) F		(c) F		(c) T		(c) F
	(d) F		(d) F		(d) T		(d) T
	(e) T		(e) F		(e) T		(e) T

16.125	(a)	F	**16.127**	(a)	F	**16.129**	(a)	T	**16.131**	(a)	T
	(b)	T		(b)	F		(b)	F		(b)	T
	(c)	T		(c)	F		(c)	F		(c)	T
	(d)	T		(d)	F		(d)	F		(d)	T
	(e)	F		(e)	T		(e)	F		(e)	F

16.126	(a)	F	**16.128**	(a)	F	**16.130**	(a)	F
	(b)	T		(b)	F		(b)	T
	(c)	T		(c)	F		(c)	T
	(d)	F		(d)	F		(d)	T
	(e)	T		(e)	F		(e)	T

Diabetes Mellitus and Other Disorders of Metabolism
Answers

17.1 (a) F
(b) T
(c) T
(d) T
(e) T

17.2 (a) F
(b) F
(c) T
(d) T
(e) T

17.3 (a) F
(b) F
(c) F
(d) F
(e) F

17.4 (a) F
(b) T
(c) T
(d) F
(e) F

17.5 (a) T
(b) T
(c) T
(d) T
(e) T

17.6 (a) T
(b) T
(c) T
(d) T
(e) T

17.7 (a) F
(b) T
(c) T
(d) T
(e) T

17.8 (a) T
(b) T
(c) F
(d) T
(e) T

17.9 (a) F
(b) T
(c) T
(d) F
(e) T

17.10 (a) T
(b) T
(c) T
(d) T
(e) T

17.11 (a) T
(b) T
(c) T
(d) F
(e) F

17.12 (a) T
(b) F
(c) T
(d) T
(e) T

17.13 (a) T
(b) T
(c) T
(d) T
(e) T

17.14 (a) T
(b) T
(c) F
(d) F
(e) T

17.15 (a) F
(b) T
(c) T
(d) T
(e) T

17.16 (a) T
(b) T
(c) T
(d) T
(e) T

17.17 (a) T
(b) T
(c) T
(d) T
(e) T

17.18 (a) T
(b) T
(c) F
(d) F
(e) T

17.19 (a) T
(b) T
(c) T
(d) T
(e) T

17.20 (a) T
(b) T
(c) T
(d) T
(e) T

17.21 (a) T
(b) F
(c) T
(d) F
(e) F

17.22 (a) T
(b) T
(c) T
(d) F
(e) F

17.23 (a) T
(b) T
(c) T
(d) T
(e) T

17.24 (a) F
(b) T
(c) T
(d) F
(e) T

17.25	(a) F	**17.33**	(a) T	**17.41**	(a) T	**17.49**	(a) T
	(b) T		(b) T		(b) T		(b) T
	(c) T		(c) T		(c) T		(c) T
	(d) T		(d) T		(d) T		(d) T
	(e) T		(e) T		(e) T		(e) T
17.26	(a) F	**17.34**	(a) F	**17.42**	(a) T	**17.50**	(a) T
	(b) T		(b) T		(b) T		(b) F
	(c) F		(c) T		(c) T		(c) F
	(d) T		(d) T		(d) T		(d) F
	(e) T		(e) T		(e) T		(e) T
17.27	(a) T	**17.35**	(a) F	**17.43**	(a) F	**17.51**	(a) T
	(b) T		(b) T		(b) T		(b) T
	(c) T		(c) F		(c) T		(c) F
	(d) T		(d) T		(d) F		(d) T
	(e) T		(e) T		(e) T		(e) F
17.28	(a) T	**17.36**	(a) T	**17.44**	(a) F	**17.52**	(a) F
	(b) T		(b) T		(b) F		(b) T
	(c) T		(c) T		(c) T		(c) T
	(d) T		(d) T		(d) T		(d) T
	(e) T		(e) T		(e) T		(e) T
17.29	(a) T	**17.37**	(a) T	**17.45**	(a) T	**17.53**	(a) F
	(b) T		(b) T		(b) T		(b) F
	(c) T		(c) T		(c) F		(c) T
	(d) T		(d) F		(d) F		(d) T
	(e) T		(e) F		(e) T		(e) T
17.30	(a) F	**17.38**	(a) F	**17.46**	(a) T	**17.54**	(a) T
	(b) T		(b) F		(b) T		(b) T
	(c) F		(c) T		(c) T		(c) T
	(d) T		(d) T		(d) F		(d) F
	(e) T		(e) T		(e) F		(e) T
17.31	(a) T	**17.39**	(a) T	**17.47**	(a) F	**17.55**	(a) T
	(b) T		(b) T		(b) T		(b) F
	(c) T		(c) T		(c) T		(c) F
	(d) T		(d) F		(d) T		(d) T
	(e) T		(e) F		(e) T		(e) T
17.32	(a) T	**17.40**	(a) F	**17.48**	(a) T	**17.56**	(a) F
	(b) T		(b) F		(b) T		(b) T
	(c) T		(c) T		(c) T		(c) F
	(d) F		(d) F		(d) F		(d) T
	(e) T		(e) F		(e) T		(e) F

17.57	(a) T	**17.65**	(a) F	**17.73**	(a) T	**17.81**	(a) F
	(b) T		(b) T		(b) T		(b) F
	(c) T		(c) F		(c) F		(c) T
	(d) T		(d) F		(d) T		(d) F
	(e) T		(e) F		(e) T		(e) T
17.58	(a) T	**17.66**	(a) T	**17.74**	(a) T	**17.82**	(a) T
	(b) T		(b) T		(b) F		(b) F
	(c) T		(c) F		(c) T		(c) T
	(d) F		(d) T		(d) T		(d) T
	(e) F		(e) T		(e) F		(e) T
17.59	(a) F	**17.67**	(a) F	**17.75**	(a) T	**17.83**	(a) F
	(b) T		(b) T		(b) T		(b) T
	(c) F		(c) T		(c) T		(c) T
	(d) T		(d) T		(d) T		(d) T
	(e) F		(e) F		(e) T		(e) F
17.60	(a) F	**17.68**	(a) T	**17.76**	(a) T	**17.84**	(a) T
	(b) T		(b) F		(b) F		(b) T
	(c) T		(c) T		(c) T		(c) T
	(d) T		(d) T		(d) T		(d) T
	(e) T		(e) T		(e) T		(e) T
17.61	(a) T	**17.69**	(a) T	**17.77**	(a) T	**17.85**	(a) T
	(b) T		(b) F		(b) T		(b) T
	(c) T		(c) T		(c) F		(c) T
	(d) T		(d) T		(d) F		(d) T
	(e) T		(e) F		(e) T		(e) T
17.62	(a) T	**17.70**	(a) T	**17.78**	(a) T	**17.86**	(a) T
	(b) T		(b) F		(b) T		(b) T
	(c) T		(c) F		(c) T		(c) T
	(d) T		(d) T		(d) F		(d) T
	(e) T		(e) T		(e) F		(e) T
17.63	(a) T	**17.71**	(a) T	**17.79**	(a) T	**17.87**	(a) T
	(b) T		(b) T		(b) F		(b) T
	(c) T		(c) T		(c) T		(c) T
	(d) T		(d) T		(d) F		(d) T
	(e) T		(e) F		(e) T		(e) F
17.64	(a) T	**17.72**	(a) F	**17.80**	(a) F	**17.88**	(a) T
	(b) T		(b) T		(b) F		(b) T
	(c) T		(c) T		(c) T		(c) F
	(d) T		(d) T		(d) F		(d) F
	(e) F		(e) T		(e) T		(e) F

17.89	(a) T	**17.93**	(a) F	**17.97**	(a) T	**17.101**	(a) T
	(b) T		(b) T		(b) T		(b) T
	(c) T		(c) T		(c) T		(c) T
	(d) T		(d) T		(d) T		(d) F
	(e) T		(e) T		(e) T		(e) F

17.90	(a) T	**17.94**	(a) F	**17.98**	(a) T	**17.102**	(a) F
	(b) T		(b) T		(b) T		(b) T
	(c) T		(c) T		(c) F		(c) T
	(d) T		(d) T		(d) T		(d) T
	(c) T		(e) T		(e) T		(e) F

17.91	(a) T	**17.95**	(a) T	**17.99**	(a) T
	(b) T		(b) T		(b) T
	(c) T		(c) T		(c) F
	(d) T		(d) T		(d) T
	(e) T		(e) T		(e) T

17.92	(a) T	**17.96**	(a) T	**17.100**	(a) T
	(b) T		(b) T		(b) T
	(c) T		(c) T		(c) T
	(d) T		(d) T		(d) T
	(e) T		(e) T		(e) T

Neurological Disease
Answers

18.1 (a) T	**18.8** (a) F	**18.15** (a) F	**18.22** (a) T
(b) T	(b) T	(b) T	(b) F
(c) T	(c) T	(c) T	(c) T
(d) T	(d) T	(d) T	(d) F
(e) T	(e) T	(e) T	(e) F
18.2 (a) T	**18.9** (a) F	**18.16** (a) T	**18.23** (a) T
(b) T	(b) F	(b) T	(b) T
(c) T	(c) T	(c) T	(c) T
(d) T	(d) T	(d) T	(d) T
(e) T	(e) T	(e) F	(e) F
18.3 (a) F	**18.10** (a) T	**18.17** (a) F	**18.24** (a) T
(b) T	(b) T	(b) F	(b) F
(c) T	(c) T	(c) F	(c) T
(d) T	(d) T	(d) T	(d) F
(e) T	(e) T	(e) F	(e) T
18.4 (a) T	**18.11** (a) F	**18.18** (a) T	**18.25** (a) F
(b) T	(b) T	(b) T	(b) T
(c) T	(c) T	(c) F	(c) T
(d) T	(d) F	(d) T	(d) T
(e) T	(e) T	(e) F	(e) F
18.5 (a) T	**18.12** (a) F	**18.19** (a) T	**18.26** (a) T
(b) T	(b) T	(b) T	(b) T
(c) T	(c) F	(c) T	(c) T
(d) T	(d) T	(d) T	(d) F
(e) F	(e) T	(e) T	(e) T
18.6 (a) F	**18.13** (a) F	**18.20** (a) T	**18.27** (a) F
(b) T	(b) T	(b) T	(b) T
(c) T	(c) T	(c) T	(c) T
(d) T	(d) T	(d) T	(d) T
(e) T	(e) T	(e) F	(e) F
18.7 (a) F	**18.14** (a) T	**18.21** (a) T	**18.28** (a) T
(b) T	(b) T	(b) T	(b) T
(c) T	(c) T	(c) T	(c) T
(d) T	(d) T	(d) T	(d) F
(e) F	(e) T	(e) F	(e) F

18.29	(a)	F	**18.37**	(a)	F	**18.45**	(a)	F	**18.53**	(a)	T
	(b)	T		(b)	T		(b)	T		(b)	T
	(c)	T		(c)	T		(c)	F		(c)	T
	(d)	T		(d)	T		(d)	T		(d)	T
	(e)	F		(e)	T		(e)	F		(e)	T

18.30	(a)	F	**18.38**	(a)	F	**18.46**	(a)	F	**18.54**	(a)	T
	(b)	F		(b)	T		(b)	F		(b)	F
	(c)	F		(c)	T		(c)	F		(c)	F
	(d)	F		(d)	F		(d)	T		(d)	T
	(e)	T		(e)	T		(e)	F		(e)	T

18.31	(a)	T	**18.39**	(a)	T	**18.47**	(a)	T	**18.55**	(a)	T
	(b)	T		(b)	T		(b)	F		(b)	T
	(c)	F		(c)	T		(c)	T		(c)	T
	(d)	T		(d)	T		(d)	F		(d)	T
	(e)	F		(e)	T		(e)	T		(e)	T

18.32	(a)	T	**18.40**	(a)	T	**18.48**	(a)	F	**18.56**	(a)	T
	(b)	T		(b)	T		(b)	T		(b)	F
	(c)	T		(c)	T		(c)	T		(c)	F
	(d)	T		(d)	T		(d)	F		(d)	T
	(e)	T		(e)	T		(e)	F		(e)	T

18.33	(a)	F	**18.41**	(a)	F	**18.49**	(a)	T	**18.57**	(a)	F
	(b)	T		(b)	T		(b)	T		(b)	T
	(c)	F		(c)	F		(c)	T		(c)	T
	(d)	T		(d)	T		(d)	T		(d)	T
	(e)	T		(e)	T		(e)	T		(e)	F

18.34	(a)	F	**18.42**	(a)	F	**18.50**	(a)	F	**18.58**	(a)	F
	(b)	T		(b)	F		(b)	F		(b)	T
	(c)	T		(c)	F		(c)	F		(c)	F
	(d)	F		(d)	T		(d)	T		(d)	F
	(e)	F		(e)	T		(e)	T		(e)	T

18.35	(a)	T	**18.43**	(a)	T	**18.51**	(a)	T	**18.59**	(a)	F
	(b)	T		(b)	T		(b)	T		(b)	T
	(c)	T		(c)	T		(c)	T		(c)	T
	(d)	T		(d)	F		(d)	T		(d)	F
	(e)	F		(e)	T		(e)	T		(e)	T

18.36	(a)	F	**18.44**	(a)	F	**18.52**	(a)	F	**18.60**	(a)	T
	(b)	T		(b)	F		(b)	T		(b)	F
	(c)	T		(c)	F		(c)	T		(c)	T
	(d)	T		(d)	T		(d)	F		(d)	T
	(e)	F		(e)	F		(e)	T		(e)	T

18.61 (a) T		**18.69** (a) F		**18.77** (a) T		**18.85** (a) T	
(b) T		(b) T		(b) F		(b) T	
(c) T		(c) T		(c) T		(c) T	
(d) T		(d) T		(d) T		(d) T	
(e) T		(e) T		(e) T		(e) T	
18.62 (a) F		**18.70** (a) T		**18.78** (a) T		**18.86** (a) F	
(b) F		(b) T		(b) T		(b) F	
(c) T		(c) T		(c) T		(c) T	
(d) T		(d) T		(d) F		(d) T	
(e) T		(e) T		(e) F		(e) T	
18.63 (a) F		**18.71** (a) F		**18.79** (a) T		**18.87** (a) F	
(b) T		(b) T		(b) T		(b) F	
(c) T		(c) T		(c) T		(c) T	
(d) T		(d) T		(d) T		(d) T	
(e) F		(e) F		(e) T		(e) F	
18.64 (a) T		**18.72** (a) F		**18.80** (a) F		**18.88** (a) T	
(b) F		(b) T		(b) F		(b) T	
(c) T		(c) T		(c) T		(c) T	
(d) F		(d) F		(d) T		(d) T	
(e) F		(e) T		(e) T		(e) T	
18.65 (a) F		**18.73** (a) T		**18.81** (a) T		**18.89** (a) T	
(b) T		(b) F		(b) T		(b) F	
(c) T		(c) T		(c) T		(c) F	
(d) F		(d) T		(d) T		(d) T	
(e) T		(e) F		(e) T		(e) T	
18.66 (a) T		**18.74** (a) F		**18.82** (a) T		**18.90** (a) T	
(b) T		(b) T		(b) T		(b) T	
(c) F		(c) F		(c) T		(c) F	
(d) T		(d) T		(d) T		(d) T	
(e) T		(e) T		(e) T		(e) F	
18.67 (a) T		**18.75** (a) F		**18.83** (a) T		**18.91** (a) F	
(b) F		(b) F		(b) T		(b) T	
(c) T		(c) T		(c) T		(c) T	
(d) F		(d) T		(d) T		(d) T	
(e) F		(e) T		(e) T		(e) T	
18.68 (a) F		**18.76** (a) T		**18.84** (a) T		**18.92** (a) F	
(b) T		(b) F		(b) T		(b) F	
(c) T		(c) T		(c) T		(c) T	
(d) T		(d) T		(d) T		(d) T	
(e) T		(e) F		(e) T		(e) T	

18.93	(a) F	**18.101**	(a) F	**18.109**	(a) F	**18.117**	(a) F
	(b) T		(b) T		(b) T		(b) T
	(c) T		(c) F		(c) T		(c) F
	(d) T		(d) F		(d) F		(d) F
	(e) T		(e) F		(e) F		(e) F
18.94	(a) F	**18.102**	(a) F	**18.110**	(a) T	**18.118**	(a) T
	(b) F		(b) T		(b) T		(b) T
	(c) T		(c) T		(c) T		(c) T
	(d) F		(d) F		(d) T		(d) T
	(e) F		(e) T		(e) T		(e) T
18.95	(a) F	**18.103**	(a) F	**18.111**	(a) T	**18.119**	(a) T
	(b) T		(b) F		(b) T		(b) T
	(c) F		(c) F		(c) F		(c) T
	(d) T		(d) F		(d) T		(d) T
	(e) T		(e) F		(e) T		(e) T
18.96	(a) T	**18.104**	(a) F	**18.112**	(a) T	**18.120**	(a) T
	(b) F		(b) F		(b) T		(b) T
	(c) F		(c) F		(c) T		(c) T
	(d) T		(d) T		(d) T		(d) T
	(e) T		(e) F		(e) T		(e) T
18.97	(a) F	**18.105**	(a) T	**18.113**	(a) F	**18.121**	(a) T
	(b) T		(b) T		(b) F		(b) F
	(c) T		(c) T		(c) F		(c) T
	(d) F		(d) T		(d) T		(d) F
	(e) F		(e) F		(e) F		(e) F
18.98	(a) T	**18.106**	(a) T	**18.114**	(a) T	**18.122**	(a) F
	(b) T		(b) F		(b) F		(b) F
	(c) T		(c) T		(c) T		(c) T
	(d) T		(d) F		(d) F		(d) T
	(e) T		(e) T		(e) F		(e) F
18.99	(a) T	**18.107**	(a) T	**18.115**	(a) F	**18.123**	(a) T
	(b) T		(b) F		(b) T		(b) T
	(c) T		(c) T		(c) T		(c) T
	(d) T		(d) T		(d) T		(d) T
	(e) T		(e) T		(e) F		(e) T
18.100	(a) T	**18.108**	(a) T	**18.116**	(a) T	**18.124**	(a) T
	(b) F		(b) T		(b) F		(b) F
	(c) T		(c) T		(c) T		(c) T
	(d) F		(d) T		(d) F		(d) F
	(e) F		(e) F		(e) F		(e) T

18.125	(a) T	18.133	(a) T	18.141	(a) T	18.149	(a) F
	(b) T		(b) T		(b) T		(b) T
	(c) F		(c) T		(c) F		(c) T
	(d) F		(d) T		(d) T		(d) F
	(e) T		(e) T		(e) T		(e) F

18.126	(a) F	18.134	(a) F	18.142	(a) T	18.150	(a) T
	(b) T		(b) T		(b) T		(b) T
	(c) T		(c) T		(c) T		(c) T
	(d) T		(d) T		(d) F		(d) T
	(e) F		(e) F		(e) T		(e) T

18.127	(a) T	18.135	(a) F	18.143	(a) T	18.151	(a) T
	(b) T		(b) F		(b) T		(b) T
	(c) T		(c) T		(c) T		(c) F
	(d) F		(d) T		(d) T		(d) T
	(e) T		(e) T		(e) T		(e) T

18.128	(a) T	18.136	(a) F	18.144	(a) F	18.152	(a) T
	(b) F		(b) T		(b) T		(b) T
	(c) F		(c) T		(c) T		(c) T
	(d) T		(d) F		(d) T		(d) T
	(e) T		(e) F		(e) F		(e) T

18.129	(a) F	18.137	(a) F	18.145	(a) F	18.153	(a) T
	(b) T		(b) T		(b) T		(b) T
	(c) T		(c) T		(c) F		(c) T
	(d) T		(d) T		(d) T		(d) F
	(e) T		(e) T		(e) T		(e) T

18.130	(a) T	18.138	(a) T	18.146	(a) F	18.154	(a) T
	(b) T		(b) T		(b) F		(b) T
	(c) T		(c) T		(c) T		(c) T
	(d) F		(d) T		(d) T		(d) T
	(e) F		(e) T		(e) T		(e) T

18.131	(a) T	18.139	(a) T	18.147	(a) F	18.155	(a) T
	(b) T		(b) T		(b) T		(b) F
	(c) T		(c) T		(c) T		(c) T
	(d) T		(d) F		(d) F		(d) T
	(e) F		(e) F		(e) T		(e) T

18.132	(a) F	18.140	(a) F	18.148	(a) T	18.156	(a) T
	(b) T		(b) F		(b) T		(b) T
	(c) F		(c) T		(c) T		(c) T
	(d) F		(d) F		(d) T		(d) T
	(e) F		(e) F		(e) T		(e) T

18.157	(a) T	18.165	(a) T	18.173	(a) F	18.181	(a) T
	(b) T		(b) T		(b) T		(b) T
	(c) T		(c) T		(c) F		(c) T
	(d) T		(d) T		(d) T		(d) T
	(e) T		(e) T		(e) T		(e) T
18.158	(a) T	18.166	(a) F	18.174	(a) T	18.182	(a) F
	(b) F		(b) T		(b) T		(b) T
	(c) T		(c) T		(c) T		(c) T
	(d) T		(d) T		(d) T		(d) T
	(e) T		(e) T		(e) T		(e) T
18.159	(a) T	18.167	(a) T	18.175	(a) T	18.183	(a) F
	(b) T		(b) T		(b) F		(b) T
	(c) T		(c) T		(c) T		(c) T
	(d) F		(d) T		(d) F		(d) T
	(e) F		(e) T		(e) F		(e) T
18.160	(a) T	18.168	(a) F	18.176	(a) F	18.184	(a) T
	(b) F		(b) T		(b) F		(b) T
	(c) T		(c) F		(c) T		(c) T
	(d) T		(d) T		(d) T		(d) T
	(e) T		(e) T		(e) T		(e) T
18.161	(a) T	18.169	(a) T	18.177	(a) T	18.185	(a) F
	(b) T		(b) T		(b) T		(b) T
	(c) T		(c) T		(c) T		(c) T
	(d) T		(d) T		(d) T		(d) T
	(e) F		(e) T		(e) T		(e) T
18.162	(a) F	18.170	(a) T	18.178	(a) T	18.186	(a) T
	(b) T		(b) T		(b) T		(b) T
	(c) F		(c) T		(c) T		(c) T
	(d) T		(d) T		(d) F		(d) T
	(e) T		(e) T		(e) T		(e) T
18.163	(a) F	18.171	(a) F	18.179	(a) T	18.187	(a) F
	(b) T		(b) F		(b) T		(b) T
	(c) F		(c) F		(c) T		(c) T
	(d) T		(d) T		(d) T		(d) T
	(e) F		(e) T		(e) T		(e) F
18.164	(a) F	18.172	(a) F	18.180	(a) F	18.188	(a) F
	(b) T		(b) T		(b) T		(b) F
	(c) T		(c) T		(c) T		(c) T
	(d) T		(d) T		(d) T		(d) T
	(e) F		(e) T		(e) F		(e) F

18.189 (a) F
(b) T
(c) T
(d) T
(e) T

18.190 (a) T
(b) T
(c) T
(d) T
(e) T

18.191 (a) F
(b) T
(c) T
(d) T
(e) F

18.192 (a) F
(b) T
(c) T
(d) F
(e) T

18.193 (a) T
(b) T
(c) T
(d) F
(e) F

18.194 (a) T
(b) T
(c) F
(d) T
(e) T

18.195 (a) T
(b) T
(c) T
(d) T
(e) F

18.196 (a) T
(b) F
(c) F
(d) F
(e) T

18.197 (a) F
(b) F
(c) T
(d) F
(e) T

18.198 (a) F
(b) T
(c) F
(d) T
(e) T

18.199 (a) T
(b) T
(c) F
(d) T
(e) T

18.200 (a) F
(b) T
(c) F
(d) T
(e) T

18.201 (a) F
(b) T
(c) F
(d) T
(e) F

18.202 (a) T
(b) F
(c) F
(d) T
(e) T

18.203 (a) F
(b) F
(c) F
(d) F
(e) F

18.204 (a) F
(b) T
(c) F
(d) F
(e) F

18.205 (a) T
(b) T
(c) T
(d) T
(e) T

Psychological Medicine
Answers

19.1 (a) T
    (b) T
    (c) T
    (d) F
    (e) T

19.2 (a) T
    (b) F
    (c) T
    (d) T
    (e) T

19.3 (a) F
    (b) F
    (c) T
    (d) T
    (e) F

19.4 (a) F
    (b) F
    (c) T
    (d) T
    (e) T

19.5 (a) F
    (b) F
    (c) T
    (d) T
    (e) T

19.6 (a) T
    (b) F
    (c) T
    (d) F
    (e) T

19.7 (a) T
    (b) F
    (c) T
    (d) F
    (e) T

19.8 (a) F
    (b) F
    (c) T
    (d) T
    (e) T

19.9 (a) T
    (b) T
    (c) T
    (d) T
    (e) T

19.10 (a) T
    (b) T
    (c) T
    (d) T
    (e) T

19.11 (a) T
    (b) T
    (c) T
    (d) T
    (e) T

19.12 (a) T
    (b) T
    (c) T
    (d) T
    (e) T

19.13 (a) T
    (b) T
    (c) T
    (d) F
    (e) T

19.14 (a) T
    (b) T
    (c) T
    (d) T
    (e) T

19.15 (a) T
    (b) F
    (c) T
    (d) F
    (e) T

19.16 (a) T
    (b) T
    (c) F
    (d) F
    (e) T

19.17 (a) T
    (b) F
    (c) T
    (d) F
    (e) T

19.18 (a) F
    (b) T
    (c) T
    (d) T
    (e) F

19.19 (a) F
    (b) T
    (c) T
    (d) F
    (e) T

19.20 (a) F
    (b) T
    (c) T
    (d) T
    (e) T

19.21 (a) F
    (b) F
    (c) T
    (d) T
    (e) F

19.22 (a) T
    (b) F
    (c) F
    (d) T
    (e) F

19.23 (a) T
    (b) T
    (c) T
    (d) T
    (e) T

19.24 (a) F
    (b) F
    (c) F
    (d) F
    (e) T

19.25 (a) F
    (b) F
    (c) F
    (d) F
    (e) T

19.26 (a) F
    (b) F
    (c) F
    (d) T
    (e) T

19.27 (a) T
    (b) T
    (c) T
    (d) F
    (e) T

19.28 (a) T
    (b) T
    (c) F
    (d) T
    (e) T

19.29 (a) T
(b) T
(c) T
(d) T
(e) F

19.30 (a) T
(b) T
(c) T
(d) T
(e) T

19.31 (a) T
(b) T
(c) T
(d) T
(e) T

19.32 (a) F
(b) F
(c) F
(d) F
(e) F

19.33 (a) T
(b) T
(c) T
(d) T
(e) T

19.34 (a) T
(b) T
(c) T
(d) T
(e) T

19.35 (a) F
(b) T
(c) F
(d) T
(e) F

19.36 (a) T
(b) T
(c) T
(d) T
(e) T

19.37 (a) F
(b) T
(c) T
(d) T
(e) F

19.38 (a) T
(b) T
(c) T
(d) T
(e) T

19.39 (a) T
(b) T
(c) T
(d) F
(e) T

19.40 (a) T
(b) F
(c) F
(d) F
(e) F

19.41 (a) T
(b) T
(c) T
(d) T
(e) T

19.42 (a) T
(b) T
(c) T
(d) T
(e) F

19.43 (a) T
(b) T
(c) T
(d) T
(e) T

19.44 (a) T
(b) T
(c) T
(d) T
(e) T

19.45 (a) T
(b) T
(c) T
(d) T
(e) T

19.46 (a) T
(b) T
(c) T
(d) T
(e) T

19.47 (a) F
(b) F
(c) F
(d) T
(e) F

19.48 (a) T
(b) F
(c) F
(d) T
(e) T

19.49 (a) T
(b) T
(c) T
(d) T
(e) T

19.50 (a) T
(b) T
(c) T
(d) T
(e) T

19.51 (a) T
(b) T
(c) T
(d) T
(e) T

19.52 (a) T
(b) T
(c) T
(d) T
(e) T

19.53 (a) T
(b) T
(c) T
(d) T
(e) T

19.54 (a) T
(b) T
(c) T
(d) T
(e) T

19.55 (a) T
(b) T
(c) T
(d) T
(e) T

19.56 (a) T
(b) T
(c) T
(d) T
(e) T

19.57 (a) T
(b) T
(c) T
(d) T
(e) F

Dermatology
Answers

20.1 (a) T	**20.8** (a) T	**20.15** (a) F	**20.22** (a) F
(b) F	(b) T	(b) F	(b) F
(c) T	(c) T	(c) T	(c) F
(d) T	(d) T	(d) F	(d) F
(e) T	(e) T	(e) T	(e) F
20.2 (a) T	**20.9** (a) T	**20.16** (a) F	**20.23** (a) F
(b) F	(b) T	(b) T	(b) T
(c) F	(c) T	(c) T	(c) T
(d) F	(d) F	(d) T	(d) T
(e) F	(e) F	(e) T	(e) T
20.3 (a) T	**20.10** (a) T	**20.17** (a) T	**20.24** (a) T
(b) T	(b) T	(b) F	(b) T
(c) F	(c) T	(c) T	(c) T
(d) T	(d) T	(d) T	(d) T
(e) T	(e) T	(e) T	(e) T
20.4 (a) T	**20.11** (a) F	**20.18** (a) F	**20.25** (a) F
(b) F	(b) F	(b) T	(b) F
(c) T	(c) T	(c) F	(c) F
(d) F	(d) T	(d) T	(d) T
(e) F	(e) T	(e) T	(e) T
20.5 (a) T	**20.12** (a) F	**20.19** (a) T	**20.26** (a) T
(b) T	(b) T	(b) T	(b) T
(c) T	(c) F	(c) T	(c) T
(d) T	(d) T	(d) T	(d) T
(e) T	(e) T	(e) T	(e) F
20.6 (a) T	**20.13** (a) T	**20.20** (a) T	**20.27** (a) T
(b) T	(b) F	(b) T	(b) T
(c) T	(c) T	(c) F	(c) T
(d) T	(d) F	(d) T	(d) T
(e) T	(e) T	(e) T	(e) T
20.7 (a) F	**20.14** (a) F	**20.21** (a) T	**20.28** (a) T
(b) T	(b) T	(b) T	(b) T
(c) F	(c) F	(c) T	(c) T
(d) T	(d) F	(d) T	(d) T
(e) T	(e) T	(e) T	(e) T

20.29	(a) F	20.37	(a) T	20.45	(a) T	20.53	(a) T
	(b) T		(b) T		(b) T		(b) T
	(c) T		(c) T		(c) T		(c) T
	(d) T		(d) T		(d) T		(d) T
	(e) T		(e) T		(e) T		(e) T

20.30	(a) F	20.38	(a) T	20.46	(a) T	20.54	(a) F
	(b) F		(b) T		(b) T		(b) F
	(c) T		(c) T		(c) T		(c) T
	(d) T		(d) T		(d) T		(d) T
	(e) T		(e) T		(e) T		(e) T

20.31	(a) F	20.39	(a) T	20.47	(a) T	20.55	(a) T
	(b) T		(b) T		(b) T		(b) T
	(c) T		(c) T		(c) T		(c) T
	(d) T		(d) T		(d) T		(d) T
	(e) F		(e) T		(e) T		(e) F

20.32	(a) F	20.40	(a) F	20.48	(a) T	20.56	(a) T
	(b) F		(b) T		(b) T		(b) F
	(c) T		(c) T		(c) T		(c) T
	(d) T		(d) T		(d) T		(d) F
	(e) T		(e) T		(e) T		(e) T

20.33	(a) F	20.41	(a) T	20.49	(a) T	20.57	(a) T
	(b) T		(b) T		(b) T		(b) T
	(c) T		(c) T		(c) T		(c) T
	(d) T		(d) T		(d) T		(d) F
	(e) F		(e) T		(e) F		(e) T

20.34	(a) T	20.42	(a) T	20.50	(a) T	20.58	(a) T
	(b) T		(b) T		(b) T		(b) T
	(c) T		(c) T		(c) T		(c) T
	(d) T		(d) T		(d) T		(d) T
	(e) T		(e) T		(e) T		(e) F

20.35	(a) T	20.43	(a) F	20.51	(a) T	20.59	(a) T
	(b) T		(b) F		(b) T		(b) T
	(c) T		(c) T		(c) T		(c) T
	(d) T		(d) T		(d) T		(d) F
	(e) T		(e) T		(e) T		(e) F

20.36	(a) T	20.44	(a) T	20.52	(a) F	20.60	(a) T
	(b) T		(b) T		(b) T		(b) T
	(c) T		(c) T		(c) T		(c) T
	(d) T		(d) T		(d) T		(d) T
	(e) T		(e) T		(e) T		(e) T

20.61	(a) F	**20.67**	(a) T	**20.73**	(a) T	**20.79**	(a) T
	(b) T		(b) F		(b) T		(b) T
	(c) F		(c) F		(c) T		(c) T
	(d) T		(d) F		(d) T		(d) T
	(e) F		(e) T		(e) F		(e) F
20.62	(a) F	**20.68**	(a) F	**20.74**	(a) T	**20.80**	(a) T
	(b) T		(b) T		(b) T		(b) T
	(c) T		(c) T		(c) T		(c) T
	(d) F		(d) T		(d) T		(d) T
	(e) T		(e) F		(e) T		(e) T
20.63	(a) T	**20.69**	(a) F	**20.75**	(a) T	**20.81**	(a) T
	(b) T		(b) T		(b) T		(b) T
	(c) T		(c) T		(c) T		(c) T
	(d) T		(d) F		(d) T		(d) T
	(e) T		(e) T		(e) T		(e) T
20.64	(a) T	**20.70**	(a) T	**20.76**	(a) T	**20.82**	(a) F
	(b) T		(b) T		(b) T		(b) T
	(c) T		(c) T		(c) T		(c) T
	(d) T		(d) T		(d) T		(d) T
	(e) T		(e) T		(e) T		(e) F
20.65	(a) T	**20.71**	(a) T	**20.77**	(a) T		
	(b) T		(b) T		(b) T		
	(c) T		(c) T		(c) T		
	(d) T		(d) T		(d) T		
	(e) T		(e) T		(e) T		
20.66	(a) T	**20.72**	(a) T	**20.78**	(a) T		
	(b) T		(b) T		(b) T		
	(c) T		(c) T		(c) T		
	(d) F		(d) T		(d) T		
	(e) F		(e) T		(e) T		